Enhancing Clinical Competence of Graduate Nurses

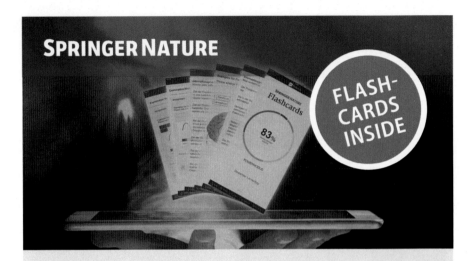

SN Flashcards Microlearning

Quick and efficient studying with digital flashcards – for work or school!

With SN Flashcards you can:

- **Learn** anytime and anywhere on your smartphone, tablet or computer
- **Master** the content of the book and test your knowledge
- **Get motivated** by using various question types enriched with multimedia components and choosing from three learning algorithms (long-term-memory mode, short-term-memory mode or exam mode)
- **Create** your own question sets to personalise your learning experience

How to access your SN Flashcards content:

1. Go to the **1st page of the 1st chapter** of this book and follow the instructions in the box to sign up for an SN Flashcards account and to access the flashcards content for this book.
2. Download the SN Flashcards mobile app from the Apple App Store or Google Play Store, open the app and follow the instructions in the app.
3. Within the mobile app or web app, select the flashcards content for this book and start learning!

If you have difficulties accessing the SN Flashcards content, please write an email to **customerservice@springernature.com** mentioning "**SN Flashcards**" and the book title in the subject line.

Kholofelo Matlhaba

Enhancing Clinical Competence of Graduate Nurses

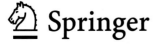 Springer

Kholofelo Matlhaba
Department of Health Studies
University of South Africa
Pretoria, South Africa

ISBN 978-3-031-81406-8   ISBN 978-3-031-81407-5   (eBook)
https://doi.org/10.1007/978-3-031-81407-5

Editorial Contact: Marie-Elia Come-Garry
This Springer imprint is published by the registered company Springer Nature Switzerland AG
The registered company address is: Gewerbestrasse 11, 6330 Cham, Switzerland

If disposing of this product, please recycle the paper.

"Dedication is the key to success, and this book is a testament to the dedication and hard work of all newly graduated nurses striving to enhance their clinical competence. It is dedicated to those who tirelessly pursue excellence in their practice, who continuously seek to learn and grow in their profession. May this book serve as a guiding light, providing knowledge, skills, and inspiration to all the new graduate nurses embarking on their journey towards becoming competent and confident nurse practitioners. Your dedication and commitment to improving your clinical skills will not go unnoticed, and I salute you for your unwavering determination to excel in your field. Moreover, this book is dedicated to nursing educators who have tirelessly imparted their knowledge and wisdom, to preceptors who have guided and supported new nurses through their transition into practice, and to experienced nurses who have served as exemplary role models and mentors. This book recognizes the dedication and hard work of all those who are committed to helping new nurses develop the

clinical competence necessary to provide safe and effective patient care. Their unwavering support and encouragement are instrumental in the success of new graduate nurses as they embark on their professional journey. Finally, I would like to dedicate this book to the memory of my late father. He was my biggest supporter and motivator throughout my journey in the nursing and academic field. Although he is no longer physically with me, his presence continues to guide me in my work in the academic world, and my passion for helping others in the nursing profession. This book is a tribute to his memory and the enduring impact he has had on my life and career. Thank you, Dad, for everything."

Preface

Entering the nursing profession as a newly graduated nurse is both an exhilarating and daunting experience. With the culmination of years of rigorous education and training, this transition from student to practitioner can be fraught with challenges and uncertainties. It is a pivotal moment that sets the trajectory for a successful nursing career. In recognition of this transformative phase, I present "Enhancing Clinical Competence of Graduate Nurses," a book dedicated to addressing the unique needs and challenges faced by new nurses as they navigate their early days in clinical settings.

This book is designed as a comprehensive guide to enrich the clinical competence of new graduate nurses. Throughout its chapters, I offer an original and conceptual framework that underscores the importance of a smooth transition from theory to practice. The foundational goal is to equip new graduates with the comprehensive clinical skills necessary to excel in their roles through a variety of innovative strategies and resources. Structured across several key themes, this book delves into critical aspects that contribute to a successful transition. First, I introduce a framework for understanding the complexities of transitioning from a student role to that of a competent practice nurse. In this section, readers will explore various strategies to navigate the challenges that often arise during this pivotal life stage. Then I address the essential clinical skills that build the foundation of effective nursing practice. The competencies outlined are not only aligned with healthcare standards but also adaptable to various clinical environments, ensuring that new graduates are well prepared to meet the demands of their roles. Additionally, mentorship plays a crucial role throughout this journey. I emphasize the importance of support systems—mentors, supervisors, and peers—who provide guidance and encouragement as new graduates acclimate to the complexities of patient care. This aspect of support is invaluable, as it fosters professional growth and enhances confidence in their nursing practice. In this technologically driven healthcare era, I also recognize the importance of integrating technology into nursing practice. The chapters explore how technology can enhance patient care, improve efficiency, and support clinical decision-making. By embracing these advancements, new graduate nurses can deliver higher quality care while remaining adaptable in an ever-evolving healthcare landscape. Furthermore, to facilitate practical learning, this book incorporates interactive online flash cards and case studies that serve as a supplementary resource. These online resources are structured to allow new graduates to engage with clinical knowledge at their own convenience. Enhanced learning tools such as these reflect my commitment to providing accessible and dynamic resources that can significantly contribute to the competency development of nursing professionals. As healthcare continues to evolve, the need for competent, confident, and skilled nurses remains a pressing priority. I believe that this book addresses not only the immediate educational needs of new graduate nurses but also the larger challenge of fostering a culture of competence and excellence within the nursing profession.

Pretoria, South Africa   Kholofelo Matlhaba

Structure of the Book

The chapters of this book offer the original conceptual and comprehensive approach during transition from a student nurse to a practice nurse (Part I), the comprehensive clinical skills needed for a new graduate nurse to excel in the clinical area (Part II), the mentorship and support needed for a new graduate nurse to transition easily and smoothly into the practice space (Part III), the integration of technology to enhance patient care and improve efficiency (Part IV), as well as the practical learning activities in the form of online flash cards and case studies for the new graduate nurses to partake in their convenient time and space (Part V).

Acknowledgments

Writing a book of this magnitude is a collaborative effort that requires the dedication and support of many individuals. I extend my heartfelt gratitude to everyone in the editorial department who has shared their expertise and insights within this volume. Your enthusiasm and commitment driving my passion to enhancing the clinical competence of new graduate nurses have been invaluable. I also wish to express my deepest appreciation to the educational institutions and healthcare organizations that continue to prioritize the training and development of new nurses. Your support and investment in nursing education create an environment where future generations of nurses can thrive. Special thanks go to the mentors and preceptors who play a crucial role in shaping the experiences of new graduate nurses. Your unwavering guidance, encouragement, and willingness to share your knowledge greatly influence the journeys of these new professionals, enabling them to build a robust foundation for their careers. Furthermore, I would like to acknowledge the contributions of my department mentor and colleague (Prof. DD Mphuthi) for proofreading the draft proposal before submission. The same gratitude goes to my academic mentor (Prof. B Khoza) for proofreading my first chapter and providing me with the tips on how to go about in this book. Your reminder that I had to stick to the publisher guidelines and your guidance words when you said that "the manuscript" must be reader friendly will forever be in my mind. All the advice, encouragement, and guidance provided me the strength to see this project through to completion. Lastly, to the language editor (Dr. M Steyn), thank you.

About the Book

This book takes a comprehensive approach to enhancing the clinical competence of newly graduated nurses. It covers a wide range of topics and provides a holistic view of the skills and knowledge required for success in the clinical setting. This book goes beyond theory and provides practical guidance for new graduate nurses. It includes practical activities at the end of each chapter and online flash cards and case study activities that allow readers to apply their knowledge and skills in a realistic clinical setting. This book encourages self-reflection and personal development in new graduate nurses. It includes exercises and activities that promote self-awareness, self-assessment, and continuous learning, empowering readers to identify their strengths and areas for improvement and take proactive steps towards professional growth. Recognizing the importance of teamwork and collaboration in healthcare, this book proposal highlights the role of interprofessional collaboration in enhancing clinical competence. It explores effective communication strategies, teamwork dynamics, and importance of building strong relationships with other healthcare professionals. One of the unique features of this book proposal is its emphasis on developing critical thinking skills in new graduate nurses. It provides tools and techniques for analyzing and solving complex clinical problems, helping readers become confident and competent decision-makers in their practice. In today's diverse healthcare landscape, cultural competence is essential for providing quality care. This book emphasizes the importance of cultural competence in nursing practice and provides strategies for developing cultural awareness, sensitivity, and competence in new graduate nurses. Recognizing the challenges faced by new graduate nurses, this book provides guidance on finding and utilizing mentorship and support networks. This book offers practical tips for building relationships with experienced nurses, seeking guidance, and navigating the transition from student to professional nurse. This book emphasizes the importance of lifelong learning and professional development in nursing. It provides resources and recommendations for further reading, aiming for empowering new graduate nurses to continue growing and evolving in their practice. This book acknowledges the increasing role of technology in healthcare and explores how new graduate nurses can effectively integrate technology into their practice. It addresses topics such as electronic health records and telehealth and provides the skills needed to navigate the digital healthcare environment. Furthermore, this book includes 50 digital study questions to test their knowledge, which can be downloaded for free from Springer Flashcards App. Finally, this book can be used by both private and public hospitals during the onboarding or orientation programs.

Contents

Abbreviations

AEDs	Automated external defibrillators
ANA	American Nurses Association
ANP	Advanced nurse practitioner
ANS	Advanced nurse specialist
APN	Advanced practice nurse
APRN	Advanced practice registered nurse
BLS	Basic life support
CNS	Clinical nurse specialist
CPR	Cardiopulmonary resuscitation
DNP	Doctor of Nursing Practice
EBP	Evidence-based practice
ED	Emergency department
EHRs	Electronic health records
eMARs	Electronic medication administration records
HAIs	Healthcare-associated infections
HIPAA	Health Insurance Portability and Accountability Act
MSN	Master of Science in Nursing
NP	Nurse practitioner
NS	Nurse specialist
PDSA	Plan-Do-Study-Act
PICO	Population, Intervention, Comparison, Outcome
PPE	Personal protective equipment
SMART	Specific, measurable, achievable, relevant, and time-bound

List of Tables

Part I

Comprehensive Approach

In this part of the book, we explore the critical phase of transitioning from being a student to becoming a competent nurse practitioner (Chap. 1). This phase marks the beginning of a new journey, where theoretical knowledge is applied in real-world clinical settings. It is a time of immense growth, learning, and self-discovery. The section begins by delving into the challenges and adjustments that new graduate nurses face during this transition. It addresses the shift in roles, responsibilities, and expectations as well as the emotional and psychological aspects of entering the professional world. By understanding and acknowledging these challenges, new graduate nurses can navigate this transition more effectively. Next, the section focuses on building a solid foundation for clinical competence (Chap. 2). It explores the essential skills, knowledge, and attitudes that new graduate nurses need to develop to provide safe and effective patient care. Topics such as critical thinking, clinical reasoning, communication, and teamwork are discussed, emphasizing their significance in delivering high-quality care. Furthermore, the section emphasizes the importance of self-reflection and personal development in the journey towards clinical competence (Chap. 3). It explores the role of self-assessment, feedback, and continuous learning in identifying strengths, weaknesses, and areas for improvement. By engaging in self-reflection, new graduate nurses can enhance their self-awareness, identify learning needs, and set goals for professional growth. The section also highlights the significance of mentorship and guidance during this transition. It discusses the role of experienced practitioners in providing support, guidance, and mentorship to new practitioners. By seeking mentorship, new graduate nurses can benefit from the wisdom and expertise of their mentors, accelerating their growth and development. Lastly, the section emphasizes the importance of maintaining a growth mindset and embracing lifelong learning. It encourages new graduate nurses to stay curious, open-minded, and adaptable to the ever-evolving healthcare landscape. By committing to continuous learning and professional development, new graduate nurses can ensure that their clinical competence remains current and relevant throughout their careers. Overall, this section provides valuable insights and guidance for new graduate nurses as they navigate the transition from student to nurse practitioners. It emphasizes the importance of building a strong foundation for clinical competence, engaging in self-reflection and personal development, seeking mentorship, and embracing lifelong learning. By embracing these principles, new graduate nurses can embark on a fulfilling and successful professional journey, making a positive impact on patient care and the nursing profession as a whole.

Transitioning from Student to Practitioner

1

Contents

Test your learning and check your understanding of this book's contents: use the "Springer Nature Flashcards" app to access questions. To use the app, please follow the instructions below:

1. Go to https://flashcards.springernature.com/login
2. Create a user account by entering your e-mail address and assigning a password.
3. Use the following link to access your SN Flashcards set: ▶ https://sn.pub/pe441e

If the link is missing or does not work, please send an e-mail with the subject "SN Flashcards" and the book title to customerservice@springer-nature.com

1.1   Key Aspects of Transitioning from a Nursing Student to a Nursing Practitioner

Understanding the transition from student hood to a professional practitioner in nursing is crucial for new graduate nurses. Matlhaba and Khunou (2022) defined transition as a period from student nurse to professional nurse. Casey et al. (2021) and Gautam et al. (2023) suggest that transitioning refers to the process of moving from one stage or role to another, often referring to the transition from being a student to a professional nurse or transitioning between different healthcare settings. Student nurse is a person who is currently enrolled in a nursing education program and is undergoing training and education to become a registered nurse (SANC 2005). A nurse practitioner refers to an advanced practice registered nurse (APRN) who has completed additional education and training beyond the registered nurse level (Savard et al. 2023; Schlunegger et al. 2023). Nurse practitioners have the authority to diagnose and treat medical conditions, prescribe medications, and provide comprehensive healthcare services.

Transitioning from a student nurse to a practice nurse is an important and exciting phase in your nursing career. The following key aspects are important to understand during the transition period:

- Role and responsibilities: As a practice nurse, you will have expanded roles and responsibilities compared to when you were a student nurse. You will provide direct patient care, manage patient assessments, administer medications, perform procedures, and collaborate with other healthcare professionals.
- Professional development: Transitioning to a practice nurse involves ongoing professional development. Take advantage of opportunities for continuing education, workshops, and certifications to enhance your knowledge and skills. Stay updated with current evidence-based practices and guidelines in your area of specialization.
- Building confidence and competence: It is normal to feel a bit overwhelmed initially. Building confidence and competence takes time and experience. Seek guidance from experienced nurses, ask questions, and actively participate in learning opportunities. Gradually, you will become more comfortable and confident in your role.
- Effective communication: Communication skills are crucial as a practice nurse. Develop effective communication techniques to interact with patients, their families, and other healthcare professionals. Practice active listening, empathy, and clear and concise communication to ensure effective collaboration and patient-centered care.
- Time management and prioritization: As a practice nurse, you will have multiple responsibilities and tasks to manage. Developing strong time management and prioritization skills is essential to ensure efficient and effective care delivery. It is essential to prioritize tasks based on patient acuity, urgency, and importance.
- Ethical and legal considerations: Understand the ethical and legal responsibilities that come with being a practice nurse. Familiarize yourself with the nursing

code of ethics, professional standards, and legal regulations governing nursing practice in your jurisdiction. Ensure that your practice aligns with these ethical and legal guidelines.

- Collaboration and teamwork: Practice nursing often involves working as part of a multidisciplinary team. Learn to collaborate effectively with other healthcare professionals, such as physicians, pharmacists, and allied health professionals. Foster a positive and respectful working relationship to provide holistic and coordinated care.
- Self-care and well-being: Transitioning to a practice nurse can be demanding both physically and emotionally. Prioritize self-care and well-being to prevent burnout. Engage in self-reflection, participate in activities that promote relaxation and stress management, and seek support from colleagues and mentors when needed.

It is important to note that transitioning from a student nurse to a practice nurse is a continuous learning process. Embrace the opportunities for growth, seek guidance when needed, and remain open to new experiences. Over time and experience, you will become more confident and proficient in your role as a practice nurse.

1.2   The Importance of Transitioning

The Significance of Transitioning from Student to Practitioner
The transition from being a student nurse to a practitioner is a significant milestone in the nursing career. The transition period increases autonomy and responsibility. Student nurses work under the direct supervision and guidance of experienced nurses. Transitioning to a practitioner means taking on more autonomy and responsibility for patient care. Practice nurses can make independent decisions, manage patient care plans, and take ownership of their nursing practice. During the transition period, the application of knowledge and skills is enhanced as student nurses have acquired theoretical knowledge and developed basic clinical skills in their training years. Transitioning to a practitioner allows new practice nurses to apply that knowledge and skills in real-world patient care settings. They can put their education into practice and make a tangible difference in the lives of patients under their care. The transition period promotes professional identity development as it further contributes to development of professional identity and growth as a nurse. New practice nurses become more confident in their role, develop a deeper understanding of the nursing profession, and align their practice with the values and ethics of nursing. The transition period provides opportunities for continual learning and professional growth. It marks the beginning of the new practice nurses' lifelong journey of learning and professional growth. New practitioners will encounter new challenges, complex patient cases, and evolving healthcare practices. Therefore, embracing these opportunities for learning and growth will help them stay current, expand their knowledge and skills, and advance in their nursing career. Transitioning to a practitioner allows you to have a greater impact on patient care. New nurses will

have the opportunity to provide direct care, develop therapeutic relationships with patients, and make clinical decisions that positively influence patient outcomes without the direct supervision of an experienced nurse. Their role as practitioners contributes to the overall quality and safety of patient care. The transition period provides new practitioners with collaboration opportunities with other healthcare professionals and opportunities to assume leadership roles within the healthcare team. They will work closely with physicians, pharmacists, and other allied health professionals to provide comprehensive and coordinated care, and this experience contributes to your professional growth and development. Transitioning to a practitioner opens doors for professional recognition and advancement. With experience and further education, new nurses can pursue advanced practice roles, such as clinical nurse specialist or nurse educator. These advanced roles offer increased responsibilities, expanded scope of practice, and opportunities for leadership and specialization in the nursing field. The transition from student nurse to practitioner is a significant step in the nursing journey. Therefore, it is essential to embrace the opportunities, challenges, and growth that accompany this transition while continually striving to provide high-quality, patient-centered care and contributing to the advancement of the nursing profession.

The Challenges and Opportunities That Come with This Transition

Transitioning from a student nurse to a practitioner comes with both challenges and opportunities. This has been previously recorded in literature globally. Below are some of the common challenges and opportunities new nurses may encounter during the transition period:

Challenges
- As practitioners, new nurses will have increased responsibility for patient care. This can be challenging as they navigate the complexities of managing multiple patients, making critical decisions, and ensuring patient safety.
- Transitioning to a practitioner requires effective time management skills. Balancing multiple tasks, prioritizing patient care, and meeting documentation requirements can be demanding. Learning to manage your time efficiently is essential to provide quality care while maintaining their own well-being.
- Building confidence in clinical skills and decision-making abilities takes time. Initially, new nurses may feel uncertain or doubt their capabilities. Overcoming self-doubt and building confidence in practice is a challenge that comes with experience and ongoing learning.
- As student nurses, they may have been primarily exposed to one clinical setting. Transitioning to a practitioner may involve adapting to new healthcare settings, such as hospitals, clinics, or community health centers. Adjusting to new workflows, policies, and team dynamics can be challenging.
- Practitioners may encounter complex ethical dilemmas that require critical thinking and decision-making. Balancing patient autonomy, beneficence, and ethical principles can be challenging. Navigating these dilemmas while upholding ethical standards is a continuous learning process.

Opportunities
- Transitioning to a practitioner opens doors for professional growth and development. New nurses can expand their knowledge, skills, and expertise through continuing education and advanced practice roles. This allows them to take on more challenging and specialized roles within the nursing profession.
- Nurses have increased autonomy in their practice. This allows them to make independent decisions, develop care plans, and contribute to the comprehensive management of patient care. The opportunity to exercise clinical judgment and decision-making skills is valuable to transitioning to a practitioner.
- Nurses are expected to build long-term therapeutic relationships with patients. This allows them to provide continuity of care, understand patients' unique needs, and positively impact their health outcomes. Building these relationships can be rewarding and fulfilling for a new nurse practitioner.
- Transitioning to a practitioner involves working collaboratively with other healthcare professionals. This provides opportunities for interdisciplinary collaboration, learning from others' expertise, and contributing to a multidisciplinary team approach to patient care, because collaborative teamwork enhances the quality and safety of patient care.
- As practitioners, new nurses are expected to assume leadership roles within the healthcare team. This includes mentoring and guiding student nurses, participating in quality improvement initiatives, and advocating for patient-centered care. Leadership roles allow them to influence and shape the nursing profession positively.

The Impact of Transition Period on Personal and Professional Growth

The transition can significantly impact personal and professional growth. The next section discusses ways in which transition can affect new nurses.

Transition to a new phase in life can serve as a catalyst for personal growth. It challenges new nurses to step out of their comfort zone, adapt to new situations, and develop new skills. It can also provide opportunities for self-reflection and self-discovery, allowing them to better understand themselves and their values. Transition to a new role or career can open new opportunities for professional growth. It may require new nurses to learn new skills, expand their knowledge base, and develop a broader perspective. It can also provide a chance to network with new people and build valuable relationships within the healthcare fraternity and beyond. Transitioning often involves a learning curve as new nurses navigate new responsibilities and expectations. This can lead to personal and professional development as they acquire new knowledge and skills. It may also involve seeking out additional training or education to enhance their capabilities. Going through a transition can build resilience and adaptability. New nurses must navigate uncertainty, overcome challenges, and embrace change. These experiences can strengthen their ability to handle future transitions and setbacks. Transition can broaden perspectives through exposure to new environments, cultures, and ways of thinking. This can enhance your creativity, problem-solving skills, and ability to work with diverse teams. The impact of a transition on personal and professional growth can be transformative. It provides an opportunity for self-improvement, learning, and development. This, in turn, can lead to a more fulfilling and successful life.

1.3   Recognizing the Differences

Recognizing the differences between nursing education and nursing practice is crucial for new graduate nurses transitioning from student to nurse practitioner. By understanding these distinctions, new graduates can better prepare themselves for the challenges of clinical practice, develop effective coping strategies, and seek guidance when faced with unfamiliar scenarios. This awareness eases their transition and fosters confidence in their abilities, ultimately leading to improved patient outcomes and professional satisfaction in their new roles. Below are some of the key differences between nursing education and nursing practice:

- Theoretical knowledge vs. practical application: Nursing education focuses on providing students with a strong foundation of theoretical knowledge. Students learn about anatomy, physiology, pharmacology, and various nursing theories. In contrast, nursing practice involves applying this theoretical knowledge in real-world clinical settings to provide direct patient care.
- Controlled environment vs. real-world complexity: Nursing education often occurs in controlled environments such as simulation labs or clinical settings with supervision. Students can practice skills and make decisions under the guidance of instructors. In nursing practice, however, nurses work in complex and dynamic healthcare settings where they must navigate various challenges, make critical decisions, and adapt to changing patient conditions.
- Limited responsibility vs. full accountability: In nursing education, students have limited responsibility for patient care. They work under the supervision of instructors or preceptors and are not held fully accountable for patient outcomes. In nursing practice, nurses have full accountability for the care they provide. They are responsible for assessing, planning, implementing, and evaluating patient care, and their decisions directly impact patient outcomes.
- Time constraints and prioritization: Nursing education allows students to focus on learning and mastering skills without the time constraints and pressures commonly found in clinical practice. In nursing practice, nurses often face time constraints and must prioritize their tasks and interventions based on the needs of multiple patients. This requires effective time management and the ability to make quick decisions.
- Collaboration and interprofessional communication: Nursing education emphasizes the importance of collaboration and communication within the healthcare team. However, in nursing practice, nurses must actively collaborate with other healthcare professionals, such as doctors, pharmacists, and therapists. Effective communication and teamwork are essential for providing safe and coordinated patient care.

- Transitioning from student to practitioner: The transition from nursing education to nursing practice involves a shift in roles and responsibilities. As a student, the focus is on learning and acquiring knowledge and skills. As a practitioner, the focus shifts to applying that knowledge and skills in real-world situations, taking on more responsibility, and making independent decisions.

It is important for nursing students to recognize these differences and be prepared for the transition from education to practice. Clinical experiences, internships, and mentorship programs can help bridge the gap between education and practice and prepare students for the realities of nursing in the healthcare setting.

Understanding the Differences Between Academic and Professional Environments

Understanding the differences between academic and professional environments is crucial for individuals transitioning from the academic setting to the professional world. Here are some key distinctions:

- Goals and objectives: In the academic environment, the primary goal is to acquire knowledge and skills through coursework, assignments, and exams. The focus is on learning and personal development. In contrast, the professional environment is driven by specific goals and objectives related to the organization's mission and the delivery of products or services. The focus is on achieving tangible outcomes and meeting the needs of clients or customers.
- Structure and hierarchy: Academic environments often have a hierarchical structure, with professors, instructors, and administrators overseeing students' progress. There are clear guidelines and expectations for coursework and assessments. There is also a hierarchical structure in professional environments, but it is typically based on job roles and responsibilities. Professionals work within teams or departments, reporting to supervisors or managers who provide guidance and direction.
- Accountability and performance: In academia, students are primarily accountable to themselves and their instructors for their academic performance. They are evaluated based on their individual achievements and progress. In the professional environment, individuals are accountable to their employers, clients, or customers. Performance is measured based on meeting organizational goals, delivering quality work, and contributing to the team or organization's success.
- Collaboration and teamwork: Academic environments often encourage student collaboration through group projects, discussions, and presentations. However, individual performance and grades are still emphasized. In professional environments, collaboration and teamwork are essential for achieving organizational objectives. Professionals work together, leveraging their diverse skills and expertise to solve problems, make decisions, and deliver results.
- Communication and professionalism: Academic communication is typically formal and structured, such as through written assignments, presentations, and classroom discussions. In the professional environment, communication is more

varied and may include formal written reports, emails, meetings, and informal conversations. Professionalism is highly valued, with expectations for punctuality, respect, and appropriate behavior in the workplace.

- Continuous learning and development: In academia, the focus is on acquiring knowledge and skills within a specific field of study. However, in the professional environment, learning and development are ongoing. Professionals are expected to stay updated on industry trends, advancements, and best practices. Continuous learning may involve attending conferences or workshops or pursuing additional certifications or advanced degrees.

Understanding these differences can help individuals navigate the transition from the academic to the professional environment more effectively. It allows them to adapt their mindset, behaviors, and expectations to thrive in their chosen profession. Seeking mentorship, networking, and participating in internships or co-op programs can also provide valuable exposure to the professional environment before fully entering the workforce.

Identifying the New Expectations and Responsibilities of a Practitioner

Identifying new expectations and responsibilities is crucial for new graduate nurses transitioning from student to nurse practitioner (NP) and their confidence and competence in professional practice. By clearly delineating their roles, these new nurses can better understand the scope of their duties, which often encompass not only patient care but also collaboration with multidisciplinary teams, adherence to evidence-based protocols, and the management of complex health situations. This clarity helps to alleviate the anxiety associated with their new positions, allowing them to focus on developing critical thinking and clinical skills rather than feeling overwhelmed by ambiguity. Moreover, recognizing expectations related to communication, leadership, and advocacy prepares them to navigate the healthcare environment more effectively, fostering a smoother transition and ultimately improving patient outcomes. As they embrace these responsibilities, new graduate nurses can cultivate a strong sense of professional identity and readiness, paving the way for their growth and success in the nursing profession. Below are the roles and expectations of the nurse practitioner:

- As an NP, you will be expected to provide advanced clinical care to patients. This includes conducting comprehensive assessments, diagnosing and treating illnesses, prescribing medications, and developing and implementing treatment plans. You will have more autonomy and independence in making clinical decisions.
- NPs often have their own patient caseload and are responsible for managing their patients' care. This involves monitoring patient progress, coordinating referrals to specialists, ordering and interpreting diagnostic tests, and providing ongoing follow-up care. You will be expected to take a holistic approach to patient management, considering physical, emotional, and social factors.

- NPs work collaboratively with other healthcare professionals, including physicians, nurses, pharmacists, and allied health professionals. You will be expected to effectively communicate and collaborate with the healthcare team to ensure coordinated and comprehensive care for patients. This may involve participating in interdisciplinary meetings, sharing information, and consulting with other providers.
- NPs play a vital role in promoting health and preventing diseases. You will be expected to educate patients on healthy lifestyle choices, provide preventive screenings and vaccinations, and offer counseling on risk reduction and health maintenance. NPs often take a proactive approach to healthcare, focusing on preventive measures to improve patient outcomes.
- As an NP, you will be more responsible for patient education. This includes explaining diagnoses, treatment options, and medication instructions to patients and their families. You will also advocate for your patients, ensuring they have access to appropriate healthcare services, resources, and support.
- NPs are often seen as leaders within the healthcare team. You may be expected to take on leadership roles, such as mentoring and precepting students, participating in quality improvement initiatives, and staying updated on the latest evidence-based practices. Professional development, such as attending conferences and continuing education courses, is also important to maintain and enhance your clinical skills and knowledge.

It's important to note that the specific expectations and responsibilities of an NP may vary depending on the healthcare setting, specialty, and state regulations. It's essential to familiarize yourself with the scope of practice and legal requirements in your specific practice area. Transitioning to the role of an NP requires ongoing learning, adaptability, and a commitment to providing high-quality patient care. Embracing these new expectations and responsibilities can lead to a rewarding and fulfilling career as a nurse practitioner.

Adapting to the Changes in Work Dynamics and Relationships
Adapting to changes in work dynamics and relationships in nursing practice is essential for a successful transition and professional growth. Strategies to help you navigate these changes include the following:

- Embrace open communication: Effective communication is crucial in any work environment, especially in nursing practice. Be open and proactive in communicating with your colleagues, supervisors, and other healthcare professionals. Listen actively, ask questions, and seek clarification when needed. Clear and open communication fosters collaboration, builds trust, and promotes a positive work environment.
- Build relationships: Take the initiative to build relationships with your colleagues and other healthcare team members. Get to know their roles, expertise, and perspectives. Building positive relationships can enhance teamwork, facilitate effective collaboration, and create a supportive work environment. Participate in

team-building activities, attend staff meetings, and engage in social interactions to foster connections.

- Seek mentorship and guidance: Find experienced nurses or nurse practitioners who can serve as mentors or guides as you navigate the changes in work dynamics. They can provide valuable insights, advice, and support. Seek their guidance on professional development, clinical decision-making, and managing challenging situations. Mentorship can help you gain confidence, expand your knowledge, and navigate the complexities of nursing practice.
- Adapt to different leadership styles: Nursing practice involves working with various leaders, such as nurse managers, physicians, and administrators. Each leader may have a different leadership style and approach. Be adaptable and flexible in understanding and working with different leadership styles. Learn from their expertise, adapt to their expectations, and contribute positively to the team under their guidance.
- Embrace interprofessional collaboration: Nursing practice often involves working closely with other healthcare professionals, including physicians, pharmacists, and therapists. Embrace interprofessional collaboration by recognizing and respecting the expertise and contributions of each team member. Foster a culture of mutual respect, effective communication, and shared decision-making. Collaborating with other professionals can enhance patient care outcomes and promote a collaborative work environment.
- Continuously learn and grow: Nursing practice is dynamic, and there are always new developments, research, and best practices emerging. Stay updated with the latest evidence-based guidelines, attend conferences, participate in continuing education programs, and engage in professional development opportunities. Continuously learning and growing will help you adapt to changes in work dynamics and relationships and provide the best possible care to your patients.

It is important to remember that adapting to changes takes time and effort. Be patient with yourself and seek support when needed. By embracing these strategies, you can successfully navigate the changes in work dynamics and relationships in nursing practice and thrive in your professional journey.

1.4   Building a Professional Network

Professional networking takes place when you build relationships with other professionals both in your career field and in other related fields. According to Roman-Fischetti (2020:185), professional networking consists of attempts by individuals to develop and maintain relationships with others who have the potential to assist you in your work environment. Building a professional network as a new graduate nurse is crucial for career advancement, mentorship, and accessing future opportunities. Strategies to help build a strong professional network include the following:

- Join professional organizations: Joining professional nursing organizations, or specialty-specific organizations, can provide valuable networking opportunities. Attend conferences, workshops, and seminars organized by these organizations to connect with other nurses, learn from experts in the field, and stay updated on industry trends.
- Attend networking events: Look for networking events specifically tailored for nurses or healthcare professionals in your area. These events can include job fairs, nursing conferences, or local meetups. Take advantage of these opportunities to meet and connect with other nurses, nurse leaders, and potential mentors.
- Utilize social media: Platforms such as LinkedIn and Twitter can serve as powerful tools for networking within the nursing profession. Establish a professional profile on LinkedIn; connect with colleagues, classmates, and nursing professionals; and actively engage in nursing-related discussions. Join nursing groups and follow influential nursing leaders on social media platforms to broaden your network.
- Seek mentorship: Identifying a mentor can offer valuable guidance, support, and valuable insights as you advance your nursing career. Reach out to experienced nurses or nurse leaders who inspire you and inquire if they would be willing to mentor you. A mentor can provide advice, share their experiences, and assist you navigating both challenges and opportunities in your career.
- Engage in professional development: Participate in continuing education programs, workshops, and seminars to develop your knowledge and skills. These events often provide opportunities to network with other healthcare professionals. Actively engaging in professional development demonstrates your commitment to growth and facilitates connections with individuals who share similar interests and goals.
- Connect with colleagues and preceptors: Stay in touch with your nursing school classmates, clinical preceptors, and colleagues from your previous clinical rotations. They can become valuable connections in your professional network. Attend alumni events or organize informal meetups to maintain these relationships and expand your network.
- Volunteer or get involved: Consider volunteering for nursing-related events, community health initiatives, or professional committees. Volunteering not only allows you to give back to the community but also offers opportunities to meet and collaborate with other healthcare professionals.
- Be proactive and genuine: Building a professional network requires proactive effort and genuine interactions. Be approachable, demonstrate interest in others, and actively listen during conversations. Be willing to offer support and assistance to others when possible. Networking is a two-way street, and building meaningful connections is based on mutual respect and support.

Building a professional network takes time and effort. Be patient and persistent in your networking endeavors. Nurture your relationships, stay connected, and continue to expand your network throughout your nursing career. A strong professional network can provide support, mentorship, and open doors to new opportunities along your nursing journey.

The Importance of Building a Professional Network

Building a professional network in nursing practice is crucial for several reasons:

1. Collaboration and support: A strong professional network allow nurses to collaborate with colleagues, share knowledge, and seek support. It provides a platform to discuss challenging cases, exchange ideas, and learn from each other's experiences. This collaboration can lead to improved patient care and better outcomes.
2. Career development: Networking opens up opportunities for career advancement. Nurses can learn about job openings, professional development programs, and continuing education opportunities through their network. They can also receive mentorship and guidance from experienced professionals, which can help them grow in their careers.
3. Access to resources: A professional network provides access to a wide range of resources, such as research articles, best practices, and clinical guidelines. Nurses can tap into this collective knowledge to enhance their practice and stay updated with the latest developments in the field.
4. Professional visibility: Networking allows nurses to establish their professional presence and build a positive reputation within the nursing community. By attending conferences, joining professional organizations, and participating in online forums, nurses can showcase their expertise and contribute to the advancement of the profession.
5. Emotional support: Nursing can be a demanding and stressful profession. Having a strong network of colleagues who understand these challenges and offer emotional support is invaluable. Nurses can share their experiences, seek advice, and find encouragement from their network, which can help them navigate the fluctuations and demands of their career.

Building a professional network in nursing practice is essential for collaboration, career development, access to resources, professional visibility, and emotional support. It can enhance the quality of patient care, promote professional growth, and contribute to the overall advancement of the nursing profession.

Strategies for Expanding Your Network

Expanding your network in nursing practice can be achieved through various strategies. Below are some effective strategies to consider:

• Attend conferences and workshops: Participating in nursing conferences, workshops, and seminars provides opportunities to meet and connect with professionals from different healthcare settings. These events often have networking sessions where you can engage in conversations, exchange contact information, and build relationships with fellow nurses and healthcare leaders.

- Join professional organizations: Joining nursing associations and professional organizations allows you to connect with like-minded individuals who share similar interests and goals. These organizations often host networking events, webinars, and online forums where you can interact with other members, learn from their experiences, and expand your professional circle.
- Utilize social media: Social media platforms, such as LinkedIn, Twitter, and Facebook, can be powerful tools for networking in nursing practice. Create a professional profile, join nursing-related groups, and actively engage in discussions. Share your knowledge, ask questions, and connect with other professionals in the field. Social media can also be a platform to showcase your expertise and build your online presence.
- Volunteer and engage in community activities: Volunteering your time and skills in healthcare-related community activities can help you meet and connect with other healthcare professionals. Look for opportunities to participate in health fairs, community outreach programs, and local nursing organizations. These activities expand your network and demonstrate your commitment to the community and the nursing profession.
- Seek mentorship and professional development opportunities: Reach out to experienced nurses or nursing leaders who can serve as mentors. They can provide guidance, support, and valuable connections in nursing. Additionally, seek out professional development opportunities, such as workshops, webinars, and continuing education programs, where you can meet and network with other nurses who are invested in their professional growth.
- Collaborate on research or quality improvement projects: Engaging in research or quality improvement projects allows you to collaborate with other healthcare professionals, including nurses, physicians, and researchers. These collaborations can lead to networking opportunities and foster relationships with individuals who share similar interests and goals.

Networking is not just about collecting business cards or adding connections on social media. It is about building meaningful relationships, fostering mutual support, and contributing to the nursing profession. Be proactive, genuine, and open to new connections, and you will gradually expand your network in nursing practice.

Leveraging Networking Opportunities to Enhance Career Prospects
Networking can be a powerful tool for enhancing career prospects as a nurse. Ways to leverage networking opportunities to advance your career include the following:

- Building relationships with colleagues: Take the time to connect with your colleagues, both within your organization and in the broader nursing community. Attend staff meetings, participate in team-building activities, and converse with your peers. Building strong relationships with colleagues can lead to valuable recommendations, referrals, and opportunities for career advancement.
- Seeking mentorship: Identify experienced nurses or nursing leaders who can serve as mentors. A mentor can guide, advise, and support as you navigate your

career. They can offer insights into career paths, help you set goals, and provide valuable connections within the nursing field. Actively seek out mentorship opportunities and maintain regular communication with your mentor.

- Attending professional development events: Take advantage of professional development events, such as conferences, workshops, and seminars. These events provide opportunities to network with professionals from various healthcare settings and learn from experts in the field. Engage in conversations, ask questions, and exchange contact information with individuals who can potentially offer career opportunities or serve as future references.
- Joining professional organizations: Joining nursing associations and professional organizations can provide access to a wide network of professionals in your field. Attend networking events organized by these organizations and actively participate in their activities. Engage in committee work, volunteer for leadership roles, and contribute to the organization's initiatives. These activities expand your network and demonstrate your commitment to professional growth and leadership.
- Utilizing online networking platforms: Leverage online networking platforms, such as LinkedIn, to connect with other professionals in the nursing field. Create a compelling profile highlighting your skills, experiences, and career goals. Join nursing-related groups and actively engage in discussions. Share relevant articles, participate in online forums, and connect with individuals who can offer career opportunities or valuable insights.
- Staying connected with alumni: Reach out to alumni from your nursing program or previous workplaces. Attend alumni events, join alumni associations, and utilize online platforms to connect with fellow alumni. Alumni networks can provide valuable connections and insights into job opportunities, career paths, and professional development resources.
- Being proactive and visible: Take initiative in networking opportunities. Attend industry conferences, present at professional meetings, and contribute to nursing publications. Actively seek out opportunities to showcase your expertise and share your knowledge. By being proactive and visible in the nursing community, you increase your chances of being recognized and considered for career advancement opportunities.

Networking is a continuous process. It requires effort, genuine engagement, and nurturing relationships over time. By leveraging networking opportunities, you can enhance your career prospects as a nurse, gain access to new opportunities, and establish yourself as a respected professional in the field.

1.5 Developing Professional Relationships

Developing professional relationships as a new graduate nurse is essential for your career growth and success. Strategies to help you build strong professional relationships include the following:

- Be open and approachable: As a new graduate nurse, it's important to be open and approachable to your colleagues. Introduce yourself, smile, and show genuine interest in getting to know your coworkers. Be friendly, respectful, and willing to learn from others.
- Seek mentorship: Look for experienced nurses who can serve as mentors. They can provide guidance, support, and valuable insights as you navigate your new role. Seek out opportunities to shadow or work closely with experienced nurses to learn from their expertise. Maintain regular communication with your mentors and seek their advice when needed.
- Participate in orientation programs: Take advantage of any orientation programs offered by your workplace. These programs are designed to help new graduate nurses transition into their roles. Attend orientation sessions, engage in discussions, and actively participate in activities. This will help you learn about the organization as well as providing the opportunities to connect with other new graduate nurses.
- Join professional organizations: Joining professional nursing organizations can provide opportunities to connect with other nurses who share similar interests and goals. Attend meetings, conferences, and networking events organized by these organizations. Engage in conversations, ask questions, and exchange contact information with fellow nurses. These connections can provide support, guidance, and potential career opportunities.
- Attend continuing education programs: Participate in continuing education programs and workshops to enhance your knowledge and skills. These programs often bring together nurses from different backgrounds and provide networking opportunities. Engage in discussions, share your experiences, and connect with other participants. Building relationships with nurses who are invested in their professional development can be beneficial for your own growth.
- Collaborate on projects: Look for opportunities to collaborate on projects or committees within your workplace. This could include quality improvement initiatives, research projects, or policy development. Working with other nurses on these projects allows you to build relationships, demonstrate your skills, and contribute to the organization's goals.
- Show appreciation and support: Acknowledge your colleagues' contributions and show appreciation for their work. Help when needed and be a team player. Building a positive and supportive work environment fosters strong professional relationships and enhances collaboration.
- Utilize social media: Utilize social media platforms, such as LinkedIn or nursing-specific online communities, to connect with other nurses. Join nursing-related groups, participate in discussions, and share your insights and experiences. Engaging in online networking will help you expand your professional network beyond your immediate workplace.

Building professional relationships takes time and effort. Be patient, be proactive, and be genuine in your interactions. Developing strong professional relationships as a new graduate nurse will support your career growth, also contributing to a positive and fulfilling work experience.

Building Meaningful Connections with Mentors

Building meaningful connections with mentors in the nursing profession can greatly benefit your career growth and professional development. Here are some strategies to help you build these connections:

- Start by identifying potential mentors within your workplace or professional networks, focusing on those whose values and experiences resonate with your own career goals.
- Approach them with genuine curiosity and a willingness to learn; express your appreciation for their expertise, and seek their guidance on navigating the transition from student to practicing nurse.
- Regularly engage in open conversations, actively listen, and ask thoughtful questions to deepen the relationship.
- Consider participating in shadowing opportunities, attending professional development workshops, or joining nursing organizations to expand your network.
- Maintaining regular communication, whether through informal check-ins or structured meetings, will solidify these connections, fostering a supportive environment that encourages both personal and professional development as you embark on your nursing career.

Building meaningful connections takes time and effort. Be proactive, maintain regular communication, and be open to learning from others. Building strong relationships with mentors can provide valuable guidance, support, and opportunities for career advancement in the nursing profession.

Nurturing Relationships for Long-Term Career Growth

Nurturing relationships for long-term career growth as a nurse is crucial for ongoing professional development and advancement. Strategies to help you nurture relationships for long-term career growth include the following:

- Maintaining regular communication: Stay in touch with your professional contacts on a regular basis. This can be through emails, phone calls, or in-person meetings. Share updates on your career progress, seek advice, and offer support when needed. Regular communication helps to strengthen the connection and keeps you on their radar.
- Showing genuine interest: Demonstrate a genuine interest in the lives and careers of your professional contacts. Ask about their work, achievements, and challenges. Show empathy and offer support when they face difficulties. By showing genuine interest, you build trust and foster a deeper connection.
- Offering support and collaboration: Be willing to offer support and collaborate with your professional contacts. This can include sharing resources, providing

project assistance, or offering expertise. By being a valuable resource to others, you strengthen your relationships and position yourself as a trusted colleague.

- Contributing to the profession: Get involved in professional organizations, committees, or research projects related to nursing. By actively contributing to the profession, you demonstrate your dedication and expertise. This involvement also provides opportunities to connect with other professionals who share similar interests and goals.
- Celebrating achievements: Acknowledge and celebrate the achievements of your professional contacts. Congratulate them on their successes, share their accomplishments with others, and offer support when they face challenges. Celebrating your achievements strengthens your relationships and creates a positive and supportive network.

Nurturing relationships for long-term career growth requires ongoing effort and genuine engagement. Be proactive, supportive, and willing to invest time and energy into building and maintaining these relationships. By nurturing strong professional connections, you create a network of support, opportunities, and growth throughout your nursing career.

Seeking Guidance and Advice from Experienced Practitioners

- Seeking guidance and advice from experienced practitioners in nursing is a valuable way to enhance your knowledge, skills, and career development. Here are some steps to help you seek guidance and advice from experienced practitioners:
- Reach out and express your interest: Once you have identified potential mentors, reach out to them and express your interest in seeking their guidance and advice. Send a polite and professional email, or request a meeting to discuss your career aspirations and ask if they would be willing to mentor you. Be clear about what you hope to gain from the mentorship relationship.
- Be prepared and respectful: When meeting with experienced practitioners, come prepared with specific questions or topics you would like to discuss. Show respect for their time and expertise by being punctual and attentive during your interactions. Listen actively and take notes to demonstrate your commitment to learning from their insights.
- Seek advice on specific challenges or goals: Use your time with experienced practitioners to seek advice on specific challenges or goals you are facing in your nursing career. Whether it's navigating a difficult situation, pursuing a particular specialty, or seeking guidance on professional development opportunities, be clear about what you need guidance on and ask for their insights and recommendations.
- Actively listen and learn: When receiving guidance and advice, be open-minded and receptive. Actively listen to the experiences and perspectives shared by experienced practitioners. Ask follow-up questions to deepen your understanding and

clarify any uncertainties. Be willing to learn from their experiences and apply their insights to your own practice.

- Maintain regular communication: Building a mentorship relationship is an ongoing process. Maintain regular communication with your mentors to update them on your progress, seek further guidance, and share your achievements. This can be through emails, phone calls, or periodic meetings. Regular communication helps to strengthen the mentorship relationship and allows for continued learning and growth.
- Show gratitude and appreciation: Express your gratitude and appreciation to the experienced practitioners who provide guidance and advice. Acknowledge the time and effort they invest in supporting your professional development. A simple thank-you note or a small token of appreciation can go a long way in nurturing the relationship.

Seeking guidance and advice from experienced practitioners is a valuable opportunity for your professional growth. Be proactive, respectful, and open to learning from their experiences. By building relationships with experienced practitioners, you can gain valuable insights, expand your knowledge, and navigate your nursing career more effectively.

1.6   Developing a Personal Brand

Personal branding is defined as the procedure whereby individuals and their vocations are set apart as brands (Pawar 2016). Developing a personal brand as a new graduate nurse is important for establishing yourself in the healthcare industry and standing out among other professionals. The following steps can assist in developing your personal brand:

- Define your values and goals: Start by identifying your core values and what you want to achieve in your nursing career. This will help you shape your personal brand and determine the message you want to convey to others.
- Identify your unique strengths: Reflect on your skills, experiences, and qualities that set you apart from other nurses. These could include your clinical expertise, communication skills, leadership abilities, or a specific area of specialization.
- Create a professional online presence: A strong online presence is crucial in today's digital age. Create a professional LinkedIn profile and consider starting a blog or website to showcase your expertise and share your insights on nursing-related topics.
- Network with professionals in the field: Attend nursing conferences, join professional organizations or associations, and connect with other healthcare professionals both online and offline. Building a strong network can help you gain visibility and open up opportunities for career growth.
- Be consistent and authentic: Your personal brand should be a reflection of who you are as a nurse. Be consistent in your messaging and ensure that your actions

align with your brand values. Authenticity is key in building trust and credibility with colleagues, patients, and employers.

- Seek feedback and continuously improve: Regularly seek feedback from colleagues, supervisors, and patients to understand how you are perceived, and identify areas for improvement. Use this feedback to refine your personal brand and enhance your professional image.

Developing a personal brand is an ongoing process. It takes time and effort to establish yourself as a new graduate nurse, but with dedication and a clear vision, you can create a strong personal brand that sets you apart in the healthcare industry.

Understanding the Concept of Personal Branding

Personal branding is creating and managing a unique professional identity and image for yourself. It involves intentionally shaping how you are perceived by others, both online and offline, to differentiate yourself and stand out in your field. Personal branding is not about creating a false persona, but rather about authentically showcasing your skills, expertise, values, and unique qualities to build a strong professional reputation. Understanding the concept of personal branding can significantly assist new graduate nurses during their transition from student to nurse practitioner by helping them articulate their unique professional identity, values, and skills in a competitive healthcare landscape. A well-defined personal brand allows these graduates to present themselves confidently to potential employers, colleagues, and patients, showcasing their strengths and distinguishing them from their peers. By actively engaging in personal branding, new nurses can develop a clear narrative around their educational background and clinical experiences, creating a cohesive story that resonates with their target audience. Additionally, a strong personal brand cultivates professional relationships and networking opportunities, essential for career advancement and mentorship in the nursing field. Emphasizing their brand on platforms such as LinkedIn or during professional interactions can enhance their visibility and reputation, ultimately easing their integration into the workforce and fostering long-term success in their nursing careers.

Here are some key aspects of personal branding:

- Self-reflection: Personal branding starts with self-reflection. You need to understand your strengths, skills, values, and passions. What makes you unique? What do you want to be known for? This self-awareness will help you define your personal brand.
- Target audience: Identify your target audience or the people you want to connect with and influence. This could be potential employers, clients, colleagues, or industry professionals. Understanding their needs and interests will help you tailor your personal brand message to resonate with them.
- Brand message: Your brand message is the core message you want to convey about yourself. It should be clear, concise, and consistent across all your communication channels. Your brand message should highlight your unique value proposition and what sets you apart from others in your field.

- Online presence: In today's digital age, having a strong online presence is crucial for personal branding. This includes having a professional website or blog, active social media profiles, and a well-crafted LinkedIn profile. Your online presence should align with your brand message and showcase your expertise and accomplishments.
- Networking: Building a strong professional network is an important aspect of personal branding. Attend industry events, join professional organizations, and connect with others in your field. Networking allows you to establish relationships, gain visibility, and create opportunities for collaboration and career growth.
- Consistency and authenticity: Consistency is key in personal branding. Ensure that your brand message, visual identity, and overall communication style are consistent across all platforms. Authenticity is also crucial. Be true to yourself and let your genuine personality shine through in your personal brand.
- Continuous learning and growth: Personal branding is an ongoing process. Stay updated with new trends in the field, enhance your skills, and seek out opportunities for professional development. Continuously refine and evolve your personal brand to stay relevant and competitive in your field.

Personal branding is not about self-promotion or creating a false image. It is about showcasing your unique qualities, expertise, and value in an authentic and intentional way. By effectively managing your personal brand, you can differentiate yourself, attract opportunities, and build a strong professional reputation.

1.7   Defining Your Professional Identity

Defining your professional identity as a nurse is important in establishing yourself in the healthcare industry and shaping your career. How to define your professional identity as a nurse:

- Nursing philosophy: Start by reflecting on your beliefs and values about nursing. What drew you to the profession? What do you believe are the core principles of nursing? Your nursing philosophy will serve as the foundation for your professional identity.
- Specialization and expertise: Consider the areas of nursing that you are passionate about and want to specialize in. This could be clinical or nonclinical specialized areas in the nursing field. Developing expertise in a specific area will help you stand out and become known for your skills and knowledge in that particular domain.
- Professional goals: Set clear professional goals for yourself. What do you want to achieve in your nursing career? Do you aspire to become a nurse leader, educator, or researcher or advance in a specific role? Having goals will give you direction and help shape your professional identity.
- Continuous learning: Nursing is a constantly evolving field, and it's important to stay updated with the latest research, advancements, and best practices. Commit

to lifelong learning and seek out opportunities for professional development, such as attending conferences, pursuing advanced certifications, or participating in continuing education programs.

- Patient-centered care: As a nurse, your primary focus should be on providing high-quality, patient-centered care. Emphasize the importance of empathy, compassion, and effective communication in your professional identity. Strive to build strong relationships with your patients and their families, and advocate for their needs and well-being.
- Collaboration and leadership: Nursing is a collaborative profession, and effective teamwork is essential for providing optimal patient care. Develop your collaboration, communication, and leadership skills to become a valuable healthcare team member. This can include taking on leadership roles in nursing organizations, participating in interdisciplinary committees, or mentoring other nurses.
- Professional ethics and integrity: Uphold the highest standards of professional ethics and integrity in your nursing practice. Adhere to the nursing code of ethics, maintain patient confidentiality, and always act in the best interest of your patients. Your commitment to ethical practice will contribute to your professional identity and reputation.

It is important to note that professional identity as a nurse is unique to individual nurse and will evolve over time as they gain experience and grow in their career. Regularly reflect on values, goals, and aspirations to ensure that professional identity aligns with who they are as a nurse and the impact they want to make in the nursing and healthcare field.

Identifying Your Unique Strengths, Skills, and Values

Identifying unique strengths, skills, and values is crucial for new graduate nurses as they transition from student to nurse practitioner because it fosters confidence and clarity in their professional identity. By recognizing their individual competencies—whether clinical skills, emotional intelligence, or critical thinking—these graduates can leverage their strengths to enhance patient care and communication within the healthcare team. Additionally, understanding their personal values allows them to align their practice with their beliefs, promoting job satisfaction and ethical decision-making. This self-awareness not only empowers new nurses to navigate the challenges of a demanding environment but also positions them to advocate for themselves and their patients effectively. Ultimately, a keen awareness of their unique attributes helps new graduate nurses establish a solid foundation for lifelong learning and professional growth in their nursing careers.

1.8 Bridging the Gap

Identifying the Skills Gap Between Academia and the Workplace

As a new graduate nurse, you may encounter a skills gap between what you learned in academia and the skills required in the workplace. This gap is common and can be addressed through various means. Here are some key areas where you may find a skills gap and suggestions on how to bridge it:

- Clinical skills: While nursing programs provide a foundation of clinical skills, the real-world healthcare setting may require additional or more advanced skills. To bridge this gap, consider seeking out additional training opportunities, such as workshops, simulation labs, or preceptorships. Take advantage of orientation programs offered by your employer to gain hands-on experience and build confidence in your clinical skills.
- Critical thinking and decision-making: Nursing practice often requires quick and effective decision-making in complex situations. While academic programs teach critical thinking skills, the workplace demands practical application. To enhance your critical thinking abilities, actively seek opportunities to participate in case studies, problem-solving exercises, and clinical discussions. Engage with experienced nurses and ask for their guidance and insights.
- Communication and collaboration: Effective communication and collaboration are essential skills in nursing practice. While nursing programs may provide some training in these areas, the workplace requires further development. Take advantage of opportunities to work in interdisciplinary teams, engage in effective handoff communication, and practice therapeutic communication with patients and their families. Seek feedback from colleagues and supervisors to improve your communication skills.
- Time management and prioritization: Balancing multiple tasks and prioritizing patient care can be challenging for new graduate nurses. Time management skills are crucial to ensure efficient and safe care delivery. To improve in this area, seek guidance from experienced nurses on effective time management strategies. Take advantage of tools and resources provided by your workplace, such as electronic health records and scheduling systems, to help you prioritize and organize your tasks.
- Professionalism and ethical decision-making: While nursing programs emphasize professionalism and ethical practice, the workplace may present unique challenges. Continuously develop your understanding of professional ethics and standards of practice. Seek out opportunities to engage in ethical discussions, participate in ethics committees, and attend professional development sessions on ethical decision-making.
- Leadership and management skills: As you progress in your nursing career, leadership and management skills become increasingly important. While academic programs may touch on these topics, further development is often required. Seek out leadership opportunities within your workplace, such as serving on committees or taking on charge nurse roles. Consider pursuing additional education or certifications in nursing leadership or management to enhance your skills in this area.

The skills gap between academia and the workplace is a normal part of transitioning into the nursing profession. Be proactive in seeking out opportunities for growth and development. Embrace a lifelong learning mindset, and continuously seek feedback and guidance from experienced nurses and mentors. With time and experience, you will bridge the skills gap and become a confident and competent nurse in the workplace.

Developing Essential Skills Required for Professional Success
Developing essential skills is crucial for professional success in nursing. Here are some key skills that are important for nurses to cultivate:

- Clinical competence: Building and maintaining clinical competence is essential for providing safe and effective patient care. Continuously update your knowledge and skills through ongoing education, attending conferences, and staying up to date with evidence-based practice. Seek out opportunities to practice and refine your clinical skills in various healthcare settings.
- Communication skills: Effective communication is vital in nursing. Develop strong verbal and written communication skills to effectively interact with patients, their families, and the healthcare team. Practice active listening, empathy, and clear and concise communication. Good communication helps build trust, ensures patient safety, and promotes collaboration.
- Critical thinking and problem-solving: Nursing require the ability to think critically and make sound decisions in complex situations. Develop your critical thinking skills by actively seeking out opportunities to analyze and solve problems. Engage in case studies, participate in clinical discussions, and seek guidance from experienced nurses. Continuously evaluate and reflect on your practice to improve your critical thinking abilities.
- Leadership and management: Leadership skills are important for nurses at all levels. Develop your leadership abilities by taking on leadership roles within your workplace, such as charge nurse or preceptor. Seek out opportunities to enhance your management skills, such as learning about resource allocation, delegation, and conflict resolution. Effective leadership and management skills contribute to improved patient outcomes and a positive work environment.
- Emotional intelligence: Emotional intelligence involves understanding and managing your own emotions and effectively relating to others. Develop self-awareness, empathy, and the ability to navigate challenging situations with emotional intelligence. This skill is crucial for building therapeutic relationships with patients, collaborating with colleagues, and managing stress in the healthcare environment.
- Cultural competence: Nursing is a diverse profession, and cultural competence is essential for providing patient-centered care. Develop an understanding and appreciation of different cultures, beliefs, and practices. Seek out opportunities to learn about cultural diversity, engage in cultural humility, and adapt your care to meet the unique needs of diverse patient populations.
- Professionalism and ethics: Upholding professionalism and ethical standards is fundamental in nursing. Demonstrate integrity, accountability, and ethical decision-making in your practice. Adhere to the nursing code of ethics, maintain

patient confidentiality, and advocate for patient rights. Continuously reflect on your professional values, and seek professional growth and development opportunities.

Developing these essential skills is an ongoing process. Embrace a lifelong learning mindset and seek out opportunities for growth and development throughout your nursing career. Continuously evaluate your skills, seek feedback from colleagues and mentors, and engage in self-reflection to enhance your professional success in nursing.

Seeking Opportunities to Enhance and Showcase Your Skills
As a new graduate nurse, seeking opportunities to enhance and showcase your skills is crucial for professional growth and advancement. Here are some strategies to consider:

- Continuing education: Pursue additional certifications, courses, or workshops to enhance your knowledge and skills in specific areas of nursing. Look for opportunities to expand your expertise in areas. Continuing education demonstrates your commitment to ongoing learning and professional development.
- Preceptorship or mentorship programs: Seek out preceptorship or mentorship programs offered by your workplace or professional organizations. These programs provide guidance and support from experienced nurses who can help you develop your skills and navigate the challenges of the nursing profession.
- Professional organizations and conferences: Join professional nursing organizations and attend conferences related to your area of interest. These events provide opportunities to network with other professionals, learn about the latest research and advancements in nursing, and showcase your skills through presentations or poster sessions.
- Volunteer or community service: Engage in healthcare-related volunteer work or community service. This not only allows you to give back to the community but also provides opportunities to develop and showcase your skills in a different setting. Volunteering can also help you build connections and expand your professional network.
- Quality improvement projects: Get involved in quality improvement initiatives within your workplace. Participate in projects to improve patient outcomes, enhance safety, or streamline processes. Involvement in these projects demonstrates your commitment to delivering high-quality care and your ability to contribute to positive change.
- Research and publications: Consider engaging in nursing research or scholarly activities. Collaborate with colleagues or mentors on research projects, and aim to publish your findings in nursing journals or present at conferences. Engaging in research demonstrates your commitment to evidence-based practice and contributes to the advancement of nursing knowledge.
- Professional portfolio: Develop a professional portfolio to showcase your skills, accomplishments, and ongoing professional development. Include copies of

certifications, letters of recommendation, examples of projects or presentations, and any other relevant documentation. A well-organized portfolio can be a valuable tool when applying for new positions or seeking advancement opportunities.

Seeking opportunities to enhance and showcase your skills requires proactive effort and a commitment to continuous learning. Be open to new experiences, seek feedback from colleagues and mentors, and actively seek out opportunities to grow and develop as a nurse. By actively engaging in these opportunities, you can enhance your skills, build your professional reputation, and open doors for future career advancement.

1.9   Overcoming Challenges

As a new graduate nurse, you may face various challenges in your role. Here are some common challenges and strategies to overcome them:

- Lack of experience: As a new graduate nurse, you may feel overwhelmed by the lack of experience. Remember that it is normal to feel this way; gaining confidence and competence takes time. Seek guidance from experienced colleagues, ask questions, and take advantage of learning opportunities to enhance your skills.
- Time management: Balancing multiple tasks and responsibilities can be challenging. Prioritize your tasks, create a schedule, and learn to delegate when appropriate. Effective time management skills will help you stay organized and meet deadlines.
- Stress and emotional demands: Nursing can be emotionally demanding, and you may encounter stressful situations. Practice self-care techniques such as exercise, mindfulness, and seeking support from colleagues or mentors. Develop healthy coping mechanisms to manage stress and maintain your well-being.
- Communication and teamwork: Effective communication and teamwork are essential in nursing. If you face challenges in this area, focus on improving your communication skills, actively listening to others, and seeking feedback. Foster a collaborative environment by building positive relationships with your colleagues and stakeholders.
- Dealing with difficult patients or families: Interacting with difficult patients or families can be challenging. Practice empathy, active listening, and effective communication techniques. Seek guidance from experienced nurses or utilize resources such as conflict resolution training to handle these situations professionally.
- Adapting to new environments: Starting a new job or working in a different healthcare setting can be overwhelming. Take the time to familiarize yourself with the policies, procedures, and culture of your workplace. Seek support from your preceptor or mentor to help you navigate the new environment.

- Continuing education and professional development: Nursing is a constantly evolving field, and it is important to stay updated with the latest evidence-based practices. To enhance your knowledge and skills, take advantage of continuing education opportunities, attend conferences, and join professional nursing organizations.
- Balancing work and personal life: Nursing can be demanding and finding a work-life balance is crucial. Set boundaries, prioritize self-care, and make time for activities outside of work that bring you joy and relaxation.

Challenges are a part of the learning process, and it's important to approach them positively. Seek support from your colleagues, mentors, and supervisors, and remember that with time and experience, you will become more confident and proficient in your role as a new graduate nurse.

1.10 Dealing with Imposter Syndrome

Understanding Imposter Syndrome and Its Impact on Professional Growth
Imposter syndrome is a psychological phenomenon where individuals doubt their abilities and have a persistent fear of being exposed as a fraud, despite evidence of their competence (Siddiqui et al. 2024). Imposter syndrome can lead to self-doubt, causing you to question your skills and knowledge as a nurse. You may feel like you don't belong or that you're not as capable as your colleagues. This self-doubt can hinder your professional growth by holding you back from taking on new challenges and opportunities. As a new graduate nurse, you may experience imposter syndrome as you transition into your professional role. Here's an understanding of imposter syndrome and its impact on professional growth:

To overcome the impact of imposter syndrome on your professional growth as a new graduate nurse, consider the following strategies:

- Recognize and acknowledge your feelings: Be aware of the signs of imposter syndrome and acknowledge when you're experiencing self-doubt or fear. Understanding that these feelings are common and not indicative of your actual abilities can help you navigate through them.
- Challenge negative self-talk: Replace negative self-talk with positive affirmations. Remind yourself of your accomplishments, skills, and the value you bring to your role as a nurse. Focus on your progress and growth rather than comparing yourself to others.
- Seek support and mentorship: Reach out to trusted colleagues, mentors, or supervisors who can provide guidance and support. Share your feelings of self-doubt and imposter syndrome with them, as they can offer reassurance and perspective.
- Set realistic goals: Break down your professional goals into smaller, achievable steps. Celebrate each milestone along the way, recognizing your progress and

growth. Setting realistic goals can help you build confidence and overcome the fear of failure.

- Embrace continuous learning: Embrace a growth mindset and view challenges as opportunities for learning and development. Seek out learning opportunities, attend workshops or conferences, and engage in professional development activities to enhance your skills and knowledge.
- Practice self-care: Prioritize self-care to maintain your physical and emotional well-being. Engage in activities that help you relax, recharge, and reduce stress. Taking care of yourself will boost your confidence and resilience in the face of imposter syndrome.

Imposter syndrome is a common experience, especially for new graduate nurses. By recognizing and addressing it, you can overcome its impact on your professional growth and thrive in your nursing career.

Strategies for Overcoming Self-Doubt and Building Confidence

- Overcoming self-doubt and building confidence as a new graduate nurse are essential for professional growth and success. Here are some strategies to help you:
- Recognize and challenge negative thoughts: Start by becoming aware of your self-doubt and negative thoughts. When you catch yourself thinking negatively, challenge those thoughts by asking yourself for evidence to support them. Replace negative thoughts with positive affirmations and focus on your strengths and accomplishments.
- Celebrate small victories: Acknowledge and celebrate your achievements, no matter how small they may seem. Recognize your progress and the positive impact you've had on patients' lives. Celebrating small victories will boost your confidence and motivate you to continue growing.
- Seek feedback and guidance: Actively seek feedback from your colleagues, mentors, and supervisors. Their input can provide valuable insights into your strengths and areas for improvement. Use their feedback as an opportunity for growth and learning.
- Set realistic goals: Set achievable goals for yourself, both short term and long term. Break them down into smaller, manageable steps. You'll gain confidence and momentum to tackle more challenging goals as you accomplish each step.
- Embrace continuous learning: Nursing is a dynamic and ever-evolving field, and continuous learning is crucial for professional growth. Engage in ongoing education, attend workshops and conferences, and stay informed with the latest research and best practices. The more knowledge and skills you acquire, the more confident you'll become in your professional abilities.
- Seek support from peers: Connect with other new graduate nurses who may be experiencing similar challenges. Share your experiences, concerns, and successes with each other. Having a support system of peers can provide encouragement and reassurance.

- Practice self-care: Taking care of your physical and emotional well-being is vital for building confidence. Make time for activities that bring you joy and relaxation. Prioritize self-care practices such as exercise, healthy eating, and getting enough rest. When you feel good physically and emotionally, your confidence will naturally improve.
- Reflect on your growth: Regularly reflect on your progress and growth as a nurse. Keep a journal or make a list of your achievements, skills you've developed, and challenges you've overcome. This reflection will remind you of how far you've come and reinforce your confidence in your abilities.
- Surround yourself with positive influences: Engage with supportive and positive individuals who have confidence in your abilities. Avoid negative or toxic environments that may contribute to self-doubt. Seek out mentors and role models who can inspire and guide you in your nursing journey.
- Practice self-compassion: Be kind and compassionate toward yourself. Remember that everyone makes mistakes and experiences setbacks. Treat yourself with the same understanding and compassion you would offer to a colleague or patient. Learn from your mistakes and use them as opportunities for growth.
- Building confidence takes time and effort, but with persistence and these strategies, you can overcome self-doubt and thrive as a new graduate nurse. Remember to be patient with yourself and celebrate your progress along the way.

1.11 Keeping Up with the Requirements of the Nursing Regulatory Body During the Transition Period

Keeping up to date with the requirements of the nursing regulatory body is crucial during the transition from student nurse to nurse practitioner. Here's why it is important:

- Nursing regulatory bodies establish and enforce standards and regulations to ensure safe and competent nursing practice. By staying updated with these requirements, nurse practitioners can ensure they are practicing within the legal and ethical boundaries of their profession.
- Nurse practitioners must obtain and maintain the necessary licensure and certification to practice. Regulatory bodies set the criteria for licensure and certification, including educational requirements, clinical experience, and examination processes. Staying informed about these requirements is essential to obtain and retain the necessary credentials.
- Nursing regulatory bodies define the scope of practice for nurse practitioners, outlining the specific activities and interventions they are authorized to perform. By staying up to date, nurse practitioners can ensure they are practicing within their authorized scope, providing safe and appropriate care to their patients.
- Regulatory bodies often require nurse practitioners to engage in continuing education to maintain their licensure and certification. Staying informed about the specific continuing education requirements allows nurse practitioners to fulfil

these obligations and stay current with the latest advancements and best practices in their field.

- Keeping up to date with the requirements of the nursing regulatory body promotes ongoing professional development. It encourages nurse practitioners to seek out opportunities for learning, growth, and skill enhancement, which ultimately benefits their patients and the quality of care they provide.
- Compliance with regulatory requirements ensures that nurse practitioners are competent and up to date with the knowledge and skills necessary to provide safe and effective care. By staying informed, nurse practitioners can contribute to uphold high standards of patient safety and quality of care.
- Staying updated with regulatory requirements demonstrates a commitment to professional accountability. It shows that nurse practitioners are aware of their professional responsibilities and are dedicated to meeting the standards set by their regulatory body.

Staying up to date with the requirements of the nursing regulatory body is essential during the transition from student nurse to nurse practitioner. It ensures compliance with regulations, facilitates licensure and certification, defines the scope of practice, promotes continuing education and professional development, enhances patient safety, and demonstrates professional accountability. By staying informed, nurse practitioners can provide safe, competent, and high-quality care to their patients.

1.12 Conclusion

Transitioning from student to practitioner is a transformative journey that requires adaptability, resilience, and continuous learning. By understanding the challenges and opportunities that come with this transition, building a strong professional network, developing a personal brand, honing essential skills, and overcoming common challenges, students can successfully navigate this transition and embark on a fulfilling and rewarding professional career. Below are the practical exercises related to this chapter.

Applied Practical Exercises
1. Self-reflection and goal setting
   (a) Take some time to reflect on your strengths, areas for improvement, and personal goals as you transition into the role of a professional nurse.
   (b) Write down three specific goals you want to achieve during your first year of practice. Consider both clinical and professional development goals.
   (c) Develop an action plan outlining the steps you will take to achieve each goal. Set timelines and identify resources or support you may need along the way.

2. Professional identity development
   (a) Conduct research on the professional values and ethics of nursing. Identify three core values that resonate with you and explain why they are important in nursing practice.
   (b) Write a personal mission statement reflecting your commitment to providing quality patient care and upholding the nursing profession's values.
   (c) Engage in a reflective journaling exercise where you document instances where you demonstrated professionalism and how it positively impacted patient care.
3. Effective communication and collaboration
   (a) Role-play scenarios that involve interdisciplinary collaboration. Practice effective communication techniques, such as active listening, clear and concise verbal communication, and respectful feedback.
   (b) Shadow a healthcare professional from a different discipline for a day. Observe their role and responsibilities and reflect on how their collaboration with nurses contributes to patient care.
   (c) Interview an experienced nurse or healthcare professional about their experiences with effective teamwork and collaboration. Discuss strategies they have found successful and apply them to your own practice.
4. Self-care and well-being
   (a) Develop a self-care plan that includes activities and strategies to promote physical, emotional, and mental well-being. Implement this plan consistently throughout your transition period.
   (b) Incorporate stress management techniques, such as deep breathing exercises, mindfulness, or engaging in hobbies or activities that bring you joy and relaxation.
   (c) Seek out a mentor or join a support group for new graduate nurses. Share experiences, challenges, and coping strategies to support each other during the transition.
5. Continuous learning and professional development
   (a) Identify three areas of nursing practice that you are particularly interested in or would like to further develop. Research professional development opportunities related to these areas, such as workshops, conferences, or online courses.
   (b) Create a professional development portfolio to track your learning and achievements. Include certificates, continuing education credits, and reflections on how these experiences have enhanced your practice.
   (c) Engage in a monthly journal club with colleagues, or join a nursing association to stay updated on the latest research and evidence-based practices. Discuss and critically analyze articles related to your area of interest.

These applied practical exercises are designed to help you actively engage with the content of the chapter and apply the concepts to your own practice. By completing these exercises, you will gain a deeper understanding of the transition process and develop practical skills to navigate the challenges and opportunities of transitioning from student to practitioner.

References

Casey K, Oja KJ, Makic MBF (2021) The lived experiences of graduate nurses transitioning to professional practice during a pandemic. Nurs Outlook 69(6):1072–1080. https://doi.org/10.1016/j.outlook.2021.06.006

Gautam S, Poudel A, Paudyal K, Prajapati MM (2023) Transition to professional practice: perspectives of new nursing graduates of Nepal. BMC Nurs 22(1):273. https://doi.org/10.1186/s12912-023-01418-2

Matlhaba KL, Khunou SH (2022) Transition of graduate nurses from student to practice during the COVID-19 pandemic: integrative review. Int J Afr Nurs Sci 17:100501. https://doi.org/10.1016/j.ijans.2022.100501

Pawar A (2016) The power of personal branding. Int J Eng Manag Res 6(2):840–847

Roman-Fischetti L (2020) Effective networking. In: Fast facts for making the most of your career in nursing, p 185. https://books.google.co.za/books?id=mvDqDwAAQBAJ&printsec=frontcover&source=gbs_ge_summary_r&cad=0

Savard I, Al Hakim G, Kilpatrick K (2023) The added value of the nurse practitioner: an evolutionary concept analysis. Nurs Open 10(4):2540–2551. https://doi.org/10.1002/nop2.1512

Schlunegger MC, Aeschlimann S, Palm R, Zumstein-Shaha M (2023) Competencies of nurse practitioners in family practices: a scoping review. J Clin Nurs 32(11–12):2521–2532. https://doi.org/10.1111/jocn.16382

Siddiqui ZK, Church HR, Jayasuriya R, Boddice T, Tomlinson J (2024) Educational interventions for imposter phenomenon in healthcare: a scoping review. BMC Med Educ 24(1):43. https://doi.org/10.1186/s12909-023-04984-w

South African Nursing Council (2005) Nursing Act (Act No. 33 of 2005). Pretoria: Government Printer

Building a Foundation for Clinical Competence

2

Contents

> Test your learning and check your understanding of this book's contents: use the "Springer Nature Flashcards" app to access questions using ▶ https://sn.pub/pe441e. To use the app, please follow the instructions in Chap. 1.

2.1 Building a Foundation for Clinical Competence of New Graduate Nurses

Clinical competency is defined as the ability to integrate knowledge, skills, attitudes, and values into a clinical situation (Hui et al. 2023). Almarwani and Alzahrani (2023) and Matlhaba and Nkoane (2024) further defined clinical competence as the ability of a nurse to effectively and safely perform clinical tasks and provide high-quality care based on their knowledge, skills, and experience.

Building a strong foundation for clinical competence is crucial for new graduate nurses as they transition into their professional nursing practice. Therefore, establishing a strong foundation for clinical practice requires an understanding of several fundamental principles and essential skills.

© The Author(s), under exclusive license to Springer Nature Switzerland AG 2024　　35
K. Matlhaba, *Enhancing Clinical Competence of Graduate Nurses*,
https://doi.org/10.1007/978-3-031-81407-5_2

- Clinical reasoning: Clinical reasoning is critical; practitioners must effectively assess patient needs, formulate diagnoses, and develop appropriate treatment plans. This is complemented by strong communication skills, facilitating clear interactions with patients and collaborative teamwork among healthcare professionals.
- Ethical practice: Ethical practice is paramount, ensuring patient confidentiality, informed consent, and the prioritization of patient welfare. Proficiency in evidence-based practice allows clinicians to integrate the best available research with clinical expertise, ensuring that interventions are both effective and up-to-date.
- Self-reflection: Ongoing self-reflection and adaptability foster continuous learning, enabling practitioners to evolve with advances in medical knowledge and changes in patient demographics or needs, thereby reinforcing the quality of care provided.

Together, these principles and skills lay the groundwork for effective, responsible, and compassionate clinical practice. Below are some key steps to help new graduate nurses develop and enhance their clinical competence:

- Orientation and preceptorship: New graduate nurses should participate in a comprehensive orientation program that provides them with the necessary knowledge and skills to practice safely and effectively. Pairing new graduates with experienced preceptors can further support their learning and development.
- Continuous learning: Encourage new graduate nurses to engage in continuous learning and professional development. This can include attending workshops, conferences, and seminars, pursuing advanced certifications, and staying updated with evidence-based practice guidelines. Encourage them to seek out learning opportunities within their clinical setting and take advantage of mentorship programs.
- Clinical skill development: New graduate nurses should focus on developing and refining their clinical skills. This includes mastering basic nursing procedures, such as medication administration, wound care, and patient assessment. Encourage them to seek opportunities to practice these skills under supervision and receive feedback to improve their proficiency.
- Critical thinking and decision-making: Help new graduate nurses develop critical thinking skills by encouraging them to analyze patient situations, consider multiple perspectives, and make informed decisions. Provide opportunities for them to participate in case discussions, problem-solving exercises, and simulation-based learning to enhance their critical thinking abilities.
- Effective communication: Effective communication is essential for clinical competence. Encourage new graduate nurses to develop strong communication skills, both verbal and written. This includes active listening, clear and concise documentation, and effective collaboration with the healthcare team. Provide feedback and guidance on communication skills to help them improve.

- Time management and organization: New graduate nurses should learn effective time management and organizational skills to prioritize tasks, manage their workload, and ensure patient safety. Teach them strategies for prioritizing and delegating tasks, managing interruptions, and maintaining accurate documentation.
- Reflective practice: Encourage new graduate nurses to engage in reflective practice, where they critically analyze their experiences, identify areas for improvement, and develop action plans for growth. This self-reflection can enhance their clinical competence by promoting self-awareness, identifying learning needs, and fostering continuous improvement.
- Support and mentorship: Provide new graduate nurses with ongoing support and mentorship. Assign them mentors who can guide and support their professional development. Regular check-ins, feedback sessions, and opportunities for open dialog can help them navigate challenges and build confidence in their clinical competence.

Building clinical competence is a continuous process that takes time and experience. Encourage new graduate nurses to embrace learning opportunities, seek guidance when needed, and remain open to feedback and self-reflection. With time and support, they will develop a strong foundation for clinical competence and excel in their nursing practice.

2.2   The Significance of Clinical Competence

Clinical competence is of utmost importance in the field of nursing. It refers to the ability of a nurse to effectively and safely perform clinical tasks and provide high-quality care to patients. Clinical competence is a multifaceted attribute that encompasses the synthesis of knowledge, skills, attitudes, and behaviors essential for healthcare professionals to provide high-quality care. This combination ensures that practitioners are not only well-versed in medical theories and evidence-based practices but also possess the technical skills necessary for effective patient assessment and intervention. Equally important are the attitudes and behaviors that reflect empathy, integrity, and a commitment to continuous learning. By integrating these elements, healthcare professionals can foster trust and rapport with patients, enhance communication within interdisciplinary teams, and adapt to the evolving challenges of the healthcare environment. Ultimately, clinical competence drives improved patient outcomes, safety, and satisfaction, highlighting its critical role in the delivery of compassionate and effective medical care. Here are some key reasons why clinical competence is significant in nursing:

- Patient safety: Clinical competence ensures that nurses have the necessary knowledge, skills, and judgment to provide safe care to patients. Competent nurses are able to accurately assess patients, identify potential risks, and implement appropriate interventions to prevent harm.

- Quality of care: Competent nurses are able to provide high-quality care that meets the standards and expectations of patients, families, and healthcare organizations. They are knowledgeable about evidence-based practices which can be effectively applied in their clinical decision-making.
- Professionalism: Clinical competence is a fundamental aspect of professionalism in nursing. Competent nurses demonstrate a commitment to lifelong learning, continuous professional development, and staying up-to-date with the latest advancements in healthcare. They also adhere to ethical standards and maintain a high level of integrity in their practice.
- Collaboration and teamwork: Competent nurses are able to effectively collaborate with other healthcare professionals, such as doctors, pharmacists, and therapists, to ensure coordinated and comprehensive care for patients. They can communicate effectively, share information, and contribute to interdisciplinary discussions and decision-making.
- Confidence and job satisfaction: Clinical competence enhances nurses' confidence in their abilities to provide safe and effective care. This confidence not only improves job satisfaction but also contributes to better patient outcomes. Competent nurses are more likely to feel fulfilled in their roles and have a positive impact on the lives of their patients.
- Professional growth and advancement: Clinical competence is essential for professional growth and advancement in nursing. Competent nurses are more likely to pursue advanced certifications, specialty areas of practice, and leadership roles. They are also better positioned to take on new challenges and adapt to changes in healthcare delivery.

Clinical competence is crucial in nursing as it ensures patient safety, quality of care, professionalism, collaboration, confidence, job satisfaction, and professional growth. It is an ongoing process that requires continuous learning, practice, and self-reflection to maintain and enhance competence throughout a nurse's career.

The Importance of Clinical Competence in Providing Safe and Effective Patient Care

Clinical competence plays a vital role in providing safe and effective patient care. Here are some key reasons why clinical competence is important in this regard:

- Patient safety: Clinical competence ensures that healthcare professionals have the necessary knowledge, skills, and abilities to provide safe care to patients. Competent healthcare professionals can accurately assess patients, identify potential risks, and implement appropriate interventions to prevent harm. They are also skilled in recognizing and responding to emergencies and adverse events promptly and effectively.
- Accurate diagnosis and treatment: Competent healthcare professionals are proficient in conducting thorough assessments, interpreting diagnostic tests, and formulating accurate diagnoses. This enables them to develop appropriate treatment plans and interventions tailored to each patient's specific needs. Clinical

competence also ensures that healthcare professionals are up-to-date with evidence-based practices, enabling them to provide the most effective treatments and interventions.

- Effective communication: Clinical competence includes effective communication skills, which are essential for safe and effective patient care. Competent healthcare professionals can communicate clearly and effectively with patients, their families, and other members of the healthcare team. This facilitates the exchange of important information, ensures patient understanding, and promotes collaborative decision-making.
- Medication safety: Competent healthcare professionals have a thorough understanding of medications, including their indications, contraindications, dosages, and potential side effects. They are skilled in medication administration and monitoring, ensuring that patients receive the right medications at the right doses and frequencies. Clinical competence also includes knowledge of medication interactions and the ability to identify and manage medication errors.
- Critical thinking and problem-solving: Clinical competence involves the ability to think critically and solve problems in complex healthcare situations. Competent healthcare professionals are skilled in analyzing information, making sound judgments, and implementing appropriate interventions. They are able to anticipate and respond to changes in patient conditions, ensuring timely and effective care.
- Continuity of care: Clinical competence ensures seamless continuity of care for patients. Competent healthcare professionals are able to effectively communicate and collaborate with other members of the healthcare team, ensuring that important information is shared and coordinated. This promotes a holistic approach to patient care and reduces the risk of errors or gaps in care.

Clinical competence is essential for providing safe and effective patient care. It encompasses a range of knowledge, skills, and abilities that enable healthcare professionals to assess, diagnose, treat, and communicate effectively with patients. By ensuring patient safety, accurate diagnosis and treatment, effective communication, medication safety, critical thinking, problem-solving, and continuity of care, clinical competence plays a crucial role in improving patient outcomes and overall healthcare quality.

The Impact of Clinical Competence on Professional Growth and Confidence
Clinical competence has a significant impact on the professional growth and confidence of new graduate nurses. Here are some ways in which clinical competence influences their development:

- Skill development: Clinical competence allows new graduate nurses to develop and refine their clinical skills. Through hands-on experience and guidance from experienced mentors, they gain proficiency in performing various nursing procedures, assessments, and interventions. This skill development enhances their confidence in their abilities and prepares them for more complex and challenging patient care situations.

- Knowledge expansion: Clinical competence requires a strong foundation of knowledge in nursing theory, evidence-based practice, and healthcare guidelines. As new graduate nurses gain clinical experience, they have the opportunity to apply and expand their theoretical knowledge in real-world scenarios. This process deepens their understanding of nursing concepts and builds their confidence in making clinical decisions.
- Critical thinking and problem-solving: Clinical competence fosters the development of critical thinking and problem-solving skills in new graduate nurses. They learn to analyze patient data, identify potential issues, and make informed decisions to provide safe and effective care. As they successfully navigate complex patient care situations, their confidence in their ability to handle challenges and solve problems grows.
- Professional networking: Clinical competence often involves working collaboratively with interdisciplinary healthcare teams. New graduate nurses have the opportunity to interact and build professional relationships with experienced nurses, physicians, and other healthcare professionals. These connections provide mentorship, guidance, and opportunities for learning and growth. Networking with professionals in the field enhances their confidence and opens doors for future career opportunities.
- Professional development opportunities: Clinical competence is a foundation for professional growth. As new graduate nurses demonstrate their competence, they may be offered opportunities for further education, specialization, and career advancement. They may pursue advanced certifications, participate in research projects, or take on leadership roles. These opportunities not only enhance their knowledge and skills but also boost their confidence in their ability to excel in their chosen career path.
- Enhanced job satisfaction: Clinical competence contributes to job satisfaction for new graduate nurses. As they gain competence and confidence in their abilities, they feel more fulfilled in their roles and experience a sense of accomplishment. This satisfaction motivates them to continue learning and growing in their profession, leading to long-term career success.

Clinical competence has a profound impact on the professional growth and confidence of new graduate nurses. It enables them to develop and refine their clinical skills, expand their knowledge, enhance critical thinking and problem-solving abilities, build professional networks, access professional development opportunities, and experience job satisfaction. By nurturing clinical competence, new graduate nurses can establish a strong foundation for a successful and fulfilling nursing career.

Recognizing the Challenges and Opportunities in Developing Clinical Competence

As a new graduate nurse, developing clinical competence can be both challenging and full of opportunities. Here are some common challenges and opportunities that new graduate nurses may encounter in their journey toward clinical competence:

Challenges

- Limited clinical experience: New graduate nurses often have limited clinical experience compared to more seasoned nurses. This can make it challenging to apply theoretical knowledge to real-world patient care situations. Overcoming this challenge requires actively seeking opportunities for hands-on experience, such as clinical rotations, internships, or preceptorship programs.
- Time management: Balancing multiple responsibilities and tasks within a fast-paced healthcare environment can be overwhelming for new graduate nurses. Learning to prioritize and manage time effectively is crucial for developing clinical competence. Seeking guidance from experienced nurses and utilizing time management strategies can help overcome this challenge.
- Confidence and self-doubt: New graduate nurses may experience self-doubt and lack confidence in their abilities. The transition from the controlled environment of nursing school to the unpredictable nature of clinical practice can be intimidating. Building confidence takes time and experience, but seeking support from mentors, participating in debriefing sessions, and reflecting on successes can help boost confidence.
- Complex patient cases: New graduate nurses may encounter complex patient cases that require advanced clinical knowledge and critical thinking skills. Managing these cases can be challenging, especially when faced with limited experience. Seeking guidance from experienced nurses, consulting with interdisciplinary team members, and engaging in continuous learning can help navigate these challenges. This section is fully explained in Chap. 7.

Opportunities

- Mentorship and preceptorship programs: Many healthcare organizations offer mentorship and preceptorship programs for new graduate nurses. These programs provide opportunities to work closely with experienced nurses who can guide and support their development. Taking advantage of these programs can accelerate the development of clinical competence.
- Continuing education and professional development: New graduate nurses have the opportunity to engage in continuing education and professional development activities. Attending workshops, conferences, and seminars, as well as pursuing advanced certifications or specialty training, can enhance clinical knowledge and skills.
- Reflective practice: Engaging in reflective practice allows new graduate nurses to critically analyze their experiences, identify areas for improvement, and develop strategies for growth. Reflective practice can be done individually or in collaboration with peers or mentors, fostering self-awareness and continuous learning.
- Interdisciplinary collaboration: Collaborating with other healthcare professionals, such as physicians, pharmacists, and therapists, provides valuable learning opportunities. Engaging in interdisciplinary discussions and participating in team-based care can broaden perspectives and enhance clinical competence.
- Feedback and evaluation: Seeking feedback from supervisors, preceptors, and colleagues is essential for growth as a new graduate nurse. Constructive feedback

helps identify strengths and areas for improvement, allowing for targeted skill development and enhanced clinical competence.

- Embracing challenges: Challenges present opportunities for growth. Embracing challenging patient cases, seeking out diverse clinical experiences, and stepping out of comfort zones can accelerate the development of clinical competence.

Developing clinical competence as a new graduate nurse comes with challenges, but it also presents numerous opportunities for growth. By actively seeking experiences, seeking mentorship, engaging in continuous learning, reflecting on practice, collaborating with interdisciplinary teams, and embracing challenges, new graduate nurses can overcome obstacles and develop the clinical competence necessary for a successful nursing career.

2.3 The Significance of Continuous Learning and Professional Development in Maintaining and Enhancing Clinical Competence Throughout One's Career

Continuous learning and professional development are crucial for nurses to maintain and enhance their clinical competence throughout their careers. As the healthcare landscape evolves due to advancements in technology, changes in patient demographics, and new medical research findings, nurses must stay current with these developments to deliver high-quality care. Ongoing education not only equips nurses with the latest evidence-based practices and skills but also fosters critical thinking and adaptability in dynamic clinical environments. Furthermore, engaging in professional development opportunities—such as workshops, certification programs, and conferences—promotes networking and collaboration among peers, enriching the nurse's practice and overall professional growth. Ultimately, a commitment to lifelong learning not only benefits individual nurses in their career trajectories but also enhances patient outcomes and contributes to the overall effectiveness of the healthcare system.

2.4 The Core Components of Clinical Competence

Clinical competence is essential in the healthcare profession, as it directly impacts patient safety and quality of care. It encompasses various components that ensure healthcare providers can deliver high-quality services. Clinical competence is a multifaceted concept that significantly influences the quality of healthcare delivery. Before we get to the core components of clinical competence, it is important that we look at the competencies new graduate nurses are expected to possess in order to render quality patient care. Table 2.1 shows the six main competencies and their descriptors as adapted from Matlhaba (2020:247–248).

Table 2.1 Six main competencies and their descriptors (adapted from Matlhaba 2020:247–248)

Competencies	Descriptors	Measures to enhance the clinical competence of new graduate nurses
1. Legal practice	Ability to identify and address legal issues based on critical reflection on the suitability of the different legal systems of the nursing and midwifery practice within the legal framework	• Stay updated on legal regulations and standards related to nursing practice • Attend workshops or courses on legal and ethical aspects of nursing • Seek guidance from experienced nurses or legal experts when faced with legal dilemmas • Adhere to professional standards and ethical guidelines to ensure legal and safe nursing practice
2. Ethics and professional practice	Ability to identify and address ethical and moral issues based on critical reflection on the suitability of different ethical value systems of the nursing and midwifery practice within the ethical and moral framework	• Participate in ethics training and discussions to develop ethical decision-making skills • Seek guidance from ethics committees or mentors when faced with ethical dilemmas • Maintain confidentiality and respect patient autonomy in all aspects of care • Engage in reflective practice to continuously evaluate and improve ethical nursing practice
3. Operational management (unit) and leadership	Ability to manage the unit from shift inception (taking over) to shift ending (handing over)	Develop leadership skills through mentorship programs or leadership courses • Take initiative in coordinating and organizing patient care activities • Collaborate with interdisciplinary teams to ensure efficient and effective care delivery • Stay updated on healthcare policies and procedures to ensure compliance and quality improvement
4. Contextual clinical and technical competence	Ability to provide holistic nursing care in different disciplines such as medical/surgical, midwifery, and mental health and within a community nursing or public health setting	• Continuously update clinical knowledge and skills through continuing education programs • Seek opportunities to practice and refine technical skills under supervision • Stay updated on evidence-based practice guidelines and incorporate them into clinical decision-making • Seek feedback from experienced nurses and clinical preceptors to improve clinical competence

(continued)

Table 2.1   (continued)

Competencies	Descriptors	Measures to enhance the clinical competence of new graduate nurses
5. Therapeutic environment	Ability to create and promote a safe and clean environment for the healthcare user under her/his care	• Create a safe and therapeutic environment for patients by maintaining privacy and dignity • Communicate effectively with patients and their families to establish trust and rapport • Collaborate with the healthcare team to ensure a holistic approach to patient care • Advocate for patient rights and preferences to promote a therapeutic environment
6. Quality nursing care	Ability to provide comprehensive/excellent nursing care for the healthcare user, family, and the community at large	• Adhere to evidence-based practice guidelines to provide high-quality care • Participate in quality improvement initiatives and contribute to data collection and analysis • Continuously evaluate patient outcomes and adjust nursing interventions as needed • Engage in interdisciplinary collaboration to ensure coordinated and comprehensive care

Below are the core components of clinical competence, which encompass knowledge, skills, and attitude or behavior.

- Clinical knowledge: At the foundation of clinical competence lies a robust body of knowledge. Nurses must possess an understanding of relevant medical information, theoretical concepts, and evidence-based practices. This includes comprehending disease processes, pharmacology, and the latest healthcare protocols. Continuous education and professional development are critical to ensure that nurses remain updated with evolving medical science and technologies, enabling them to make informed decisions that positively impact patient outcomes.
- Practical skills: Practical skills are another core component of clinical competence. These skills encompass both technical abilities, such as administering injections and performing assessments, and soft skills, including communication and teamwork. Proficiency in these areas ensures that nurses can perform tasks effectively while collaborating with multidisciplinary teams. Practical simulations and hands-on training are essential elements in developing these skills, enabling nurses to gain confidence and proficiency in clinical tasks that are often executed under pressure.
- Attitude or behavior: The attitude or behavior of a nurse significantly affects their interactions with patients and colleagues. A positive attitude fosters a

supportive environment, enhancing teamwork and patient satisfaction. Core attributes such as empathy, compassion, and resilience are paramount, as they influence the quality of patient care and the nurse's ability to handle the challenges inherent in clinical settings. Moreover, a commitment to lifelong learning and professional ethics should inform the attitudes of nurses, driving them to strive for excellence in their practice.

Clinical competence encompasses a harmonious blend of clinical knowledge, practical skills, and attitude or behavior. For new graduate nurses, developing these core components is essential. It equips them to navigate the complexities of modern healthcare effectively, ultimately promoting a holistic approach to patient care. As the healthcare landscape continues to evolve, ongoing education and reflective practices will be crucial in sustaining clinical competence throughout their careers.

2.5   Critical Thinking in Clinical Decision-Making

Critical thinking plays a crucial role in clinical decision-making as nurses must carefully assess and analyze various factors to make the best choices for their patients. By utilizing critical thinking skills, clinicians are able to consider multiple viewpoints, weigh evidence, and determine the most effective course of action. This process involves gathering information, assessing its validity and relevance, identifying potential biases, and making informed decisions based on the best available evidence. A lack of critical thinking in clinical decision-making can lead to errors in diagnosis, treatment, and patient care. Therefore, nurses must continuously hone their critical thinking skills to provide the highest quality of care to their patients.

2.5.1   The Importance of Critical Thinking in Clinical Decision-Making

Critical thinking is foundational in clinical decision-making, as it enables healthcare professionals to analyze complex information, evaluate evidence, and make informed choices that directly affect patient outcomes.

2.5.2   Strategies to Enhance Critical Thinking Skills

- Engaging in reflective practice, which involves reviewing past experiences and outcomes to identify areas for improvement.
- Collaborative discussions with colleagues can also foster diverse perspectives, encouraging deeper analysis of clinical scenarios.
- Incorporating structured problem-solving frameworks, such as the plan-do-study-act (PDSA) cycle, can help clinicians systematically approach challenges.

- Regularly participating in simulation training can further enhance clinical reasoning abilities by allowing practitioners to navigate real-world scenarios in a controlled environment.

By embracing these strategies, new graduate nurses can significantly improve their problem-solving skills, ultimately leading to better patient care and more effective clinical practices.

2.5.3 Strategies to Improve Problem-Solving Skills and Enhance Clinical Reasoning Abilities

Improving problem-solving skills and enhancing clinical reasoning abilities are crucial for new graduate nurses. Here are some strategies to help develop these skills:

- Stay updated with the latest evidence-based practices, guidelines, and research in nursing. Attend workshops, conferences, and seminars to enhance your knowledge and skills.
- Find experienced nurses or nurse educators who can guide and mentor you in developing your problem-solving and clinical reasoning abilities. They can provide valuable insights and help you navigate complex patient care situations.
- Take time to reflect on your clinical experiences. Analyze the challenges you faced, the decisions you made, and the outcomes. Reflective practice helps you identify areas for improvement and develop better problem-solving strategies.
- Develop critical thinking skills by questioning assumptions, analyzing information, and considering alternative perspectives. This will help you make informed decisions and solve problems effectively.
- Engage in collaborative practice with other healthcare professionals. Interacting with physicians, pharmacists, and other team members can broaden your understanding of patient care and help you develop comprehensive problem-solving approaches.
- Work on case studies that simulate real-life patient scenarios. Analyze the information, identify the problem, and develop a plan of action. This will help you apply your clinical reasoning skills in a controlled environment.
- Familiarize yourself with clinical decision-making tools such as clinical algorithms, flowcharts, and evidence-based guidelines. These tools can assist you in making systematic and evidence-based decisions.
- Request feedback from your preceptors, colleagues, and patients. Feedback provides valuable insights into your problem-solving abilities and helps you identify areas for improvement.
- Participate in simulation-based training programs that replicate real-life patient care scenarios. Simulations allow you to practice problem-solving and clinical reasoning skills in a safe and controlled environment.

- Reflect on mistakes: Learn from your mistakes and use them as opportunities for growth. Analyze what went wrong, identify the contributing factors, and develop strategies to prevent similar errors in the future.

Developing problem-solving skills and enhancing clinical reasoning abilities are an ongoing process. Continuously seek opportunities to learn, practice, and reflect on your experiences to become a proficient nurse.

2.6 Evidence-Based Practice in Clinical Competence

Evidence-based practice in clinical competence is vital for ensuring that nurses deliver the highest quality of care to their patients. By integrating the most current research and scientific evidence, nurses can make well-informed decisions regarding patient care and treatment options. This approach not only enhances the effectiveness of healthcare interventions but also helps to minimize risks and improve patient outcomes. It requires nurses to continuously update their knowledge and skills, staying abreast of the latest advancements in their field. Ultimately, evidence-based practice in clinical competence is essential for promoting patient safety and achieving the best possible results in healthcare settings.

2.6.1 The Significance of Evidence-Based Practice in Clinical Competence

Evidence-based practice (EBP) plays a crucial role in enhancing clinical competence, as it integrates the best available research, clinical expertise, and patient values into healthcare decision-making. By emphasizing the importance of using empirical evidence to guide treatment protocols and patient interactions, EBP not only improves patient outcomes but also fosters a culture of continuous learning and adaptation among healthcare professionals. This approach empowers clinicians to critically appraise and apply research findings in their practice, thereby enabling them to stay current with advancements in medical knowledge and technology. Furthermore, the consistent application of evidence-based strategies leads to standardized care, reduces variability in treatment outcomes, and ultimately enhances the overall quality of healthcare delivery. Thus, practicing evidence-based methods is fundamental for clinicians striving to achieve excellence in their professional competencies while providing safe and effective patient care.

2.6.2 The Principles of Evidence-Based Practice, Including the Steps Involved in Conducting Research

Evidence-based practice (EBP) is an essential framework in healthcare that integrates the best available research evidence with clinical expertise and patient values to guide decision-making. The process begins with formulating a clear, answerable clinical question often framed using the Population, Intervention, Comparison, Outcome (PICO) model. Following this, systematic research is conducted to gather relevant evidence from credible sources, such as randomized controlled trials, systematic reviews, and practice guidelines. Once evidence is gathered, it is critically appraised for its validity, reliability, and applicability to the specific clinical context, ensuring that the findings are robust and relevant. This appraisal includes assessing the quality of the studies, understanding the statistical significance of results, and identifying any potential biases. Finally, the appraised evidence is applied to clinical decision-making by integrating it with the clinician's expertise and considering patient preferences, leading to informed, patient-centered care that enhances outcomes and promotes safety. EBP not only fosters a culture of continuous improvement among healthcare professionals but also empowers patients by involving them in their own care decisions.

2.6.3   The Importance of Staying Up-to-Date with the Latest Research and Utilizing Evidence to Improve Patient Outcomes

As new nurses enter the healthcare field, staying up-to-date with the latest research and utilizing evidence-based practices are crucial for enhancing patient outcomes. The healthcare landscape is constantly evolving, with advancements in technology, treatments, and understanding of diseases emerging regularly. By engaging with current literature and clinical guidelines, new nurses can apply the most effective interventions and make informed decisions that directly impact patient care. Furthermore, familiarity with evidence-based practices fosters critical thinking and encourages a culture of lifelong learning, enabling nurses to adapt to changing protocols and improve their clinical skills. Ultimately, by integrating the latest research into their practice, new nurses not only uphold the standards of modern healthcare but also advocate for their patients, ensuring they receive the highest quality of care possible.

Measures for New Graduate Nurses to Stay Up-to-Date with the Latest Research
Staying up-to-date with the latest research and utilizing evidence-based practice are crucial for new graduate nurses to improve patient outcomes. New graduate nurses can stay up-to-date by

- Participating in continuing education programs, workshops, and conferences to stay updated on the latest research and evidence-based practices in nursing. Many organizations offer online courses and webinars that can be accessed from anywhere.
- Subscribing to nursing journals and publications that focus on evidence-based practice. Reading research articles and staying informed about current studies will help nurses stay up-to-date with the latest findings.

- Joining professional nursing organizations provides access to resources, networking opportunities, and educational events. These organizations often publish newsletters and journals that highlight the latest research and evidence-based practices.
- Taking advantage of online resources such as nursing websites, research databases, and online forums. These platforms provide access to a wealth of information, research articles, and discussions on evidence-based practice.
- Engaging in discussions and collaborating with colleagues to share knowledge and experiences. Participate in journal clubs or research groups to critically analyze research articles and discuss their implications for practice.
- Finding a mentor who is experienced in evidence-based practice and research. A mentor can guide and support new graduate nurses in understanding and applying research findings to improve patient outcomes.
- Actively incorporating evidence-based practice into daily nursing care. Use research findings to guide decision-making, develop protocols, and implement best practices that are supported by evidence.
- Consider participating in research studies or quality improvement projects. Involvement in research allows nurses to contribute to the advancement of nursing knowledge and gain firsthand experience in utilizing evidence to improve patient outcomes.
- Regularly reviewing and staying updated on clinical guidelines and protocols issued by professional organizations and regulatory bodies. These guidelines are often based on the latest research and evidence-based practices.
- Continuously reflecting on nursing practice and evaluating the effectiveness of interventions. By critically analyzing outcomes and seeking feedback, nurses can identify areas for improvement and adjust their practice accordingly.

By actively engaging in these measures, new graduate nurses can stay up-to-date with the latest research and effectively utilize evidence-based practice to improve patient outcomes.

2.7 Conclusion

In conclusion, we are saying building a strong foundation for clinical competence is essential for new graduate nurses as they transition from the classroom to the clinical setting. It is crucial for them to develop critical thinking skills, effective communication, and a strong knowledge base to provide safe and competent care to patients. By focusing on acquiring these skills and continuously seeking opportunities for learning and growth, new graduate nurses can boost their confidence and improve their performance as healthcare professionals. Building a strong foundation for clinical competence not only benefits the nurses themselves but also enhances patient outcomes and ensures the delivery of high-quality care in healthcare settings.

Applied Practical Exercises

1. Critical thinking scenario: Present a complex clinical scenario to the readers and ask them to analyze the situation using critical thinking skills. Encourage them to identify potential problems, consider alternative solutions, and make evidence-based decisions. Provide guiding questions to help them navigate through the scenario and reflect on their decision-making process.

2. Communication skills role-play: Divide readers into pairs and assign them different roles, such as a healthcare professional and a patient or a healthcare professional and a colleague. Provide them with a specific communication challenge, such as delivering bad news or resolving a conflict. Ask them to role-play the scenario, focusing on applying effective communication skills. Afterward, encourage them to reflect on their performance and discuss strategies for improvement.

3. Interdisciplinary collaboration case study: Provide a case study that involves a complex patient scenario requiring collaboration among different healthcare professionals. Ask readers to analyze the case study and identify the key stakeholders involved. Then, prompt them to develop a collaborative care plan, considering each professional's expertise and perspectives. Encourage them to reflect on the challenges and benefits of interdisciplinary collaboration.

4. Evidence-based practice research project: Assign readers a research project related to a clinical topic of their choice. Ask them to conduct a literature review, critically appraise the evidence, and develop recommendations for clinical practice based on their findings. Encourage them to reflect on the process of conducting research, the challenges encountered, and the implications of their findings for patient care.

5. Self-reflection and goal setting: Ask readers to engage in a self-reflection exercise where they assess their current clinical competence and identify areas for improvement. Encourage them to set specific, measurable, achievable, relevant, and time-bound (SMART) goals for their professional development. Provide a template or framework for them to structure their reflections and goals.

6. Case-based decision-making: Present readers with a series of case scenarios that require clinical decision-making. Ask them to analyze each case, consider the available evidence, and make a decision based on their clinical competence. Encourage them to reflect on their decision-making process, including any uncertainties or ethical considerations they encountered.

These applied practical exercises provide readers with opportunities to apply the concepts and skills discussed in "Building a Foundation for Clinical Competence" to real-world scenarios. By engaging in these exercises, readers can enhance their critical thinking, communication, collaboration, evidence-based practice, and self-reflection skills, ultimately strengthening their clinical competence.

References

Almarwani AM, Alzahrani NS (2023) Factors affecting the development of clinical nurses' competency: a systematic review. Nurse Educ Pract 73:103826. https://doi.org/10.1016/j.nepr.2023.103826

Hui T, Zakeri MA, Soltanmoradi Y, Rahimi N, Hossini Rafsanjanipoor SM, Nouroozi M, Dehghan M (2023) Nurses' clinical competency and its correlates: before and during the COVID-19 outbreak. BMC Nurs 22(1):156. https://doi.org/10.1186/s12912-023-01330-9

Matlhaba KL (2020) Development of an evaluation tool for clinical competence of community service nurses in North West Province, South Africa. Doctoral dissertation, North-West University (South-Africa). https://repository.nwu.ac.za/bitstream/handle/10394/35085/21377146%20Matlhaba%20KL.pdf?sequence=1&isAllowed=y

Matlhaba KL, Nkoane NL (2024) Factors influencing clinical competence of new graduate nurses employed in selected public hospitals of North West Province: Operational Managers' perspectives. Int J Afr Nurs Sci 20:100683. https://doi.org/10.1016/j.ijans.2024.100683

Self-Reflection and Personal Development

3

Contents

Test your learning and check your understanding of this book's contents: use the "Springer Nature Flashcards" app to access questions using ▶ https://sn.pub/pe441e. To use the app, please follow the instructions in Chap. 1.

3.1   Self-Reflection

Self-reflection in nursing is an essential practice that allows nurses to evaluate their own thoughts, actions, and behaviors in order to improve their practice and patient care. It involves looking back on experiences, challenging assumptions, and identifying areas for growth and development. By taking the time for self-reflection, nurses can gain insight into their strengths and weaknesses, enhance their clinical skills, and develop a deeper understanding of the impact they have on their patients and colleagues. Ultimately, self-reflection in nursing helps nurses to continuously learn and evolve in their profession, contributing to positive outcomes for both patients and healthcare systems.

© The Author(s), under exclusive license to Springer Nature Switzerland AG 2024   53
K. Matlhaba, *Enhancing Clinical Competence of Graduate Nurses*,
https://doi.org/10.1007/978-3-031-81407-5_3

3.1.1   Understanding Self-Reflection

Self-reflection is the process of examining and analyzing one's thoughts, feelings, actions, and experiences (Reljić et al. 2019). It involves introspection and self-awareness to gain insight and understanding about oneself (Falon et al. 2021). Self-reflection is a valuable tool for personal growth, learning, and development. This process will allow new nurses to gain insights into their strengths, weaknesses, and areas for improvement. Self-reflection will also help them to identify patterns in their behavior and make conscious decisions on how to approach challenges in the future. As they transition into the role of a practice nurse, self-reflection becomes even more crucial as they navigate new responsibilities, relationships with colleagues and patients, and the fast-paced environment of a healthcare setting. By continuously engaging in self-reflection, new nurses can adapt to their new role, grow professionally, and provide optimal care to patients under their care.

Here are some key aspects of understanding self-reflection:

- Purpose: Self-reflection serves the purpose of gaining a deeper understanding of oneself, including one's thoughts, emotions, values, beliefs, strengths, weaknesses, and motivations. It allows individuals to examine their experiences and actions to learn from them and make positive changes.
- Introspection: Self-reflection involves looking inward and examining one's internal experiences, such as thoughts, emotions, and reactions. It requires individuals to take a step back and objectively observe themselves without judgment.
- Self-awareness: Self-reflection promotes self-awareness, which is the ability to recognize and understand one's own thoughts, emotions, and behaviors. It helps individuals become more conscious of their patterns, biases, and triggers, enabling them to make more intentional choices and responses.
- Critical thinking: Self-reflection encourages critical thinking, which involves analyzing and evaluating one's thoughts, actions, and experiences. It helps individuals question their assumptions, challenge their beliefs, and consider alternative perspectives. Critical thinking through self-reflection can lead to deeper insights and personal growth.
- Learning and growth: Self-reflection is a powerful tool for learning and personal growth. By reflecting on past experiences, individuals can identify what worked well, what didn't, and what lessons they can take away. This self-awareness and learning can guide future actions and decision-making.
- Goal-setting and improvement: Self-reflection allows individuals to identify areas for improvement and set goals for personal and professional development. By recognizing strengths and weaknesses, individuals can focus on enhancing their strengths and addressing areas that need improvement.
- Emotional intelligence: Self-reflection contributes to the development of emotional intelligence, which is the ability to recognize, understand, and manage one's own emotions and the emotions of others. By reflecting on their own emotions and reactions, individuals can develop empathy, self-regulation, and better interpersonal skills.

- Continuous process: Self-reflection is an ongoing process that requires regular practice. It is not a one-time event but rather a habit that individuals can cultivate to deepen their self-understanding and personal growth.

Self-reflection is a valuable practice that allows individuals to gain insight into themselves, learn from their experiences, and make positive changes. It promotes self-awareness, critical thinking, and personal growth, leading to improved decision-making, relationships, and overall well-being.

3.1.2   Self-Improvement

Self-improvement is the idea of continually working on oneself to grow and become a better version of oneself. It involves setting goals, making positive changes, and developing skills to enhance one's overall well-being and success. Self-improvement can encompass various aspects of life, including personal development, physical health, mental well-being, and professional growth. By engaging in self-improvement, individuals can increase their self-awareness, boost their confidence, and create a more fulfilling and purposeful life. Embracing the concept of self-improvement can lead to greater personal satisfaction, improved relationships, and a more fulfilling and meaningful life journey.

The Importance of Self-Reflection as a Tool for Self-Improvement
Self-reflection is a crucial tool for new graduate nurses during their transition period as they enter the workforce. Taking the time to reflect on their experiences, interactions with patients, and their own performance can help them identify areas for improvement and growth. Through self-reflection, nurses can gain a better understanding of their strengths and weaknesses, allowing them to set goals for personal and professional development. It also provides an opportunity for new nurses to process challenging situations and learn from their mistakes. By taking the time to reflect on their practice, new graduate nurses can become more confident and competent in their roles, ultimately leading to better patient outcomes and job satisfaction.

3.1.3   The Role of Self-Reflection in Nursing Practice

Self-reflection plays a crucial role in nursing practice as it allows nurses to examine their thoughts, actions, and experiences to enhance their professional growth and improve patient care. Here are some key aspects of the role of self-reflection in nursing practice:

- Personal growth and self-awareness: Self-reflection helps nurses develop self-awareness by examining their beliefs, values, strengths, and areas for improvement. It allows them to gain insight into their emotions, biases, and reactions, which can positively impact their interactions with patients, colleagues, and the healthcare team.

- Critical thinking and decision-making: Self-reflection encourages nurses to critically analyze their clinical experiences and decisions. By reflecting on their actions and outcomes, nurses can identify areas where they can improve their critical thinking skills and make more informed decisions in future situations.
- Continuous learning and professional development: Self-reflection promotes a mindset of continuous learning and professional development. Nurses can reflect on their experiences, identify knowledge gaps, and seek opportunities for further education or training to enhance their skills and knowledge base.
- Emotional intelligence and empathy: Self-reflection helps nurses develop emotional intelligence and empathy. By reflecting on their own emotions and experiences, nurses can better understand and empathize with the emotions and experiences of their patients. This can lead to improved patient-centered care and stronger therapeutic relationships.
- Identifying strengths and areas for improvement: Self-reflection allows nurses to identify their strengths and areas for improvement. By recognizing their strengths, nurses can leverage them to provide high-quality care. Similarly, by identifying areas for improvement, nurses can set goals and take steps to enhance their skills and knowledge in those areas.
- Quality improvement and patient safety: Self-reflection plays a role in quality improvement and patient safety. By reflecting on their practice, nurses can identify potential errors, near misses, or areas where patient safety could be compromised. This reflection can lead to changes in practice, implementation of best practices, and improved patient outcomes.
- Professional accountability and ethical practice: Self-reflection promotes professional accountability and ethical practice. Nurses can reflect on their adherence to professional standards, ethical principles, and codes of conduct. This reflection helps nurses maintain their professional integrity and make ethical decisions in challenging situations.

Self-reflection is a valuable tool for nurses to enhance their practice, improve patient care, and foster personal and professional growth. It allows nurses to continuously learn, adapt, and provide the best possible care to their patients.

Exploring the Significance of Self-Reflection in Nursing Practice
Self-reflection plays a significant role in nursing practice as it allows nurses to gain insights into their own thoughts, actions, and emotions. Here are some key points that highlight the significance of self-reflection in nursing practice:

- Enhancing self-awareness: Self-reflection helps nurses develop a deeper understanding of their own values, beliefs, strengths, and weaknesses. By examining their thoughts, feelings, and behaviors, nurses can gain insight into how these factors influence their interactions with patients, colleagues, and the healthcare team.

- Improving patient care: Self-reflection enables nurses to critically evaluate their practice and identify areas for improvement. By reflecting on their experiences, nurses can recognize patterns, identify gaps in knowledge or skills, and make necessary adjustments to enhance the quality of patient care.
- Promoting professional growth: Self-reflection is a powerful tool for professional growth and development. It allows nurses to identify their professional goals, strengths, and areas for improvement. By engaging in self-reflection, nurses can set meaningful goals, seek out learning opportunities, and continuously strive to enhance their knowledge and skills.
- Fostering empathy and compassion: Self-reflection helps nurses develop empathy and compassion toward their patients. By reflecting on their own experiences, nurses can better understand the emotions and challenges faced by their patients. This understanding enables nurses to provide more compassionate and patient-centered care.
- Building resilience: Nursing can be emotionally and physically demanding. Self-reflection helps nurses recognize and manage their own emotions, stressors, and burnout. By reflecting on their experiences, nurses can develop strategies to cope with challenges, build resilience, and maintain their well-being.
- Strengthening interprofessional collaboration: Self-reflection allows nurses to reflect on their interactions and collaborations with other healthcare professionals. By examining their communication styles, teamwork skills, and contributions to the healthcare team, nurses can identify areas for improvement and enhance their ability to work effectively with others.
- Ethical decision-making: Self-reflection plays a crucial role in ethical decision-making. By reflecting on their own values, biases, and ethical frameworks, nurses can make more informed and ethical decisions in complex situations. Self-reflection helps nurses consider the impact of their decisions on patients, families, and the broader healthcare system.

Self-reflection is a valuable practice in nursing as it enhances self-awareness, improves patient care, promotes professional growth, fosters empathy and compassion, builds resilience, strengthens collaboration, and supports ethical decision-making. By engaging in self-reflection, nurses can continuously improve their practice and provide high-quality, patient-centered care.

Understanding How Self-Reflection Contributes to Personal and Professional Growth

Self-reflection contributes significantly to both personal and professional growth. Here are some ways in which self-reflection supports personal and professional development:

- Self-awareness: Self-reflection allows individuals to develop a deeper understanding of their thoughts, emotions, values, and beliefs. By reflecting on their experiences and actions, individuals gain insight into their strengths, weaknesses, and areas for improvement. This self-awareness is crucial for personal growth as it helps individuals identify their goals, values, and aspirations.

- Identifying strengths and areas for improvement: Through self-reflection, individuals can recognize their strengths and leverage them to enhance their performance. It also helps identify areas for improvement, allowing individuals to focus on developing specific skills or knowledge. By understanding their strengths and weaknesses, individuals can make informed decisions about their professional development and seek opportunities to grow.
- Learning from experiences: Self-reflection enables individuals to learn from their experiences, both positive and negative. By reflecting on past situations, individuals can identify what worked well and what could have been done differently. This learning process helps individuals refine their approaches, develop new strategies, and make better-informed decisions in the future.
- Goal-setting and action planning: Self-reflection provides individuals with the opportunity to set meaningful goals for personal and professional growth. By reflecting on their aspirations and areas for improvement, individuals can establish clear objectives and develop action plans to achieve them. This goal-setting process helps individuals stay focused, motivated, and accountable for their own development.
- Enhancing critical thinking and problem-solving skills: Self-reflection encourages individuals to think critically about their experiences, actions, and outcomes. It promotes a deeper understanding of the underlying factors contributing to success or challenges. Through self-reflection, individuals can develop their problem-solving skills, analyze situations from different perspectives, and make more informed decisions.
- Building resilience and adaptability: Self-reflection fosters resilience by helping individuals understand their reactions to challenges and setbacks. By reflecting on how they have overcome obstacles in the past, individuals can develop strategies to cope with adversity and bounce back stronger. Self-reflection also promotes adaptability by encouraging individuals to learn from change and adjust their approaches accordingly.
- Enhancing interpersonal skills: Self-reflection supports the development of interpersonal skills by encouraging individuals to reflect on their interactions with others. By examining their communication styles, listening skills, and ability to collaborate, individuals can identify areas for improvement and work toward building stronger relationships with colleagues, clients, and stakeholders.

Self-reflection is a powerful tool for personal and professional growth. It fosters self-awareness, helps individuals identify strengths and areas for improvement, facilitates learning from experiences, supports goal-setting and action planning, enhances critical thinking and problem-solving skills, builds resilience and adaptability, and promotes the development of interpersonal skills. By engaging in regular self-reflection, individuals can continuously evolve and grow both personally and professionally.

Recognizing the Impact of Self-Awareness on Patient Care and Professional Relationships
Self-awareness has a significant impact on patient care and professional relationships in the following ways:

- Enhanced empathy and patient-centered care: Self-awareness allows healthcare professionals to understand their own biases, emotions, and perspectives. By recognizing their own experiences and beliefs, they can better empathize with patients and provide more patient-centered care. Self-awareness helps healthcare professionals to be more attuned to the needs and preferences of their patients, leading to improved communication, trust, and overall patient satisfaction.
- Effective communication: Self-awareness enables healthcare professionals to recognize their communication styles, nonverbal cues, and the impact they have on others. By understanding their own communication patterns, they can adapt their approach to effectively communicate with patients, colleagues, and other members of the healthcare team. This leads to clearer and more meaningful interactions, reducing misunderstandings and enhancing collaborative relationships.
- Self-regulation and emotional intelligence: Self-awareness helps healthcare professionals recognize and manage their own emotions, stressors, and reactions. By understanding their emotional triggers, they can regulate their responses in challenging situations. This self-regulation promotes professionalism, empathy, and effective decision-making, even in high-pressure environments. It also contributes to a positive work environment and fosters healthy professional relationships.
- Reflective practice and continuous improvement: Self-awareness encourages healthcare professionals to engage in reflective practice, examining their own actions, decisions, and outcomes. By reflecting on their experiences, they can identify areas for improvement and make necessary adjustments to their practice. This commitment to continuous improvement enhances the quality of patient care and contributes to professional growth.
- Building trust and collaboration: Self-awareness fosters trust and collaboration in professional relationships. When healthcare professionals are self-aware, they are more open to feedback, willing to acknowledge their limitations, and receptive to different perspectives. This creates an environment of trust and mutual respect, enabling effective teamwork and collaboration among healthcare professionals. It also promotes a culture of learning and innovation.
- Ethical decision-making: Self-awareness plays a crucial role in ethical decision-making. By understanding their own values, biases, and ethical frameworks, healthcare professionals can make more informed and ethical choices. Self-awareness helps them recognize potential conflicts of interest, navigate ethical dilemmas, and act in the best interest of their patients. This contributes to maintaining professional integrity and upholding ethical standards in patient care.

Self-awareness has a profound impact on patient care and professional relationships. It enhances empathy, promotes effective communication, supports self-regulation and emotional intelligence, encourages reflective practice and continuous improvement, builds trust and collaboration, and facilitates ethical decision-making. By cultivating self-awareness, healthcare professionals can provide high-quality, patient-centered care and foster positive teamwork and collaboration.

Strategies for Self-Reflection

Self-reflection is a valuable practice for nurses to enhance their professional growth and improve patient care. Here are some strategies for self-reflection in nursing:

- Schedule dedicated time: Set aside dedicated time for self-reflection on a regular basis. This can be daily, weekly, or monthly, depending on individual preferences and availability. Treat this time as a nonnegotiable commitment to yourself.
- Find a quiet and comfortable space: Choose a quiet and comfortable space where you can reflect without distractions. This could be a private office, a peaceful corner in your home, or a nearby park. Create an environment that promotes relaxation and focus.
- Use reflection prompts or questions: Utilize reflection prompts or questions to guide your self-reflection process. These prompts can help you explore your thoughts, emotions, and experiences. Examples of reflection prompts include "What went well today? What could have been improved? How did I contribute to the team's success?".
- Keep a reflective journal: Maintain a reflective journal to record your thoughts, insights, and reflections. Write freely and honestly about your experiences, challenges, and successes. Review your journal periodically to track your progress and identify patterns or areas for improvement.
- Seek feedback from others: Request feedback from colleagues, mentors, or supervisors to gain different perspectives on your performance and areas for growth. Actively listen to their feedback and reflect on how you can incorporate it into your practice.
- Engage in peer reflection: Collaborate with peers to engage in reflective discussions. Share experiences, challenges, and lessons learned. Peer reflection can provide valuable insights and support in your self-reflection journey.
- Use technology tools: Explore technology tools that can facilitate self-reflection, such as mobile apps or online platforms designed for reflection and journaling. These tools can provide prompts, reminders, and organization features to enhance your self-reflection practice.
- Attend reflective workshops or seminars: Participate in workshops or seminars that focus on self-reflection in nursing. These events can provide guidance, techniques, and opportunities for interactive reflection exercises.
- Set goals for improvement: Identify specific areas for improvement based on your self-reflection. Set SMART goals to guide your professional development. Regularly assess your progress toward these goals.
- Celebrate successes: Acknowledge and celebrate your achievements and successes resulting from your self-reflection efforts. Recognize the positive impact

of your growth and improvement on patient care and your professional development.

Self-reflection is a continuous process. Be open to learning, embrace feedback, and be kind to yourself throughout the journey. By incorporating these strategies into your nursing practice, you can enhance your self-awareness, improve your skills, and provide better care to your patients.

Journaling and Writing Reflections

Journaling and writing reflections are powerful tools for self-reflection in nursing. Here are some strategies to effectively use journaling and writing reflections:

- Make it a habit: Set a regular time and place for journaling and writing reflections. Consistency is key to developing a habit. It could be at the end of each shift, at the beginning or end of the day, or during designated reflection time.
- Choose a journaling format: Decide on the format that works best for you. It could be a traditional paper journal, a digital journaling app, or an online platform. Choose a format that is convenient and accessible for you.
- Write freely and honestly: When journaling, write freely and honestly about your experiences, thoughts, and emotions. Don't worry about grammar or structure. The goal is to capture your authentic reflections.
- Use reflection prompts: Utilize reflection prompts to guide your writing. These prompts can help you delve deeper into specific aspects of your nursing practice. Examples of prompts include "What was a challenging situation I encountered today? How did I handle it? What could I have done differently?".
- Reflect on both positive and negative experiences: It's important to reflect on both positive and negative experiences. Celebrate your successes and achievements, but also explore areas where you faced challenges or made mistakes. Reflecting on both helps you learn and grow.
- Focus on learning and improvement: Use your journaling and reflections as a tool for learning and improvement. Identify areas where you can enhance your skills, knowledge, or communication. Set goals for improvement based on your reflections.
- Seek feedback and guidance: Share your reflections with trusted colleagues, mentors, or supervisors. Seek their feedback and guidance to gain different perspectives and insights. This can deepen your self-reflection and provide valuable input for growth.
- Review and revisit your reflections: Periodically review and revisit your previous reflections. This allows you to track your progress, identify patterns, and assess your growth over time. It also helps you identify areas that may require further attention.
- Use writing as a therapeutic outlet: Writing can be a therapeutic outlet for processing emotions and stress. Use your journaling as a way to express and release any emotional burdens or challenges you may have encountered during your nursing practice.

- Celebrate milestones and achievements: Celebrate milestones and achievements that you have documented in your reflections. Recognize the progress you have made and the positive impact you have had on patient care and your professional development.

Journaling and writing reflections are personal and individual practices. Find a style and approach that resonates with you. Embrace the process of self-reflection and allow it to guide your growth as a nurse.

Utilizing Journaling as a Tool for Self-Reflection
Journaling is a powerful tool for self-reflection as it allows you to explore your thoughts, emotions, and experiences in a structured and introspective way. Here are some strategies to effectively utilize journaling as a tool for self-reflection:

- Set aside dedicated time: Schedule regular time for journaling in your routine. It could be daily, weekly, or whenever you feel the need to reflect. Consistency is key to developing the habit of journaling.
- Create a conducive environment: Find a quiet and comfortable space where you can focus and reflect without distractions. This could be a peaceful corner in your home, a park, or a cosy café. Make sure you have the necessary tools, such as a journal and pen or a digital device.
- Start with a prompt or question: Begin each journaling session with a prompt or question to guide your reflection. This can help you delve deeper into specific aspects of your nursing practice or personal experiences. Some prompts could be "What challenges did I face today? How did I handle them? What did I learn from them?".
- Write freely and honestly: When journaling, write freely and honestly without judgment. Allow your thoughts and emotions to flow onto the pages. Don't worry about grammar or structure. The goal is to capture your authentic reflections.
- Reflect on both positive and negative experiences: Explore both positive and negative experiences in your journaling. Celebrate your successes and achievements, but also reflect on challenges, mistakes, or areas for improvement. This balanced approach helps you learn and grow.
- Focus on self-awareness: Use journaling as a tool to enhance self-awareness. Reflect on your thoughts, feelings, and reactions in different situations. Identify patterns, triggers, and areas where you can develop greater self-understanding.
- Explore lessons learned: Reflect on the lessons you have learned from your experiences. Identify what worked well and what could have been done differently. Consider how you can apply these lessons to future situations to improve your nursing practice.
- Set goals for growth: Based on your reflections, set specific and actionable goals for personal and professional growth. These goals can be related to improving specific skills, enhancing communication, or developing a better work-life balance. Regularly review and update your goals as you progress.

- Seek feedback and guidance: Share your journal entries with trusted colleagues, mentors, or supervisors. Seek their feedback and guidance to gain different perspectives and insights. Their input can provide valuable support and help you gain new insights.
- Celebrate progress: Celebrate milestones and progress you have made based on your reflections. Acknowledge your growth, achievements, and positive changes in your nursing practice. Celebrating progress can motivate and inspire you to continue your self-reflection journey.

Journaling is a personal practice, and there is no right or wrong way to do it. Find a style and approach that works best for you. Embrace the process of self-reflection through journaling, and allow it to deepen your self-awareness, enhance your nursing practice, and support your personal growth.

Writing Reflections on Clinical Experiences, Challenges, and Successes
Writing reflections on clinical experiences, challenges, and successes is an effective way to gain insights, learn from your experiences, and promote personal and professional growth. Here are some strategies to help you write meaningful reflections:

- Start with a specific experience: Choose a specific clinical experience, challenge, or success that you want to reflect upon. It could be a particular patient interaction, a complex case, a difficult decision, or a positive outcome.
- Describe the experience: Begin by describing the experience in detail. Include relevant information such as the setting, the people involved, the actions taken, and the emotions you experienced. Paint a clear picture of the situation.
- Reflect on your thoughts and emotions: Explore your thoughts and emotions during the experience. What were your initial reactions? How did you feel? What were your concerns or uncertainties? Reflecting on your emotions can help you gain insights into your reactions and decision-making process.
- Analyze the challenges faced: If the experience involved challenges, analyze them in-depth. What were the specific challenges? What factors contributed to these challenges? Reflect on how you approached and managed the challenges. Consider what you learned from them and how you could handle similar situations differently in the future.
- Identify successes and achievements: Acknowledge and celebrate your successes and achievements in the experience. Reflect on what went well, the positive outcomes, and the impact you had on the patient's care or the team. Recognize your strengths and the skills you utilized effectively.
- Consider the lessons learned: Reflect on the lessons you learned from the experience. What insights did you gain? What knowledge or skills did you acquire or improve? How can you apply these lessons to future clinical situations? Reflecting on lessons learned helps you grow and develop as a nurse.
- Connect to broader concepts or theories: Consider how the experience relates to broader concepts or theories in nursing. Reflect on how it aligns with

evidence-based practice, ethical considerations, or professional standards. This helps you contextualize your experience within the larger nursing framework.

- Set goals for improvement: Based on your reflections, identify areas for improvement or further development. Set specific and actionable goals that can help you enhance your skills, knowledge, or approach to patient care. Regularly review and update these goals as you progress.
- Seek feedback and guidance: Share your reflections with trusted colleagues, mentors, or supervisors. Seek their feedback and guidance to gain different perspectives and insights. Their input can provide valuable support and help you gain new insights.
- Write with honesty and authenticity: Write your reflections with honesty and authenticity. Be open about your thoughts, emotions, and challenges. This allows for a genuine reflection and helps you gain a deeper understanding of yourself and your nursing practice.

The purpose of writing reflections is to learn and grow. Embrace the opportunity to reflect on your clinical experiences, challenges, and successes, and use them as steppingstones for continuous improvement in your nursing practice.

Using Reflective Writing to Identify Areas for Growth and Improvement
Reflective writing is a valuable tool for self-assessment and personal development. By engaging in reflective writing, you can gain insights into your thoughts, feelings, and experiences and identify areas for growth and improvement. Here are some steps to help you use reflective writing to identify areas for growth:

- Set aside dedicated time: Find a quiet and comfortable space where you can focus on your thoughts without distractions. Set aside a specific time for reflective writing, whether it's daily, weekly, or monthly.
- Choose a prompt or question: Start by selecting a prompt or question that will guide your reflection. This could be a general question like "What have I learned recently?" or a specific prompt related to a particular experience or challenge you faced.
- Reflect on your experiences: Take some time to think deeply about the prompt or question. Consider your thoughts, feelings, and reactions to the experiences you've had. Reflect on both positive and negative aspects, as both can provide valuable insights.
- Write freely and honestly: Begin writing without judgment or self-censorship. Let your thoughts flow freely onto the paper or screen. Be honest with yourself and explore your thoughts and emotions without holding back.
- Analyze your reflections: Once you have written your thoughts, take some time to analyze and interpret them. Look for patterns, recurring themes, or commonalities in your reflections. Consider the underlying reasons behind your thoughts and feelings.
- Identify areas for growth: Based on your analysis, identify specific areas for growth and improvement. These could be skills you want to develop, habits you

want to change, or attitudes you want to cultivate. Be specific and realistic in your identification.

- Set goals and create an action plan: Once you have identified areas for growth, set goals that are specific, measurable, achievable, relevant, and time-bound (SMART goals). Create an action plan outlining the steps you will take to work toward these goals.
- Reflect on your progress: Regularly revisit your reflective writing and assess your progress. Reflect on how your actions and efforts have contributed to your growth and improvement. Celebrate your successes and make adjustments as needed.

Remember, reflective writing is a continuous process. It is important to make it a habit and regularly engage in self-reflection to identify new areas for growth and improvement.

3.1.4 Self-Awareness

Self-awareness is the ability to recognize and understand one's own thoughts, feelings, and behaviors. It involves being in tune with our own internal experiences and the impact we have on others. This concept allows individuals to have a deeper understanding of themselves, their motivations, and their values. Self-awareness plays a crucial role in personal growth and development, as it enables people to make more informed choices and take control of their lives. By being self-aware, individuals can improve their relationships, communication skills, and overall well-being. Ultimately, self-awareness is a powerful tool for self-improvement and achieving personal fulfillment.

Using Self-Awareness as a Tool to Identify Strengths, Weaknesses, Values, and Goals
Self-awareness is a valuable tool for new graduate nurses to identify their strengths, weaknesses, values, and goals. Here's how they can use self-awareness in each of these areas:

- Strengths
  - Reflect on your clinical experiences during nursing school and identify areas where you excelled. This could include skills such as effective communication, critical thinking, or leadership abilities.
  - Seek feedback from preceptors, mentors, and colleagues to gain insights into your strengths as perceived by others.
  - Consider your personal qualities, such as empathy, compassion, or resilience, which contribute to your effectiveness as a nurse.
- Weaknesses
  - Reflect on areas where you feel less confident or need improvement. This could be related to specific clinical skills, time management, or communication techniques.

- Seek feedback from preceptors, mentors, and colleagues to identify areas for growth and development.
- Be open to constructive criticism and view weaknesses as opportunities for learning and improvement.
- Values
  - Reflect on your personal values and how they align with the values of the nursing profession. Consider what motivates you to be a nurse and the principles that guide your practice.
  - Identify the values that are important to you in providing patient-centered care, such as respect, integrity, or advocacy.
  - Consider how your values influence your decision-making and interactions with patients, families, and the healthcare team.
- Goals
  - Set short-term and long-term goals for your nursing career. These goals can be related to professional development, clinical skills, leadership, or further education.
  - Consider your strengths, weaknesses, and values when setting goals to ensure they align with your personal and professional aspirations.
  - Break down larger goals into smaller, achievable steps and create a plan to work toward them.

To enhance self-awareness in these areas, new graduate nurses might consider the following strategies:

- Engage in self-reflection exercises, such as journaling or meditation, to gain insights into your thoughts, emotions, and behaviors.
- Seek feedback from trusted individuals who can provide honest and constructive assessments of your strengths, weaknesses, and areas for growth.
- Take advantage of self-assessment tools or personality assessments that can provide insights into your strengths, preferences, and areas for development.
- Engage in ongoing professional development and continuing education to enhance your knowledge and skills in areas of weakness or interest.
- Regularly revisit and reassess your goals to ensure they remain aligned with your values and aspirations.

Self-awareness is a continuous process that requires reflection, feedback, and a willingness to grow. Embrace the journey of self-discovery, and use it as a foundation for personal and professional development as a new graduate nurse.

Engaging in Introspection to Identify Strengths, Weaknesses, Values, and Goals

New graduate nurses can engage in introspection to identify their strengths, weaknesses, values, and goals through the following steps:

- Create a quiet and reflective space: Find a quiet and comfortable space where you can engage in introspection without distractions. This could be a peaceful corner in your home, a park, or any place where you feel calm and focused.
- Set aside dedicated time: Schedule dedicated time for introspection. It could be a few minutes each day or a longer period once a week. Consistency is key to developing a habit of self-reflection.
- Reflect on past experiences: Think about your experiences during nursing school, clinical rotations, and any healthcare-related experiences you have had. Consider the tasks or situations where you felt confident and performed well. Reflect on the qualities and skills that contributed to your success in those situations.
- Identify strengths: Based on your reflections, identify your strengths as a nurse. These could be clinical skills, such as wound care or medication administration, or personal qualities like empathy, communication, or leadership abilities. Consider the feedback you have received from preceptors, mentors, and colleagues to gain insights into your strengths.
- Recognize weaknesses: Reflect on areas where you feel less confident or need improvement. This could be related to specific clinical skills, time management, communication techniques, or any other aspect of nursing practice. Be honest with yourself and acknowledge areas where you can grow and develop.
- Explore personal values: Consider your personal values and how they align with the values of the nursing profession. Reflect on what motivates you to be a nurse and the principles that guide your practice. Identify the values that are important to you in providing patient-centered care, such as respect, integrity, or advocacy.
- Set goals: Based on your self-reflection, set short-term and long-term goals for your nursing career. These goals can be related to professional development, clinical skills, leadership, or further education. Consider your strengths, weaknesses, and values when setting goals to ensure they align with your personal and professional aspirations.
- Write it down: Journaling can be a powerful tool for introspection. Write down your reflections, strengths, weaknesses, values, and goals. This helps to solidify your thoughts and provides a reference for future self-assessment and growth.
- Seek feedback: Engage in conversations with preceptors, mentors, and colleagues to gain additional perspectives on your strengths, weaknesses, values, and goals. Their insights can provide valuable feedback and help you gain a more comprehensive understanding of yourself.
- Revisit and revise: Regularly revisit and revise your reflections, strengths, weaknesses, values, and goals. As you gain more experience and grow as a nurse, your self-awareness will evolve. Continuously reassess and adjust your self-perception to align with your current reality.

Engaging in introspection requires time, patience, and a willingness to be honest with yourself. By regularly engaging in self-reflection, new graduate nurses can gain a deeper understanding of themselves and their strengths, weaknesses, values, and goals. This self-awareness serves as a foundation for personal and professional growth throughout their nursing career.

Enhancing Self-Awareness, Empathy, and Effective Communication Skills
Enhancing self-awareness, empathy, and effective communication skills is crucial
for new graduate nurses. Here are some strategies to help in these areas:

- Self-awareness
  - Engage in self-reflection exercises, such as journaling or mindfulness, to increase self-awareness. Take time to reflect on your thoughts, emotions, and reactions in different situations.
  - Seek feedback from preceptors, mentors, and colleagues to gain insights into your strengths, weaknesses, and areas for improvement.
  - Regularly assess your own performance and identify areas where you can grow and develop.
  - Engage in ongoing professional development and continuing education to enhance your knowledge and skills.
- Empathy
  - Practice active listening to truly understand and empathize with patients, their families, and colleagues. Give them your full attention, maintain eye contact, and show genuine interest in their concerns.
  - Put yourself in the patient's shoes and try to understand their perspective, emotions, and needs.
  - Practice empathy through verbal and nonverbal communication. Use comforting gestures, facial expressions, and tone of voice to convey empathy and understanding.
  - Seek opportunities to learn about different cultures, backgrounds, and experiences to enhance your ability to empathize with diverse populations.
- Effective communication
  - Develop strong verbal communication skills by using clear and concise language. Avoid medical jargon and explain information in a way that patients and their families can understand.
  - Practice active listening by giving your full attention, asking clarifying questions, and summarizing information to ensure understanding.
  - Use nonverbal communication effectively by maintaining open body language, making appropriate eye contact, and using facial expressions that convey empathy and understanding.
  - Develop written communication skills by ensuring your documentation is accurate, concise, and organized.
  - Seek feedback from colleagues and patients to improve your communication skills and adapt your approach as needed.
- Role-play and simulation
  - Engage in role-playing exercises or simulations to practice effective communication and empathy in various healthcare scenarios.
  - Work with colleagues or educators to simulate challenging situations, and practice responding with empathy and effective communication techniques.
  - Use these opportunities to receive feedback and identify areas for improvement.

- Seek mentorship and feedback
  - Find an experienced nurse who can serve as a mentor and provide guidance on enhancing self-awareness, empathy, and communication skills.
  - Seek feedback from preceptors, mentors, and colleagues on your communication style and empathy levels. Use this feedback to make necessary adjustments and improvements.
- Continuous learning
  - Engage in continuing education opportunities that focus on communication skills, empathy, and self-awareness.
  - Attend workshops, conferences, or webinars that provide strategies and techniques for effective communication and empathy in healthcare settings.

Enhancing self-awareness, empathy, and effective communication skills is an ongoing process. Be patient with yourself, seek opportunities for growth, and continuously strive to improve these essential skills as a new graduate nurse.

Recognizing the Impact of Self-Awareness on Patient Care and Professional Relationships

New graduate nurses can recognize the impact of self-awareness on patient care and professional relationships in the following ways:

- Improved communication: Self-awareness allows nurses to understand their own communication style, including strengths and weaknesses. By being aware of their own biases, emotions, and reactions, nurses can communicate more effectively with patients, families, and colleagues. This leads to clearer and more empathetic communication, which enhances patient understanding, trust, and satisfaction.
- Enhanced empathy: Self-awareness helps nurses recognize their own emotions and experiences, which in turn allows them to empathize with patients and their families. By understanding their own feelings, nurses can better understand and connect with the emotions and experiences of others. This empathy fosters a therapeutic relationship, improves patient-centered care, and promotes better health outcomes.
- Self-regulation: Self-awareness enables nurses to recognize and manage their own emotions, stress levels, and reactions in challenging situations. By understanding their triggers and stressors, nurses can respond to difficult situations in a calm and professional manner. This self-regulation promotes a positive and supportive environment for patients and colleagues, leading to better teamwork and collaboration.
- Personal growth and professional development: Self-awareness allows nurses to identify their strengths, weaknesses, and areas for improvement. By recognizing their own limitations, nurses can seek opportunities for growth, continuing education, and professional development. This ongoing self-reflection and improvement positively impact patient care by ensuring nurses are continuously enhancing their knowledge and skills.

- Building trust and rapport: Self-awareness helps nurses build trust and rapport with patients and colleagues. By being aware of their own values, beliefs, and biases, nurses can approach interactions with an open mind and without judgment. This fosters a safe and inclusive environment where patients and colleagues feel respected, heard, and valued.
- Conflict resolution: Self-awareness allows nurses to recognize their own role in conflicts and take responsibility for their actions. By understanding their own communication and conflict resolution styles, nurses can approach conflicts with empathy, active listening, and a willingness to find common ground. This promotes effective resolution of conflicts and maintains positive professional relationships.
- Patient advocacy: Self-awareness enables nurses to advocate for their patients effectively. By understanding their own values and beliefs, nurses can align their actions with the best interests of their patients. This includes advocating for patient rights, informed decision-making, and ensuring their voices are heard in the healthcare setting.

By recognizing the impact of self-awareness on patient care and professional relationships, new graduate nurses can actively cultivate self-awareness through reflection, feedback, and ongoing personal and professional development. This, in turn, leads to improved patient outcomes, enhanced teamwork, and a more fulfilling nursing practice.

3.1.5 Self-Care and Well-being

The concept of self-care and well-being focuses on the importance of taking care of oneself in a holistic manner, including physical, mental, and emotional well-being. It emphasizes the need to prioritize self-care practices such as exercise, healthy eating, relaxation techniques, and seeking support when needed. The idea behind self-care is to maintain a healthy balance in life, reduce stress, and prevent burnout. By practicing self-care regularly, individuals can improve their overall well-being, increase their resilience to life's challenges, and enhance their quality of life. It is essential to recognize the importance of self-care and make it a priority in our daily lives to ensure that we are taking care of ourselves in the best possible way.

Importance of Self-Care
Self-care is essential for maintaining overall well-being and improving the quality of life. Here are some reasons why self-care is important:

- Physical health: Taking care of yourself physically is crucial for your overall health. Engaging in regular exercise, eating nutritious food, getting enough sleep, and practicing good hygiene can help prevent illness, boost your immune system, and increase your energy levels.

- Mental health: Self-care plays a vital role in maintaining good mental health. Taking time for activities that bring you joy, practicing relaxation techniques, and engaging in hobbies can help reduce stress, anxiety, and depression. It allows you to recharge and rejuvenate your mind.
- Emotional well-being: Self-care helps you to connect with your emotions and understand your needs. It allows you to prioritize your emotional well-being by engaging in activities that bring you happiness, practicing self-compassion, and setting boundaries in relationships.
- Increased productivity: When you prioritize self-care, you are better equipped to handle daily challenges and responsibilities. Taking breaks, setting realistic goals, and managing your time effectively can improve your productivity and prevent burnout.
- Improved relationships: When you take care of yourself, you are better able to show up for others in your life. Self-care helps you maintain healthy boundaries, communicate effectively, and foster positive relationships with others.
- Self-reflection and personal growth: Engaging in self-care activities provides an opportunity for self-reflection and personal growth. It allows you to explore your values, beliefs, and goals and make necessary changes to align your life with your true desires.

Self-care is important because it promotes physical and mental well-being, enhances productivity, improves relationships, and fosters personal growth. It is a necessary practice for maintaining a balanced and fulfilling life.

Prioritize Physical, Mental, and Emotional Well-Being
Self-care and well-being are crucial for new graduate nurses to maintain their physical, mental, and emotional health while navigating the demands of their profession. Here are some strategies to prioritize self-care and well-being:

- Establish healthy habits: Maintain a balanced diet, engage in regular exercise, and get enough sleep. These foundational habits support your overall well-being and provide you with the energy and resilience needed for your nursing practice.
- Practice mindfulness and stress management: Incorporate mindfulness techniques, such as deep breathing exercises or meditation, into your daily routine. These practices can help reduce stress, increase self-awareness, and promote mental well-being.
- Set boundaries: Learn to set boundaries between work and personal life. Avoid overworking and make time for activities that bring you joy and relaxation. Prioritize self-care activities, hobbies, and spending time with loved ones.
- Seek support: Build a support system of colleagues, friends, and family who understand the challenges of nursing. Share your experiences, concerns, and successes with them. Consider joining support groups or seeking professional counseling if needed.

- Practice self-compassion: Be kind to yourself and acknowledge that you are doing your best. Avoid self-criticism and negative self-talk. Celebrate your achievements and learn from your mistakes without being too hard on yourself.
- Take breaks: Allow yourself regular breaks during your shifts to rest, recharge, and refocus. Use these breaks to engage in activities that help you relax and rejuvenate, such as taking a walk, listening to music, or practicing deep breathing exercises.
- Engage in activities that bring joy: Make time for activities that bring you joy and fulfilment outside of work. Engaging in hobbies, pursuing creative outlets, or participating in activities that you enjoy can help reduce stress and enhance your overall well-being.
- Practice work-life balance: Strive to maintain a healthy work-life balance. Prioritize your personal life and make time for activities that are important to you. Avoid excessive overtime and learn to delegate tasks when necessary.
- Practice self-reflection: Regularly reflect on your experiences, emotions, and challenges as a new graduate nurse. Journaling or engaging in self-reflection exercises can help you process your thoughts and emotions, leading to increased self-awareness and personal growth.
- Seek professional development opportunities: Invest in your professional growth and development. Pursue continuing education, certifications, and specialized training that align with your interests and career goals. This can enhance your confidence and job satisfaction.

Self-care is not selfish but essential for your overall well-being and ability to provide quality care to your patients. Prioritizing self-care as a new graduate nurse will help you navigate the challenges of your profession and promote a sustainable and fulfilling nursing career.

Recognizing the Importance of Self-Care in Maintaining Clinical Competence
Recognizing the importance of self-care in maintaining clinical competence is crucial for new graduate nurses. Here's why self-care is essential for maintaining clinical competence:

- Physical well-being: Taking care of your physical health is vital for maintaining clinical competence. When you prioritize self-care activities such as getting enough sleep, eating nutritious meals, and engaging in regular exercise, you have the energy and stamina needed to perform your nursing duties effectively. Physical well-being also reduces the risk of burnout and helps you stay focused and alert during your shifts.
- Mental and emotional well-being: Self-care plays a significant role in maintaining your mental and emotional well-being. Nursing can be emotionally demanding, and it's essential to take care of your mental health to provide quality care to your patients. Engaging in activities that reduce stress, such as practicing mindfulness, seeking support from colleagues or therapists, and engaging in hobbies

or relaxation techniques, can help you manage the emotional challenges of nursing and maintain your clinical competence.

- Preventing burnout: Burnout is a common issue among healthcare professionals, including new graduate nurses. It can negatively impact your clinical competence and overall job performance. By prioritizing self-care, you can prevent burnout and maintain your passion for nursing. Taking breaks, setting boundaries, and engaging in activities that bring you joy and fulfilment can help you recharge and prevent burnout from affecting your clinical competence.
- Enhancing critical thinking and decision-making: Self-care activities that promote relaxation and stress reduction can enhance your critical thinking and decision-making skills. When you are well-rested and mentally refreshed, you can think more clearly, analyze situations effectively, and make sound clinical judgments. This is essential for maintaining clinical competence and providing safe and effective patient care.
- Continuous learning and professional development: Self-care is not just about physical and mental well-being; it also includes investing in your professional growth and development. By engaging in self-care activities, you create space for continuous learning, attending educational programs, and seeking opportunities for professional development. This ongoing learning and growth contribute to your clinical competence and keep you updated with the latest evidence-based practices.
- Role modeling for patients and colleagues: As a new graduate nurse, practicing self-care and maintaining clinical competence set a positive example for your patients and colleagues. When you prioritize self-care, you demonstrate the importance of taking care of oneself to provide the best possible care to others. By role modeling self-care, you inspire and encourage others to prioritize their well-being, contributing to a healthier and more competent nursing workforce.

Self-care is not a luxury but a necessity for maintaining clinical competence as a new graduate nurse. By prioritizing self-care, you can enhance your physical and mental well-being, prevent burnout, enhance critical thinking, and continue your professional growth. Ultimately, self-care allows you to provide the best possible care to your patients and maintain your clinical competence throughout your nursing career.

Strategies to Prioritizing Physical, Mental, and Emotional Well-Being
Self-care and well-being are crucial for new graduate nurses to maintain their physical, mental, and emotional health while navigating the demands of their profession. Here are some strategies to prioritize self-care and well-being:

- Establish healthy habits: Maintain a balanced diet, engage in regular exercise, and get enough sleep. These foundational habits support your overall well-being and provide you with the energy and resilience needed for your nursing practice.
- Practice mindfulness and stress management: Incorporate mindfulness techniques, such as deep breathing exercises or meditation, into your daily routine. These practices can help reduce stress, increase self-awareness, and promote mental well-being.

- Set boundaries: Learn to set boundaries between work and personal life. Avoid overworking and make time for activities that bring you joy and relaxation. Prioritize self-care activities, hobbies, and spending time with loved ones.
- Seek support: Build a support system of colleagues, friends, and family who understand the challenges of nursing. Share your experiences, concerns, and successes with them. Consider joining support groups or seeking professional counseling if needed.
- Practice self-compassion: Be kind to yourself and acknowledge that you are doing your best. Avoid self-criticism and negative self-talk. Celebrate your achievements and learn from your mistakes without being too hard on yourself.
- Take breaks: Allow yourself regular breaks during your shifts to rest, recharge, and refocus. Use these breaks to engage in activities that help you relax and rejuvenate, such as taking a walk, listening to music, or practicing deep breathing exercises.
- Engage in activities that bring joy: Make time for activities that bring you joy and fulfilment outside of work. Engaging in hobbies, pursuing creative outlets, or participating in activities that you enjoy can help reduce stress and enhance your overall well-being.
- Practice work-life balance: Strive to maintain a healthy work-life balance. Prioritize your personal life and make time for activities that are important to you. Avoid excessive overtime and learn to delegate tasks when necessary.
- Practice self-reflection: Regularly reflect on your experiences, emotions, and challenges as a new graduate nurse. Journaling or engaging in self-reflection exercises can help you process your thoughts and emotions, leading to increased self-awareness and personal growth.
- Seek professional development opportunities: Invest in your professional growth and development. Pursue continuing education, certifications, and specialized training that align with your interests and career goals. This can enhance your confidence and job satisfaction.

Self-care is not selfish but essential for your overall well-being and ability to provide quality care to your patients. Prioritizing self-care as a new graduate nurse will help you navigate the challenges of your profession and promote a sustainable and fulfilling nursing career.

Recognizing the Importance of Self-Care in Maintaining Clinical Competence
Recognizing the importance of self-care in maintaining clinical competence is crucial for new graduate nurses. Here's why self-care is essential for maintaining clinical competence:

- Physical well-being: Taking care of your physical health is vital for maintaining clinical competence. When you prioritize self-care activities such as getting enough sleep, eating nutritious meals, and engaging in regular exercise, you have the energy and stamina needed to perform your nursing duties effectively. Physical well-being also reduces the risk of burnout and helps you stay focused and alert during your shifts.

- Mental and emotional well-being: Self-care plays a significant role in maintaining your mental and emotional well-being. Nursing can be emotionally demanding, and it's essential to take care of your mental health to provide quality care to your patients. Engaging in activities that reduce stress, such as practicing mindfulness, seeking support from colleagues or therapists, and engaging in hobbies or relaxation techniques, can help you manage the emotional challenges of nursing and maintain your clinical competence.
- Preventing burnout: Burnout is a common issue among healthcare professionals, including new graduate nurses. It can negatively impact your clinical competence and overall job performance. By prioritizing self-care, you can prevent burnout and maintain your passion for nursing. Taking breaks, setting boundaries, and engaging in activities that bring you joy and fulfilment can help you recharge and prevent burnout from affecting your clinical competence.
- Enhancing critical thinking and decision-making: Self-care activities that promote relaxation and stress reduction can enhance your critical thinking and decision-making skills. When you are well-rested and mentally refreshed, you can think more clearly, analyze situations effectively, and make sound clinical judgments. This is essential for maintaining clinical competence and providing safe and effective patient care.
- Continuous learning and professional development: Self-care is not just about physical and mental well-being; it also includes investing in your professional growth and development. By engaging in self-care activities, you create space for continuous learning, attending educational programs, and seeking opportunities for professional development. This ongoing learning and growth contributes to your clinical competence and keeps you updated with the latest evidence-based practices.
- Role modeling for patients and colleagues: As a new graduate nurse, practicing self-care and maintaining clinical competence sets a positive example for your patients and colleagues. When you prioritize self-care, you demonstrate the importance of taking care of oneself to provide the best possible care to others. By role modeling self-care, you inspire and encourage others to prioritize their well-being, contributing to a healthier and more competent nursing workforce.

Self-care is not a luxury but a necessity for maintaining clinical competence as a new graduate nurse. By prioritizing self-care, you can enhance your physical and mental well-being, prevent burnout, enhance critical thinking, and continue your professional growth. Ultimately, self-care allows you to provide the best possible care to your patients and maintain your clinical competence throughout your nursing career.

3.1.6 Challenges and Obstacles That New Graduate Nurses May Encounter in Their Personal and Professional Lives

New graduate nurses may encounter various challenges and obstacles in their personal and professional lives. Common challenges and strategies to overcome them will be discussed in detail in the next sections. NB: Some of the strategies might apply for more than one challenge.

- Transitioning to the workforce: Adjusting to the demands and expectations of the professional nursing environment.
- Time management: Balancing work responsibilities, personal life, and self-care.
- Dealing with stress and burnout: High workload, emotional demands, and challenging patient situations can lead to stress and burnout.
- Building confidence and competence: Feeling overwhelmed and lacking confidence in clinical skills and decision-making.
- Communication and collaboration: Effective communication with patients, families, and interdisciplinary healthcare teams.
- Handling ethical dilemmas: Facing ethical dilemmas and making difficult decisions in patient care.
- Work-life balance: Balancing work commitments with personal life and maintaining a healthy lifestyle.

Strategies for Adjusting to the Demands and Expectations of the Professional Nursing Environment

Adjusting to the demands and expectations of the professional nursing environment can be challenging for new graduate nurses. Here are some strategies to help with this transition:

- Seek mentorship: Find an experienced nurse who can serve as a mentor and guide you through the initial stages of your nursing career. They can provide valuable insights, advice, and support.
- Participate in orientation programs: Take advantage of any orientation programs offered by your workplace. These programs are designed to help new nurses acclimate to the organization's policies, procedures, and culture.
- Embrace continuous learning: Nursing is a constantly evolving field, so it's important to stay updated with the latest evidence-based practices and advancements. Engage in continuous learning through workshops, conferences, online courses, and professional development opportunities.
- Develop time management skills: Effective time management is crucial in the nursing profession. Learn to prioritize tasks, delegate when appropriate, and organize your schedule to ensure you can meet the demands of your role.
- Build strong communication skills: Effective communication is essential in nursing. Practice active listening, develop clear and concise verbal and written communication skills, and learn to adapt your communication style to different individuals and situations.
- Be open to feedback: Constructive feedback is a valuable tool for growth and improvement. Be open to receiving feedback from your preceptors, mentors, and colleagues, and use it as an opportunity to enhance your skills and knowledge.

- Take care of yourself: Nursing can be physically and emotionally demanding. Prioritize self-care activities such as exercise, healthy eating, adequate sleep, and stress management techniques. Taking care of yourself will help you maintain your well-being and perform at your best.
- Foster professional relationships: Build positive relationships with your colleagues, interdisciplinary healthcare team members, and other healthcare professionals. Collaboration and teamwork are essential in providing quality patient care.
- Develop critical thinking skills: Nursing requires strong critical thinking skills to make sound clinical judgments and decisions. Continuously work on developing your critical thinking abilities through case studies, simulations, and real-life patient scenarios.
- Stay organized: Develop organizational skills to keep track of patient information, medications, and tasks. Utilize tools such as electronic health records, checklists, and calendars to stay organized and ensure nothing falls through the cracks.

Strategies for Managing Stress and Prevent Burnout

Implementing strategies to manage stress and prevent burnout is crucial for new graduate nurses. Here are some strategies to help you effectively manage stress and prevent burnout:

- Prioritize self-care: Make self-care a priority in your daily routine. Engage in activities that promote relaxation, such as exercise, meditation, deep breathing exercises, or hobbies that bring you joy. Set aside time for yourself to recharge and rejuvenate.
- Set boundaries: Establish clear boundaries between work and personal life. Avoid overworking and learn to say no when necessary. Set realistic expectations for yourself and communicate your limits to your colleagues and supervisors.
- Practice time management: Develop effective time management skills to prioritize tasks and avoid feeling overwhelmed. Break down your workload into manageable chunks, and create a schedule or to-do list to stay organized. Delegate tasks when appropriate and seek support from your team.
- Seek support: Build a support system of colleagues, friends, and family who understand the challenges of nursing. Share your experiences, concerns, and successes with them. Seek guidance and support from mentors or join support groups for new graduate nurses.
- Practice stress reduction techniques: Explore stress reduction techniques that work for you, such as deep breathing exercises, progressive muscle relaxation, guided imagery, or journaling. Engage in activities that help you unwind and reduce stress.
- Practice mindfulness: Incorporate mindfulness practices into your daily routine. Mindfulness involves being fully present in the moment and nonjudgmentally

observing your thoughts and feelings. This can help reduce stress and increase resilience.

- Take breaks: Allow yourself regular breaks during your shifts to rest and recharge. Use these breaks to engage in activities that help you relax and rejuvenate, such as taking a walk, listening to music, or practicing mindfulness exercises.
- Seek professional development opportunities: Invest in your professional growth and development. Pursue continuing education, certifications, and specialized training that align with your interests and career goals. This can enhance your confidence and job satisfaction.
- Practice healthy communication: Develop effective communication skills to express your needs, concerns, and boundaries. Communicate openly with your colleagues and supervisors about your workload, stressors, and any challenges you may be facing.
- Reflect and learn from experiences: Regularly reflect on your experiences, both positive and challenging. Identify areas for growth and learning. Seek feedback from colleagues and supervisors to improve your skills and enhance your confidence.

Managing stress and preventing burnout are an ongoing process. It's important to be proactive in implementing these strategies and adjusting them as needed. By taking care of yourself and managing stress effectively, you can maintain your well-being, prevent burnout, and thrive as a new graduate nurse.

Seeking Support and Utilizing Resources for Personal and Professional Well-Being

As a new graduate nurse, there are several resources and support systems available to help you with your personal and professional well-being such as the following:

- Mentorship programs: Look for mentorship programs offered by your workplace or professional nursing organizations. Having a mentor can provide guidance, support, and help you navigate the challenges of being a new nurse.
- Continuing education: Stay updated with the latest advancements in nursing by participating in continuing education programs. Many hospitals and healthcare organizations offer educational opportunities for their staff. Additionally, professional nursing organizations often provide webinars, conferences, and workshops that can enhance your knowledge and skills.
- Employee assistance programs (EAPs): EAPs are confidential counseling services provided by many employers. They can help you with personal issues, stress management, and work-life balance. Check with your employer to see if they offer an EAP and how to access it.
- Support groups: Joining a support group for new graduate nurses can provide a safe space to share experiences, ask questions, and receive support from others who are going through similar challenges. Look for local or online support groups specifically tailored for new nurses.

- Self-care: Taking care of your own well-being is crucial. Make sure to prioritize self-care activities such as exercise, healthy eating, getting enough sleep, and engaging in hobbies or activities that bring you joy and relaxation. Remember to set boundaries and take breaks when needed.
- Professional nursing organizations: Joining professional nursing organizations can provide networking opportunities, access to resources, and opportunities for professional development. These organizations often have special interest groups or sections dedicated to new graduate nurses.
- Seek feedback and reflect: Actively seek feedback from your colleagues, preceptors, and supervisors. Reflect on your experiences, identify areas for improvement, and set goals for your professional growth. Regularly reviewing your progress can help you stay motivated and focused.

Transitioning from a student to a professional nurse can be challenging, but with the right support and resources, you can thrive in your new role. Do not hesitate to reach out for help when needed and take advantage of the available resources.

Strategies When Facing Ethical Dilemmas and Making Difficult Decisions in Patient Care

- Familiarize yourself with ethical principles and guidelines: Develop a strong understanding of ethical principles such as autonomy, beneficence, non-maleficence, and justice. Familiarize yourself with the ethical guidelines and policies of your healthcare organization.
- Seek guidance from experienced nurses or ethics committees: Consult with experienced nurses, nurse educators, or ethics committees within your organization. They can provide guidance and support and help you navigate complex ethical situations.
- Engage in ethical discussions: Participate in ethical discussions with colleagues, mentors, and interdisciplinary healthcare team members. Sharing perspectives and engaging in dialog can help broaden your understanding of ethical issues and potential solutions.
- Utilize ethical decision-making models: Use ethical decision-making models, such as the "four-box method" or "principle-based approach," to systematically analyze ethical dilemmas. These models provide a structured framework to consider the ethical principles, values, and potential consequences involved.
- Consider the patient's perspective: Take into account the patient's values, beliefs, and preferences when making ethical decisions. Engage in open and honest communication with the patient and their family to understand their wishes and involve them in the decision-making process whenever possible.
- Consult ethical resources: Utilize ethical resources such as professional codes of ethics, ethical guidelines, and scholarly literature to inform your decision-making process. These resources can provide valuable insights and guidance in navigating ethical dilemmas.
- Reflect on personal values and beliefs: Reflect on your own values, beliefs, and biases that may influence your decision-making. Recognize and manage any

conflicts between your personal values and the ethical principles guiding nursing practice.

- Document the decision-making process: Document the ethical dilemma, the considerations taken into account, and the decision made in the patient's medical record. This ensures transparency, accountability, and continuity of care.
- Seek supervision and support: If you are unsure or overwhelmed by an ethical dilemma, seek supervision and support from your preceptor, mentor, or a trusted colleague. They can provide guidance, help you explore options, and offer emotional support during challenging times.
- Engage in continuing education: Stay updated with current ethical issues and debates in nursing through continuing education opportunities. Attend workshops, conferences, or webinars that focus on ethics in healthcare to enhance your knowledge and skills in ethical decision-making.

Ethical dilemmas can be complex and there may not always be a clear-cut solution. It's important to approach these situations with empathy, respect, and a commitment to patient-centered care. Seek support, engage in ethical discussions, and continuously strive to enhance your ethical decision-making skills.

Strategies for Managing Maintaining Work-Life Balance

Managing work-life balance as a new graduate nurse can be challenging, but it's essential for your overall well-being and long-term success.

- Set boundaries: Establish clear boundaries between work and personal life. Define specific times for work and nonwork activities. Avoid bringing work-related stress or tasks into your personal time. Communicate your boundaries to your colleagues and supervisors, and respectfully decline or delegate tasks that others can handle.
- Plan and organize: Plan and organize your time effectively. Use tools such as calendars, to-do lists, or time management apps to prioritize tasks, and allocate time for both work and personal activities. This will help you stay organized and ensure that you have dedicated time for yourself and your loved ones.
- Delegate and ask for help: Don't hesitate to delegate tasks or ask for help when needed. Recognize that you can't do everything on your own. Collaborate with your colleagues and utilize the resources available to you. Delegating tasks will help lighten your workload and create more time for personal activities.
- Practice effective time management: Develop strong time management skills to optimize your productivity and efficiency. Prioritize tasks based on urgency and importance. Break down larger tasks into smaller, manageable steps. Avoid procrastination and minimize distractions during work hours to maximize your productivity, and create more time for personal activities.
- Communicate with your support system: Maintain open communication with your support system, including family, friends, and loved ones. Let them know about your work schedule and commitments and discuss your needs and

expectations. They can provide understanding, support, and help you maintain a healthy work-life balance.

- Take advantage of flexible scheduling options: Explore flexible scheduling options, if available, such as part-time work, job-sharing, or flexible shifts. These options can provide more control over your work hours and allow for better work-life integration.
- Practice self-compassion: Be kind to yourself and avoid self-judgment. Understand that achieving a perfect work-life balance is not always possible, and there will be times when work demands more of your attention. Practice self-compassion and forgive yourself for any perceived imbalances. Strive for progress, not perfection.
- Regularly evaluate and adjust: Regularly evaluate your work-life balance and make adjustments as needed. Assess whether your current schedule and commitments align with your priorities and values. Be willing to make changes and adapt as necessary to maintain a healthy balance.

Work-life balance is a continuous process that requires ongoing effort and adjustment. As a new graduate nurse, you can achieve a healthier work-life balance by prioritizing self-care, setting boundaries, and practicing effective time management. In addition to the mentioned strategies, prioritize self-care and engage in activities that help you relax and recharge, such as exercise, hobbies, spending time with loved ones, or practicing mindfulness and meditation.

Setting Boundaries and Prioritizing Self-Care
Setting boundaries and prioritizing self-care as a new graduate nurse are essential for maintaining your well-being and preventing burnout. Here are some strategies to help you:

- Define your limits: Take the time to identify your personal and professional boundaries. Determine what you are comfortable with in terms of workload, working hours, and responsibilities. Communicate these boundaries to your colleagues and supervisors so they are aware of your limitations.
- Learn to say no: It's important to learn to say no when you are overwhelmed or a task or request goes beyond your boundaries. Remember that it's okay to prioritize your well-being and not take on more than you can handle. Be assertive and communicate your reasons for declining politely.
- Create a self-care routine: Develop a self-care routine that includes activities that help you relax, recharge, and take care of yourself. This can include exercise, meditation, reading, spending time with loved ones, pursuing hobbies, or engaging in activities that bring you joy. Schedule regular self-care activities into your routine and make them nonnegotiable.
- Prioritize rest and sleep: Adequate rest and sleep are crucial for your physical and mental well-being. Make sure to prioritize getting enough sleep each night and allow yourself time to rest and recharge. Avoid sacrificing sleep for work-related tasks and establish a consistent sleep schedule.

- Take breaks during work: Take regular breaks during your workday to rest and recharge. Use this time to step away from your work environment, engage in activities that help you relax, or simply take a few moments to breathe and clear your mind. Taking breaks can help reduce stress and improve focus and productivity.
- Disconnect from work: When you are not at work, consciously disconnect from work-related activities. Avoid checking work emails or messages during your time off. Set boundaries around your personal time and prioritize activities that help you unwind and recharge.
- Seek support: Reach out for support when you need it. Talk to your colleagues, mentors, or supervisors about any challenges or stressors you are facing. They can provide guidance, advice, and support. Additionally, consider seeking support from friends, family, or professional organizations where you can connect with other nurses who may be experiencing similar challenges.

Setting boundaries and prioritizing self-care are a continuous process. Regularly reassess your boundaries and self-care routine to ensure they align with your needs and well-being. By taking care of yourself, you will be better equipped to provide quality patient care and thrive in your nursing career.

Seeking Support and Utilizing Resources for Personal and Professional Well-Being

As a new graduate nurse, there are several resources and support systems available to help you with your personal and professional well-being. Here are some suggestions:

- Mentorship programs: Look for mentorship programs offered by your workplace or professional nursing organizations. Having a mentor can provide guidance and support and help you navigate the challenges of being a new nurse.
- Continuing education: Stay updated with the latest advancements in nursing by participating in continuing education programs. Many hospitals and healthcare organizations offer educational opportunities for their staff. Additionally, professional nursing organizations often provide webinars, conferences, and workshops that can enhance your knowledge and skills.
- Employee assistance programs (EAPs): EAPs are confidential counseling services provided by many employers. They can help you with personal issues, stress management, and work-life balance. Check with your employer to see if they offer an EAP and how to access it.
- Support groups: Joining a support group for new graduate nurses can provide a safe space to share experiences, ask questions, and receive support from others who are going through similar challenges. Look for local or online support groups specifically tailored for new nurses.
- Self-care: Taking care of your own well-being is crucial. Make sure to prioritize self-care activities such as exercise, healthy eating, getting enough sleep, and engaging in hobbies or activities that bring you joy and relaxation. Remember to set boundaries and take breaks when needed.

- Professional nursing organizations: Joining professional nursing organizations can provide networking opportunities, access to resources, and opportunities for professional development. These organizations often have special interest groups or sections dedicated to new graduate nurses.
- Seek feedback and reflect: Actively seek feedback from your colleagues, preceptors, and supervisors. Reflect on your experiences, identify areas for improvement, and set goals for your professional growth. Regularly reviewing your progress can help you stay motivated and focused.

Transitioning from a student to a professional nurse can be challenging, but with the right support and resources, you can thrive in your new role. Don't hesitate to reach out for help when needed and take advantage of the available resources.

Recognizing the Importance of Self-Care for Personal Well-Being and Professional Effectiveness

Recognizing the importance of self-care for personal well-being and professional effectiveness is crucial for new graduate nurses. Here's why:

- Physical and mental well-being: Self-care is essential for maintaining good physical and mental health. As new graduate nurses transition into their professional roles, they may experience increased stress, long working hours, and emotional demands. Engaging in self-care activities such as exercise, getting enough sleep, and practicing relaxation techniques can help prevent burnout, reduce stress levels, and promote overall well-being.
- Enhanced job performance: Taking care of oneself directly impacts job performance. When new graduate nurses prioritize self-care, they are better equipped to handle the demands of their profession. They can think more clearly, make sound decisions, and provide quality care to their patients. Self-care also helps prevent fatigue and improves concentration, leading to increased productivity and effectiveness in their roles.
- Emotional resilience: Nursing can be emotionally challenging, especially for new graduate nurses who are still adjusting to the demands of the profession. Engaging in self-care activities helps build emotional resilience, allowing nurses to better cope with stress, manage their emotions, and maintain a positive mindset. This resilience enables them to provide compassionate care while protecting their own emotional well-being.
- Work-life balance: Self-care promotes a healthy work-life balance, which is essential for new graduate nurses to prevent burnout and maintain satisfaction in their personal and professional lives. By setting boundaries, prioritizing personal time, and engaging in activities outside of work, nurses can recharge and maintain a sense of fulfilment and happiness.
- Role modeling for patients and colleagues: As healthcare professionals, new graduate nurses serve as role models for their patients and colleagues. By practicing self-care, they demonstrate the importance of prioritizing well-being and

taking care of oneself. This can inspire others to do the same and create a positive culture of self-care within the healthcare setting.

To prioritize self-care as a new graduate nurse, consider the following:

- Establish a self-care routine: Schedule regular self-care activities and make them a priority in your daily or weekly schedule.
- Set boundaries: Learn to say no to excessive work demands and create boundaries to protect your personal time and well-being.
- Seek support: Build a support network of colleagues, mentors, and friends who can provide guidance, advice, and emotional support.
- Practice stress management techniques: Engage in activities such as exercise, meditation, deep breathing, or hobbies that help you relax and reduce stress.
- Take breaks: Allow yourself regular breaks during shifts to rest, recharge, and refocus.
- Engage in activities that bring joy: Make time for activities that bring you happiness and fulfilment outside of work.

Self-care is not selfish but essential for your personal well-being and professional effectiveness as a new graduate nurse. By taking care of yourself, you can provide the best care to your patients and thrive in your nursing career.

Implementing Self-Care Strategies to Prevent Burnout and Promote Work-Life Balance

Implementing self-care strategies is crucial for new graduate nurses to prevent burnout and promote work-life balance. Here are some strategies to consider:

- Prioritize self-care: Make self-care a nonnegotiable part of your routine. Set aside dedicated time for activities that promote relaxation, rejuvenation, and personal well-being. This can include exercise, hobbies, spending time with loved ones, or engaging in activities that bring you joy and fulfilment.
- Set boundaries: Establish clear boundaries between work and personal life. Learn to say no to excessive work demands that may encroach on your personal time. Communicate your boundaries to colleagues and supervisors, and advocate for your own well-being.
- Practice stress management techniques: Develop and practice stress management techniques that work for you. This can include deep breathing exercises, mindfulness or meditation practices, journaling, or engaging in activities that help you relax and unwind. Find what works best for you and incorporate it into your daily routine.
- Take breaks: Take regular breaks during your shifts to rest and recharge. Use this time to engage in activities that help you relax and refocus. Even short breaks can make a significant difference in preventing burnout and maintaining productivity.

- Seek support: Build a support network of colleagues, mentors, and friends who can provide guidance, advice, and emotional support. Share your experiences and challenges with trusted individuals who can offer perspective and understanding. Don't hesitate to seek professional support if needed.
- Practice self-compassion: Be kind and compassionate toward yourself. Recognize that you are human and that it's okay to make mistakes or have limitations. Treat yourself with the same care and compassion you provide to your patients.
- Engage in regular self-reflection: Take time to reflect on your experiences, emotions, and challenges. Regular self-reflection can help you identify areas of improvement, recognize signs of burnout, and make necessary adjustments to your self-care routine.
- Utilize resources and support programs: Take advantage of resources and support programs available to you. Many healthcare organizations offer employee assistance programs, counseling services, or wellness initiatives. Explore these resources and utilize them as needed.
- Practice work-life integration: Instead of striving for a perfect work-life balance, aim for work-life integration. Find ways to incorporate activities that bring you joy and fulfilment into your work and personal life. This can include finding meaning in your work, engaging in hobbies or activities during your free time, or setting aside dedicated time for self-care.

Self-care is an ongoing process and requires commitment. It's important to regularly assess and adjust your self-care strategies based on your needs and circumstances. By prioritizing self-care, you can prevent burnout, promote work-life balance, and thrive in your nursing career as a new graduate nurse.

Seeking Support and Utilizing Resources for Self-Care and Mental Health
Seeking support and utilizing available resources for self-care and mental health are crucial for new graduate nurses. Here are some ways to do so:

- Employee assistance programs (EAPs): Many healthcare organizations offer EAPs that provide confidential counseling services, mental health support, and resources for employees. Take advantage of these programs to seek professional help and guidance when needed.
- Peer support: Connect with fellow nurses or colleagues who can provide support and understanding. Share your experiences, challenges, and concerns with trusted peers who may have gone through similar situations. Peer support can be invaluable in navigating the ups and downs of nursing practice.
- Professional organizations and networks: Join professional nursing organizations or networks that focus on mental health and well-being. These organizations often provide resources, educational materials, and networking opportunities that can support your self-care and mental health journey.
- Counseling services: Consider seeking counseling services from licensed therapists or counselors who specialize in healthcare professionals' mental health.

They can provide a safe space to discuss your challenges, emotions, and concerns and offer guidance and coping strategies.

- Mindfulness and meditation: Practice mindfulness and meditation techniques to promote mental well-being and reduce stress. There are numerous apps, websites, and guided meditation resources available that can help you incorporate these practices into your daily routine.
- Wellness initiatives: Take advantage of wellness initiatives offered by your healthcare organization. These may include workshops, seminars, or classes on stress management, resilience building, and self-care. Participating in these initiatives can provide valuable tools and strategies for maintaining your mental health.
- Online resources and support groups: Explore online resources and support groups specifically tailored to healthcare professionals' mental health. These platforms offer a wealth of information, self-help resources, and opportunities to connect with others who may be facing similar challenges.
- Supervision and mentorship: Seek guidance and support from experienced nurses or mentors who can provide insights and advice on managing stress, maintaining work-life balance, and prioritizing self-care. Regular supervision or mentorship sessions can be beneficial for your professional and personal growth.
- Personal support network: Lean on your personal support network, including family and friends, for emotional support and understanding. Share your experiences and challenges with them, and allow them to provide encouragement and a listening ear.

Seeking support and utilizing resources are a sign of strength, not weakness. Prioritizing your mental health and well-being is essential for your personal and professional growth as a new graduate nurse. Don't hesitate to reach out for help when needed, as it can make a significant difference in your overall well-being.

3.2   Emotional Intelligence and Self-Care

Raghubir (2018) defines emotional intelligence as ones' ability to manage own emotions and emotions of others. As defined by Slemon et al. (2021), self-care in nursing involve nurses' practices for promoting their own health and well-being and managing the stressors of the profession. As new graduate nurses enter the healthcare field, it is essential for them to prioritize emotional intelligence and self-care in order to maintain their well-being, cope with stress, and provide effective patient care. Emotional intelligence allows nurses to understand and manage their own emotions, as well as empathize with the emotions of their patients. By developing this skill, new nurses can better navigate the challenges of the healthcare environment and build strong connections with patients. Additionally, practicing self-care is crucial for relieving stress and preventing burnout. This can include activities such as mindfulness, exercise, and seeking support from colleagues or counselors.

By taking care of their mental and physical well-being, new graduate nurses can ensure they are in a strong position to provide the best possible care to their patients.

Strategies for Developing Emotional Intelligence and Practicing Self-Care

- Develop self-awareness: Take time to reflect on your emotions, strengths, and areas for growth. Understand how your emotions impact your thoughts, behaviors, and interactions with others. Self-awareness is the foundation of emotional intelligence.
- Practice empathy: Empathy is the ability to understand and share the feelings of others. Cultivate empathy by actively listening to patients, colleagues, and their concerns. Put yourself in their shoes and strive to understand their perspectives.
- Manage stress: Nursing can be a demanding and stressful profession. Develop healthy coping mechanisms to manage stress effectively. This may include engaging in relaxation techniques, such as deep breathing exercises, mindfulness, or engaging in hobbies and activities that bring you joy.
- Build strong relationships: Foster positive relationships with colleagues, mentors, and support networks. Seek opportunities for collaboration, teamwork, and open communication. Building strong relationships can provide emotional support and create a positive work environment.
- Practice self-care: Prioritize self-care activities to maintain your physical, mental, and emotional well-being. This may include getting enough sleep, eating nutritious meals, engaging in regular exercise, and taking breaks when needed. Set boundaries to ensure a healthy work-life balance.
- Develop emotional regulation skills: Learn to manage and regulate your emotions effectively. Practice techniques such as deep breathing, mindfulness, and reframing negative thoughts. This can help you respond to challenging situations with composure and resilience.
- Seek support and debriefing: Nursing can involve emotionally challenging situations. Seek support from colleagues, mentors, or professional counselors to process and debrief after difficult experiences. Sharing your feelings and experiences can help prevent burnout and promote emotional well-being.
- Continuously learn and grow: Engage in ongoing professional development to enhance your knowledge and skills. This can boost your confidence and competence, leading to increased emotional intelligence. Attend workshops, conferences, and educational programs that focus on emotional intelligence and self-care.
- Practice self-reflection: Regularly reflect on your emotions, actions, and interactions with others. Consider how you can improve your emotional intelligence and self-care practices. Journaling or engaging in reflective exercises can help deepen your self-awareness.
- Seek feedback and learn from experiences: Be open to feedback from colleagues, supervisors, and patients. Use feedback as an opportunity for growth and learning. Reflect on your experiences, and identify areas for improvement in your emotional intelligence and self-care practices.

Remember, emotional intelligence and self-care are ongoing practices. Prioritize your well-being and invest in developing your emotional intelligence skills. By taking care of yourself, you can provide better care to your patients and thrive in your nursing career.

3.2.1   Developing Emotional Intelligence

Developing emotional intelligence is crucial for new graduate nurses to effectively navigate the complex and emotionally demanding healthcare environment. Here are some strategies to develop emotional intelligence:

- Self-awareness: Start by developing self-awareness, which involves recognizing and understanding your own emotions, strengths, and areas for growth. Pay attention to your thoughts, feelings, and reactions in different situations.
- Reflect on emotions: Take time to reflect on your emotions and the underlying reasons behind them. Consider how your emotions may impact your interactions with patients, colleagues, and other healthcare professionals.
- Practice empathy: Empathy is the ability to understand and share the feelings of others. Practice putting yourself in the shoes of patients and their families, and try to understand their perspectives and emotions. This can help you provide compassionate and patient-centered care.
- Active listening: Develop active listening skills to truly understand and connect with others. Pay attention to both verbal and nonverbal cues and show genuine interest in what others are saying. This can help you build rapport and establish trust with patients and colleagues.
- Manage stress: Nursing can be a stressful profession, so it's important to develop healthy coping mechanisms. Find stress management techniques that work for you, such as deep breathing exercises, mindfulness, physical activity, or engaging in hobbies. Managing stress effectively can help you maintain emotional balance.
- Develop emotional regulation skills: Learn to manage and regulate your own emotions in challenging situations. Practice techniques such as deep breathing, positive self-talk, and reframing negative thoughts. This can help you respond to stressors with composure and resilience.
- Build strong relationships: Foster positive relationships with colleagues, mentors, and support networks. Seek opportunities for collaboration, teamwork, and open communication. Building strong relationships can provide emotional support and create a positive work environment.
- Seek feedback: Be open to feedback from colleagues, supervisors, and patients. Actively seek feedback on your communication skills, empathy, and emotional intelligence. Use feedback as an opportunity for growth and improvement.
- Continuous learning: Engage in ongoing learning and professional development to enhance your emotional intelligence. Attend workshops, seminars, or courses that focus on emotional intelligence, communication skills, and self-awareness.

- Reflect and learn from experiences: Regularly reflect on your experiences and interactions with patients and colleagues. Consider how you could have handled situations differently and identify areas for improvement. Reflective practice can help deepen your emotional intelligence.

Remember, developing emotional intelligence is a lifelong journey. Be patient with yourself and embrace opportunities for growth and learning. By developing your emotional intelligence, you can enhance your relationships, provide better patient care, and thrive in your nursing career.

Understanding the Importance of Emotional Intelligence in Nursing Practice
Emotional intelligence is crucial in nursing practice for several reasons:

- Building rapport with patients: Nurses with high emotional intelligence can effectively connect with patients on an emotional level. This helps to establish trust, comfort, and open communication, which are essential for providing quality care.
- Empathy and understanding: Emotional intelligence enables nurses to understand and empathize with the emotions and experiences of their patients. This allows them to provide compassionate care and support, which can greatly enhance the patient's overall well-being.
- Managing stress and emotions: Nursing can be a highly demanding and stressful profession. Nurses with strong emotional intelligence are better equipped to manage their own stress and emotions, which helps them stay calm and focused on challenging situations. This, in turn, allows them to provide better care to their patients.
- Conflict resolution: Nurses often encounter conflicts and disagreements in the healthcare setting. Emotional intelligence helps nurses navigate these conflicts by understanding the perspectives of others, effectively communicating, and finding mutually beneficial solutions.
- Teamwork and collaboration: Nursing is a team-based profession, and effective teamwork is essential for providing safe and efficient care. Emotional intelligence helps nurses work well with others, understand and respect different viewpoints, and effectively communicate and collaborate with colleagues.

Overall, emotional intelligence plays a vital role in nursing practice by enhancing patient care, promoting positive relationships, and improving the overall healthcare experience for both patients and healthcare professionals.

Enhancing Self-Awareness, Empathy, and Effective Communication Skills
Enhancing self-awareness, empathy, and effective communication skills is essential for healthcare professionals, including nurses. Here's why:

- Self-awareness: Self-awareness is the ability to recognize and understand one's own emotions, thoughts, and behaviors (Jebur et al. 2024). It is crucial for nurses to be self-aware as it helps them understand how their emotions and actions can impact their patients and colleagues. By being self-aware, nurses can regulate their emotions, manage stress, and maintain professionalism in challenging situations.

- Empathy: Empathy is the ability to understand and share the feelings of others (Shahzad et al. 2023). It is a key component of patient-centered care. Nurses who are empathetic can connect with their patients on a deeper level, understand their needs and concerns, and provide compassionate care. Empathy also helps nurses build trust and rapport with patients, leading to better patient outcomes.
- Effective communication: Effective communication is vital in nursing practice as it ensures clear and accurate exchange of information between healthcare professionals, patients, and their families (Zaga et al. 2023). Nurses with strong communication skills can convey complex medical information in a way that patients can understand, actively listen to patients' concerns, and provide emotional support. Effective communication also helps nurses collaborate with other healthcare team members, leading to better coordination of care.

To enhance these skills, nurses can

- Engage in self-reflection and self-assessment to identify their strengths and areas for improvement.
- Seek feedback from colleagues, supervisors, and patients to gain insights into their communication and empathy skills.
- Participate in training programs or workshops that focus on emotional intelligence, empathy, and communication.
- Practice active listening, which involves giving full attention to the speaker, understanding their perspective, and responding appropriately.
- Engage in role-playing exercises to practice effective communication and empathy in different scenarios.
- Read books or articles on emotional intelligence, empathy, and effective communication to gain knowledge and insights.

By continuously working on self-awareness, empathy, and effective communication skills, nurses can provide high-quality, patient-centered care and contribute to positive healthcare experiences for their patients.

Managing Emotions and Building Resilience in Challenging Situations
Managing emotions and building resilience are crucial skills for nurses to navigate challenging situations in their practice. Here are some strategies to help with this:

- Recognize and acknowledge emotions: It's important for nurses to be aware of their emotions and recognize when they are experiencing stress, frustration, or other challenging emotions. By acknowledging these emotions, nurses can better understand their impact on their thoughts and actions.

- Practice self-care: Taking care of oneself is essential for managing emotions and building resilience. Nurses should prioritize self-care activities such as exercise, getting enough sleep, eating well, and engaging in hobbies or activities that bring joy and relaxation. Self-care helps to recharge and reduce stress levels.
- Seek support: It's important for nurses to have a support system in place. This can include colleagues, friends, family, or professional support networks. Sharing experiences, seeking advice, or simply venting can help nurses process their emotions and gain perspective.
- Develop coping strategies: Nurses can develop healthy coping strategies to manage their emotions in challenging situations. This can include deep breathing exercises, mindfulness or meditation practices, journaling, or engaging in activities that promote relaxation and stress reduction.
- Reflect and learn from experiences: Reflecting on challenging situations and learning from them can help nurses build resilience. By analyzing what went well and what could have been done differently, nurses can develop strategies to handle similar situations in the future.
- Seek professional development opportunities: Continuous learning and professional development can enhance nurses' skills and knowledge, which in turn can boost their confidence and resilience. Attending workshops and conferences or pursuing advanced certifications can provide nurses with new tools and strategies to manage emotions in challenging situations.
- Maintain a positive mindset: Adopting a positive mindset can help nurses approach challenging situations with resilience. Focusing on strengths, finding silver linings, and practicing gratitude can help shift perspective and build resilience.

Building resilience takes time and practice. It's important for nurses to be patient with themselves and seek support when needed. By managing emotions and building resilience, nurses can navigate challenging situations more effectively and provide the best possible care to their patients.

3.2.2 Developing a Culture of Self-Reflection

Developing a culture of self-reflection is essential for new graduate nurses to enhance their clinical competence. By encouraging new nurses to regularly reflect on their experiences, actions, and decisions, they can gain valuable insights into their strengths and areas for improvement. This process allows them to identify patterns in their practice, learn from mistakes, and continuously strive for personal and professional growth. Through self-reflection, nurses can enhance their critical thinking skills, develop greater self-awareness, and make more informed decisions in their clinical practice. By creating a supportive environment that values self-reflection, new graduate nurses can cultivate a culture of continuous learning and improvement, ultimately leading to better patient outcomes and increased job satisfaction.

Promoting a Culture of Self-Reflection Within Healthcare Organizations

Promoting a culture of self-reflection for new graduate nurses within healthcare organizations is crucial for their professional growth and development. Here are some strategies that can help in fostering this culture:

- Encourage regular self-reflection: Healthcare organizations can encourage new graduate nurses to engage in regular self-reflection by providing dedicated time and resources for this purpose. This can be done through workshops, seminars, or online platforms that facilitate self-reflection.
- Provide mentorship and guidance: Assigning experienced nurses as mentors to new graduate nurses can greatly support their self-reflection process. Mentors can provide guidance and feedback and help new nurses identify areas for improvement and growth.
- Incorporate self-reflection in performance evaluations: Including self-reflection as a component of performance evaluations can encourage new graduate nurses to actively engage in this practice. This can be done by asking nurses to reflect on their strengths, weaknesses, and areas for improvement.
- Create a safe and supportive environment: It is important to create a safe and supportive environment where new graduate nurses feel comfortable sharing their thoughts and experiences. This can be achieved by promoting open communication, active listening, and nonjudgmental feedback.
- Provide resources for self-reflection: Healthcare organizations can provide resources such as journals, reflection prompts, or online platforms that facilitate self-reflection. These resources can help new graduate nurses structure their thoughts and promote deeper self-awareness.
- Encourage peer collaboration: Encouraging new graduate nurses to engage in peer collaboration and discussion can enhance their self-reflection process. This can be done through group activities, case studies, or regular meetings where nurses can share their experiences and learn from each other.
- Recognize and celebrate growth: Healthcare organizations should recognize and celebrate the growth and development of new graduate nurses who actively engage in self-reflection. This can be done through awards, certificates, or public acknowledgments, which can further motivate nurses to continue their self-reflection journey.

By implementing these strategies, healthcare organizations can create a culture of self-reflection that supports the professional growth and development of new graduate nurses.

Encouraging Self-Reflection as a Tool for Continuous Improvement

Encouraging self-reflection as a tool for continuous improvement is essential for personal and professional growth. Here are some ways to promote self-reflection as a means of continuous improvement:

- Set clear goals: Encourage individuals to set clear and specific goals for themselves. These goals can be related to their personal or professional development.

By having clear goals, individuals can reflect on their progress and identify areas for improvement.

- Provide time and space for reflection: Create an environment that allows individuals to have dedicated time and space for self-reflection. This can be done by scheduling regular reflection sessions or providing quiet areas where individuals can reflect without distractions.
- Use reflection prompts or questions: Provide individuals with reflection prompts or questions to guide their self-reflection process. These prompts can help individuals think deeply about their experiences, actions, and outcomes and identify areas where they can improve.
- Encourage journaling: Encourage individuals to keep a journal where they can record their thoughts, experiences, and reflections. Journaling allows individuals to reflect on their actions, emotions, and thoughts and gain insights into their strengths and areas for improvement.
- Foster a culture of feedback: Create a culture where giving and receiving feedback is encouraged and valued. Feedback from others can provide individuals with different perspectives and insights, helping them identify areas for improvement and growth.
- Provide resources and support: Offer resources such as books, articles, or online courses that promote self-reflection and continuous improvement. Additionally, provide support through coaching or mentoring programs to help individuals navigate their self-reflection journey.
- Celebrate growth and progress: Recognize and celebrate individuals' growth and progress resulting from their self-reflection efforts. This can be done through acknowledgment, rewards, or opportunities for advancement, which can motivate individuals to continue their self-reflection journey.
- Lead by example: Leaders should lead by example and demonstrate the importance of self-reflection for continuous improvement. When leaders actively engage in self-reflection and share their experiences, it encourages others to do the same.

By promoting self-reflection as a tool for continuous improvement, individuals can gain valuable insights, identify areas for growth, and make positive changes in their personal and professional lives.

Overcoming Barriers to Self-Reflection in the Nursing Profession
Self-reflection is a valuable practice in the nursing profession, but there can be barriers that hinder its implementation. Here are some common barriers to self-reflection in the nursing profession and strategies to overcome them:

- Time constraints: Nurses often have demanding work schedules, leaving little time for self-reflection. To overcome this barrier, healthcare organizations can prioritize and allocate dedicated time for self-reflection. This can be done by incorporating it into nurses' schedules or providing designated spaces for reflection during breaks.
- Lack of awareness: Some nurses may not fully understand the benefits of self-reflection or how to engage in the practice. To address this, healthcare

organizations can provide education and training on the importance of self-reflection and offer guidance on how to effectively engage in the process. This can be done through workshops, seminars, or online resources.

- Fear of judgment: Nurses may be hesitant to engage in self-reflection due to a fear of being judged or criticized. To overcome this barrier, healthcare organizations can foster a culture of psychological safety, where nurses feel comfortable sharing their thoughts and experiences without fear of negative consequences. This can be achieved through open communication, nonjudgmental feedback, and supportive leadership.
- Lack of support: Nurses may feel unsupported or isolated in their self-reflection efforts. To address this, healthcare organizations can provide mentorship programs or peer support groups where nurses can discuss their reflections, share experiences, and receive guidance and feedback. This can create a supportive environment that encourages self-reflection.
- Heavy workload and burnout: Nurses experiencing high workloads and burnout may find it challenging to engage in self-reflection. To overcome this barrier, healthcare organizations should prioritize nurse well-being and work-life balance. By implementing strategies to reduce workload, provide adequate staffing, and promote self-care, nurses will have more energy and mental space for self-reflection.
- Lack of structure: Some nurses may struggle with the process of self-reflection if they don't have a clear structure or framework to follow. Healthcare organizations can provide resources such as reflection templates, prompts, or guidelines to help nurses structure their reflections and guide their thinking process.
- Limited feedback and evaluation: Without feedback and evaluation, nurses may find it difficult to assess their progress and identify areas for improvement. Healthcare organizations can incorporate regular performance evaluations that include self-reflection as a component. This allows nurses to receive feedback, set goals, and track their growth over time.

By addressing these barriers and implementing strategies to overcome them, healthcare organizations can create an environment that supports and encourages self-reflection in the nursing profession. This, in turn, can lead to improved professional development, enhanced patient care, and increased job satisfaction among nurses.

3.3   Personal Development

Transitioning from a new graduate nurse to a practicing nurse is a crucial period of personal development. During this time, new nurses are not only learning clinical skills and procedures, but they are also gaining confidence in their abilities and honing their critical thinking skills. This transition requires adapting to the fast-paced and demanding environment of healthcare, as well as building relationships with patients, colleagues, and other healthcare professionals. It is a time of growth, reflection, and self-discovery as new nurses navigate the complexities of the health-care setting and find their place within the profession. Personal development during this transition involves embracing challenges, seeking feedback, and continuously learning and improving in order to become a competent and confident practice nurse.

3.3.1   Understanding the Difference Between Personal and Professional Development

Personal development and professional development are two distinct yet intercon-nected aspects of growth and improvement. Personal development focuses on self-improvement, self-awareness, and self-discovery, encompassing areas such as emotional intelligence, communication skills, and resilience. It involves reflecting on one's beliefs, values, and behaviors and striving to become a better version of oneself. On the other hand, professional development pertains to advancing skills and knowledge in a specific career or field, such as attending workshops, pursuing further education, or gaining certifications. While personal development enhances overall well-being and fulfilment, professional development aims to enhance per-formance and success in the workplace. Both are crucial for achieving personal and career goals, and striking a balance between the two is essential for holistic growth and success.

Importance of Setting Personal and Professional Goals
Setting personal and professional goals is important for several reasons:

- Clarity and focus: Setting goals helps you gain clarity about what you want to achieve in your personal and professional life. It provides a clear direction and focus, allowing you to prioritize your efforts and make better decisions.
- Motivation and drive: Goals provide motivation and drive to work toward some-thing meaningful. When you have a clear goal in mind, you are more likely to stay motivated and take consistent action to achieve it.
- Measurement of progress: Goals act as a benchmark to measure your progress. They help you track your achievements and evaluate how far you have come. This measurement of progress can boost your confidence and provide a sense of accomplishment.
- Personal growth and development: Setting goals pushes you out of your comfort zone and encourages personal growth and development. It challenges you to acquire new skills, expand your knowledge, and overcome obstacles, leading to self-improvement.
- Time management: Goals help you manage your time effectively. When you have specific goals, you can prioritize tasks and allocate your time accordingly. This prevents procrastination and ensures that you are working toward your goals consistently.
- Increased success and achievement: Setting goals increases your chances of suc-cess and achievement. By setting clear objectives and working toward them, you

are more likely to accomplish what you set out to do. This sense of achievement can boost your self-confidence and satisfaction.

- Accountability: Goals provide a sense of accountability. When you set goals, you are more likely to hold yourself accountable for your actions and decisions. This accountability can help you stay focused and committed to your goals.

Setting personal and professional goals is essential for personal growth, success, and fulfilment. It provides direction, motivation, and a framework for continuous improvement.

Significance of Ongoing Learning and Personal Development
New graduate nurses face a significant transition period as they enter the workforce, and ongoing learning and personal development play a crucial role during this time. The healthcare field is constantly evolving with new technologies, treatments, and best practices emerging. Therefore, it is essential for new nurses to commit to life-long learning to stay current and provide the best care for their patients. Additionally, personal development is equally important as it helps new nurses build confidence, resilience, and critical thinking skills to navigate the challenges they may encounter in their roles. By continuously seeking opportunities to learn and grow, new graduate nurses can make a smooth transition into their careers and establish a strong foundation for their future success in the healthcare field.

Areas to focus on for personal development as a new graduate nurse are as follows:

- Continuous learning: Nursing is a dynamic field, and there is always something new to learn. Commit to lifelong learning by staying updated on evidence-based practices, attending conferences or workshops, and seeking out opportunities for professional development. This will help you enhance your knowledge and skills as a nurse.
- Time management and organization: Develop effective time management and organizational skills to handle the demands of your nursing responsibilities. Prioritize tasks, create schedules, and utilize tools such as to-do lists or digital calendars to stay organized and ensure timely completion of tasks.
- Communication skills: Effective communication is essential in nursing. Work on developing strong verbal and written communication skills to effectively interact with patients, families, and healthcare team members. Practice active listening, empathy, and clarity in your communication.
- Critical thinking and problem-solving: Nursing often require quick thinking and decision-making. Enhance your critical thinking skills by actively seeking opportunities to analyze complex situations, anticipate potential issues, and develop effective problem-solving strategies. Seek guidance from experienced nurses and engage in case studies or simulations to sharpen your critical thinking abilities.
- Self-care and stress management: Nursing can be physically and emotionally demanding. Prioritize self-care to maintain your well-being. Practice stress

management techniques such as exercise, mindfulness, and seeking support from colleagues or mentors. Take breaks when needed and establish a healthy work-life balance.

- Professional networking: Build professional relationships and networks within the nursing community. Attend nursing conferences, join professional organizations, and engage in online nursing communities. Networking can provide opportunities for mentorship, collaboration, and career advancement.
- Cultural competence: Develop cultural competence to provide patient-centered care to individuals from diverse backgrounds. Seek to understand different cultural beliefs, values, and practices to deliver culturally sensitive care. Embrace diversity and strive for inclusivity in your nursing practice.
- Reflective practice: Engage in reflective practice to continuously improve your nursing skills and knowledge. Regularly reflect on your experiences, identify areas for growth, and set goals for improvement. Consider keeping a reflective journal or participating in reflective discussions with colleagues or mentors.
- Professional ethics and integrity: Uphold professional ethics and integrity in your nursing practice. Adhere to ethical standards, maintain patient confidentiality, and advocate for patient rights. Seek guidance from your nursing code of ethics, and consult with experienced nurses or mentors when faced with ethical dilemmas.

Personal development is a lifelong journey. Embrace opportunities for growth, seek feedback from experienced nurses, and be open to continuous learning. By investing in your personal development as a new graduate nurse, you can enhance your skills, confidence, and overall effectiveness in providing quality patient care.

Setting Personal and Professional Goals
Setting personal and professional goals is an important step in personal development and career growth. Here are some steps to help you set effective goals:

- Reflect on your values and aspirations: Start by reflecting on your values, passions, and long-term aspirations. Consider what is truly important to you in both your personal and professional life. This self-reflection will help you align your goals with your core values and create a sense of purpose.
- Identify specific areas for improvement: Assess your current strengths and weaknesses in both personal and professional domains. Identify areas where you want to improve or develop new skills. This could include areas such as communication, leadership, technical skills, or personal well-being.
- Make your goals SMART: Ensure that your goals are specific, measurable, achievable, relevant, and time-bound (SMART). Specific goals clearly define what you want to achieve. Measurable goals have clear criteria to track progress. Achievable goals are realistic and within your reach. Relevant goals align with your values and aspirations. Time-bound goals have a specific timeline for completion.
- Prioritize your goals: Determine which goals are most important to you and prioritize them accordingly. Focus on a few key goals at a time to avoid feeling

overwhelmed. Prioritization will help you allocate your time and resources effectively.

- Break goals into actionable steps: Break down each goal into smaller, actionable steps. This will make them more manageable and help you track progress. Assign deadlines to each step to maintain momentum and accountability.
- Seek support and accountability: Share your goals with a trusted mentor, colleague, or friend who can provide support and hold you accountable. Regularly update them on your progress and seek their guidance when needed. Consider joining professional networks or support groups to connect with like-minded individuals who can offer support and encouragement.
- Monitor and evaluate your progress: Regularly monitor your progress toward your goals. Assess what is working well and what needs adjustment. Celebrate milestones and achievements along the way. If necessary, revise your goals or action steps based on new insights or changing circumstances.
- Adapt and embrace challenges: Be open to adapting your goals as you gain new experiences and insights. Embrace challenges as opportunities for growth and learning. View setbacks as learning experiences and adjust your approach accordingly.
- Celebrate achievements and set new goals: Once you have achieved a goal, take time to celebrate your accomplishment. Reflect on what you have learned and how you have grown. Then, set new goals to continue your personal and professional development journey.

Goal-setting is an ongoing process. Regularly review and revise your goals as you progress and evolve. Stay motivated, stay focused, and stay committed to your personal and professional growth.

Identifying Personal and Professional Goals for Growth and Development
Identifying personal and professional goals for growth and development is an important step in your journey toward self-improvement. Here are some areas to consider when setting personal and professional goals:

Personal Goals
- Health and well-being: Set goals related to your physical and mental health. This could include exercising regularly, eating a balanced diet, getting enough sleep, practicing mindfulness or meditation, or seeking therapy or counseling if needed.
- Personal relationships: Focus on nurturing and strengthening your relationships with family, friends, and loved ones. Set goals to spend quality time with them, improve communication, or resolve conflicts.
- Personal growth and learning: Set goals to expand your knowledge and skills in areas that interest you. This could involve reading books, taking courses or workshops, learning a new hobby or skill, or pursuing personal interests and passions.
- Work-life balance: Strive for a healthy work-life balance by setting goals to prioritize self-care, establish boundaries, and allocate time for activities outside of work that bring you joy and fulfilment.

Professional Goals

- Career advancement: Set goals related to your career growth and advancement. This could include acquiring new certifications or qualifications, seeking promotions or leadership roles, or expanding your professional network.
- Skill development: Identify specific skills you want to develop or improve in your professional role. This could be enhancing your communication skills, becoming proficient in new technologies or software, or developing leadership or project management skills.
- Continuing education: Set goals to pursue ongoing professional development and education. This could involve attending conferences, workshops, or seminars, participating in webinars or online courses, or seeking mentorship or coaching opportunities.
- Networking and professional relationships: Set goals to expand your professional network and build meaningful relationships within your industry. This could involve attending networking events, joining professional organizations, or seeking mentorship from experienced professionals.
- Contribution and impact: Set goals to make a positive impact in your professional field or community. This could involve volunteering, participating in community service projects, or taking on leadership roles in initiatives that align with your values and interests.

Remember to make your goals SMART (specific, measurable, achievable, relevant, and time-bound), and break them down into actionable steps. Regularly review and assess your progress, make adjustments as needed, and celebrate your achievements along the way. By setting personal and professional goals, you can actively work toward your growth and development in all aspects of your life.

3.3.2 Creating SMART (Specific, Measurable, Achievable, Relevant, Time-Bound) Goals

SMART goals are a framework for setting objectives that are specific, measurable, achievable, relevant, and time-bound. By following this framework, you can create goals that are clear and actionable and have a higher chance of success. Here's how you can create SMART goals:

- Specific: Clearly define what you want to achieve. Be specific about the outcome you want to see.
- Measurable: Set criteria to measure your progress and determine when you have achieved your goal. This helps you track your progress and stay motivated.
- Achievable: Ensure that your goal is realistic and attainable. Consider your resources, skills, and limitations when setting your goal.
- Relevant: Make sure your goal is aligned with your overall objectives and priorities. It should be relevant to your personal or professional growth.

- Time-bound: Set a deadline or timeline for achieving your goal. This creates a sense of urgency and helps you stay focused.

An example of a SMART goal to enhance the clinical competence of new graduate nurses is as follows:

Goal: To complete 20 h of online courses in areas such as critical care, medication administration, or wound care within the first 6 months of starting their new nursing job.

Specific: 20 h and the specific topics.

Measurable: Keeping records of completed courses.

Achievable: Accessibility of online courses and ability to complete around work schedules.

Relevant: Gaining additional knowledge and skills in these areas will directly enhance their clinical competence.

Time-bound: Achieve the goal within the next 6 months.

SMART goals provide a clear roadmap for success and help you stay motivated and focused on your objectives. By setting and achieving this SMART goal, new graduate nurses can improve their clinical skills and provide better care to their patients.

Developing Action Plans to Achieve Set Goals

Developing an action plan is crucial for achieving your set goals. It helps you break down your goals into actionable steps and provides a roadmap to follow. Here's a step-by-step guide to developing an action plan:

- Identify the specific actions: Break down your goal into smaller, actionable tasks. Identify the specific actions you need to take to achieve your goal.
- Prioritize the actions: Determine the order in which you need to complete the actions. Prioritize them based on their importance and dependencies.
- Set deadlines: Assign deadlines to each action. This helps create a sense of urgency and keeps you accountable.
- Allocate resources: Determine the resources you need to accomplish each action. This includes time, money, tools, and support from others.
- Create a timeline: Create a timeline or schedule for completing each action. This helps you stay organized and track your progress.
- Assign responsibilities: Determine who will be responsible for each action. Assign tasks to individuals or teams based on their skills and availability.
- Monitor and track progress: Regularly monitor and track your progress toward each action. This helps you stay on track and make adjustments if needed.
- Evaluate and adjust: Periodically evaluate your action plan and make adjustments if necessary. This allows you to adapt to changing circumstances and ensure your plan remains effective.
- Stay motivated and focused: Keep yourself motivated and focused on your action plan. Celebrate small victories along the way to maintain momentum.

An action plan is a dynamic document that may require adjustments as you progress. Regularly review and update your plan to ensure it remains relevant and effective in helping you achieve your goals.

Significance of Regularly Reviewing and Adjusting Set Goals to Ensure Progress and Growth
Regularly reviewing and adjusting set goals is crucial for new graduate nurses to ensure progress and growth in their careers. As they navigate through the challenges and responsibilities of being a nurse, it is important for them to regularly assess their goals and make necessary adjustments to stay on track. By reviewing their goals, new graduate nurses can identify areas where they may be falling short and make any necessary changes to align their actions with their long-term objectives. This process allows them to track their progress, stay motivated, and continue to develop their skills and knowledge in the field of nursing. Ultimately, regularly reviewing and adjusting goals can help new graduate nurses to achieve success in their careers and make a positive impact on patient care.

3.3.3   Challenges and Obstacles That New Graduate Nurses May Encounter in Their Personal and Professional Lives

New graduate nurses may encounter various challenges and obstacles in both their personal and professional lives. Some of these challenges include the following:

- Transitioning to the professional role: New graduate nurses may find it challenging to transition from the role of a student to that of a professional nurse. They may struggle with the increased responsibilities, decision-making, and accountability that come with the job.
- Lack of experience: As new graduates, nurses may have limited clinical experience, which can make it difficult for them to handle complex patient cases and make critical decisions. They may feel overwhelmed and unsure of themselves in certain situations.
- Time management: Balancing multiple responsibilities, such as patient care, documentation, and administrative tasks, can be challenging for new graduate nurses. They may struggle with prioritizing tasks and managing their time effectively.
- Dealing with difficult patients and families: New graduate nurses may encounter challenging situations where they have to deal with difficult patients or families. This can include managing conflicts, addressing emotional needs, and providing patient education effectively.
- Workplace dynamics: Adjusting to the dynamics of the healthcare team and establishing professional relationships with colleagues can be a challenge for new graduate nurses. They may face issues such as communication barriers, conflicts, or feeling like an outsider in an established team.

- Emotional stress and burnout: Nursing can be emotionally demanding, and new graduate nurses may experience high levels of stress and burnout. They may struggle with managing their own emotions while providing care to patients who are suffering or in critical conditions.
- Continuing education and professional development: New graduate nurses need to continuously update their knowledge and skills to provide quality care. Keeping up with the latest evidence-based practices and pursuing further education can be a challenge while juggling work and personal life.
- Work-life balance: Finding a balance between work and personal life can be challenging for new graduate nurses, especially when they are adjusting to the demands of their new profession. Long working hours, shift work, and irregular schedules can impact their personal relationships and well-being.

It is important for new graduate nurses to seek support from mentors, colleagues, and professional organizations to navigate these challenges successfully. Continuous learning, self-care, and seeking guidance can help them overcome these obstacles and thrive in their personal and professional lives.

Strategies to Overcome Abovementioned Challenges and Obstacles
New graduate nurses can overcome the challenges and obstacles they face by implementing the following strategies:

- Seek mentorship and guidance: Finding a mentor who can provide guidance and support can be invaluable for new graduate nurses. Mentors can offer advice, share their experiences, and help navigate the challenges of transitioning to the professional role.
- Take advantage of orientation and training programs: Many healthcare facilities offer orientation and training programs specifically designed for new graduate nurses. These programs provide additional support, education, and hands-on experience to help them build confidence and competence in their roles.
- Continuously update knowledge and skills: New graduate nurses should prioritize continuing education and professional development. They can attend workshops, conferences, and seminars or pursue advanced certifications to enhance their knowledge and skills. Staying updated with evidence-based practices will help them provide quality care.
- Develop effective time management skills: Learning to prioritize tasks, delegate when appropriate, and manage time efficiently is crucial for new graduate nurses. They can use tools such as to-do lists, calendars, and time-blocking techniques to stay organized and meet deadlines.
- Build strong communication skills: Effective communication is essential in nursing practice. New graduate nurses should focus on developing strong communication skills, both verbal and written. They should actively listen, ask questions, and seek clarification when needed. Building rapport with patients, families, and colleagues will help in navigating difficult situations.

- Practice self-care and stress management: New graduate nurses should prioritize self-care to prevent burnout. They can engage in activities that promote physical and mental well-being, such as exercise, meditation, hobbies, and spending time with loved ones. Seeking support from friends, family, or professional counselors can also be beneficial.
- Embrace a growth mindset: It is important for new graduate nurses to approach challenges with a growth mindset. They should view obstacles as opportunities for learning and growth rather than as failures. Embracing a positive attitude and being open to feedback will help them overcome setbacks and continuously improve.
- Seek support from colleagues and professional organizations: Building a network of supportive colleagues and joining professional organizations can provide new graduate nurses with a sense of community and resources. They can participate in peer support groups, attend networking events, and engage in discussions to share experiences and seek advice.

By implementing these strategies and seeking support, new graduate nurses can overcome the challenges and obstacles they encounter and thrive in their personal and professional lives.

3.4   Reflective Practice in Ethical Decision-Making

Reflective practice plays a crucial role in ethical decision-making in nursing. It involves a thoughtful and critical examination of one's actions, values, and beliefs in order to improve practice and make ethical decisions. Here's how reflective practice supports ethical decision-making in nursing:

- Self-awareness: Reflective practice helps nurses develop self-awareness by examining their own values, biases, and assumptions. This self-awareness is essential in recognizing potential ethical dilemmas and understanding how personal beliefs may influence decision-making.
- Identifying ethical issues: Reflective practice allows nurses to identify and analyze ethical issues that arise in their practice. By reflecting on their experiences, nurses can recognize situations where ethical principles, such as autonomy, beneficence, non-maleficence, and justice, may be at stake.
- Examining alternative perspectives: Reflective practice encourages nurses to consider alternative perspectives and viewpoints. This includes considering the perspectives of patients, families, and other healthcare professionals involved in the ethical dilemma. By examining different viewpoints, nurses can gain a more comprehensive understanding of the situation and make informed decisions.
- Ethical reasoning and decision-making: Reflective practice supports nurses in developing their ethical reasoning skills. It involves critically analyzing the ethical principles and values at play, weighing the potential consequences of

different actions, and making decisions that align with ethical standards and professional guidelines.

- Learning from experiences: Reflective practice allows nurses to learn from their experiences, both positive and challenging. By reflecting on past ethical dilemmas and decisions, nurses can identify areas for improvement, develop strategies to address similar situations in the future, and enhance their ethical decision-making skills.
- Continuous professional development: Reflective practice is an ongoing process that supports nurses in their continuous professional development. It encourages lifelong learning, self-reflection, and growth in ethical decision-making. By engaging in reflective practice, new graduate nurses can continually refine their ethical reasoning skills and stay updated with evolving ethical standards and guidelines.

To engage in reflective practice for ethical decision-making, nurses can

- Set aside dedicated time for reflection, either individually or as part of a reflective practice group.
- Use reflective models or frameworks, such as Gibbs' reflective cycle (1988) or the Johns model of structured reflection (2000), to guide the reflection process.
- Document reflections in a journal or reflective diary to track personal growth and learning.
- Seek feedback from colleagues, mentors, or ethics committees to gain different perspectives on ethical dilemmas.
- Engage in ethical case discussions or participate in ethics committees to enhance ethical reasoning skills.
- Stay updated with ethical guidelines, codes of ethics, and professional standards to inform decision-making.

By incorporating reflective practice into their routine, new graduate nurses can enhance their ethical decision-making skills, promote patient-centered care, and uphold the ethical principles of the nursing profession.

3.4.1   Applying Reflective Practice in Ethical Dilemmas

Reflective practice is a valuable tool for nurses when faced with ethical dilemmas. It involves critically analyzing and evaluating one's actions, decisions, and beliefs to improve practice and enhance ethical decision-making. Here are some steps to apply reflective practice in ethical dilemmas in nursing:

- Identify the ethical dilemma: Begin by clearly identifying the ethical dilemma you are facing. This could involve conflicting values, moral principles, or professional responsibilities.

- Gather information: Collect all relevant information about the situation, including the patient's medical history, cultural background, and any legal or institutional guidelines that may apply.
- Reflect on personal values and beliefs: Take time to reflect on your own values, beliefs, and biases that may influence your decision-making. Consider how these factors may impact your ability to provide ethical care.
- Consider ethical principles and theories: Familiarize yourself with ethical principles such as autonomy, beneficence, non-maleficence, and justice. Apply these principles to the specific situation and consider different ethical theories that may guide your decision-making.
- Seek different perspectives: Engage in discussions with colleagues, supervisors, and other healthcare professionals to gain different perspectives on the ethical dilemma. This can help broaden your understanding and challenge your own assumptions.
- Analyze the consequences: Consider the potential consequences of different courses of action. Evaluate the potential benefits and harms to the patient, their family, and other stakeholders involved.
- Make a decision: Based on your reflection, analysis, and consideration of ethical principles, make a decision on how to proceed. Ensure that your decision aligns with your professional responsibilities and ethical obligations.
- Evaluate and learn: After implementing your decision, reflect on the outcomes and evaluate whether your actions were effective in addressing the ethical dilemma. Identify any areas for improvement and learn from the experience to enhance your future practice.

Reflective practice is an ongoing process that requires continuous self-reflection and learning. By applying reflective practice in ethical dilemmas, nurses can enhance their ethical decision-making skills and provide compassionate and patient-centered care.

Using Self-Reflection to Navigate Ethical Dilemmas in Nursing Practice
Self-reflection is a powerful tool that can help nurses navigate ethical dilemmas in their practice. Here are some ways new graduate nurses can use self-reflection in ethical decision-making:

- Pause and reflect: When faced with an ethical dilemma, take a moment to pause and reflect on the situation. Step back from the immediate pressures and emotions and create a space for self-reflection.
- Identify your emotions and biases: Recognize and acknowledge your own emotions, biases, and personal values that may influence your decision-making. Reflect on how these factors may impact your ability to provide ethical care.
- Examine your beliefs and values: Reflect on your own beliefs and values related to nursing, healthcare, and ethics. Consider how these beliefs may align or conflict with the ethical dilemma at hand. This self-awareness will help you make decisions that are consistent with your values.

- Consider the patient's perspective: Put yourself in the patient's shoes and try to understand their perspective. Reflect on their values, preferences, and goals of care. This empathetic approach will help you make decisions that prioritize the patient's well-being.
- Seek feedback and guidance: Engage in discussions with colleagues, mentors, or ethics committees to seek feedback and guidance. Share your thoughts and concerns and listen to different perspectives. This external input can provide valuable insights and challenge your own assumptions.
- Analyze the situation: Analyze the ethical dilemma by considering the relevant ethical principles, laws, and professional guidelines. Reflect on the potential consequences of different courses of action and evaluate the risks and benefits involved.
- Explore alternative solutions: Engage in creative thinking and explore alternative solutions to the ethical dilemma. Reflect on the potential impact of each solution on the patient, their family, and other stakeholders. Consider the ethical implications of each option.
- Make a decision: Based on your self-reflection, analysis, and consideration of ethical principles, make a decision on how to proceed. Ensure that your decision is aligned with your professional responsibilities and ethical obligations.
- Reflect on the outcome: After implementing your decision, reflect on the outcome and evaluate whether your actions were effective in addressing the ethical dilemma. Consider the lessons learned and identify areas for improvement in your future practice.

Self-reflection is an ongoing process that requires continuous self-awareness and learning. By using self-reflection in ethical decision-making, nurses can navigate complex ethical dilemmas with integrity and provide patient-centered care.

Considering Personal Values and Ethical Frameworks in Decision-Making
Considering personal values and ethical frameworks is crucial in decision-making, especially when faced with ethical dilemmas. Here's how new graduate nurses can incorporate them into your decision-making process:

- Identify your personal values: Start by identifying your own personal values. These are the principles and beliefs that guide your behavior and shape your worldview. Reflect on what matters most to you in terms of patient care, professional integrity, and ethical conduct.
- Understand ethical frameworks: Familiarize yourself with different ethical frameworks or theories that can provide guidance in ethical decision-making. Some common frameworks include deontology, utilitarianism, virtue ethics, and principlism. Learn about their principles and how they can be applied to ethical dilemmas.
- Analyze the ethical dilemma: Analyze the ethical dilemma you are facing by considering the facts, values, and principles involved. Reflect on how the

situation aligns or conflicts with your personal values and the ethical frameworks you are familiar with.

- Evaluate the potential consequences: Consider the potential consequences of different courses of action. Reflect on how each option may impact the patient, their family, and other stakeholders. Assess whether the outcomes align with your personal values and the ethical frameworks you adhere to.
- Seek different perspectives: Engage in discussions with colleagues, mentors, or ethics committees to gain different perspectives on the ethical dilemma. Listen to their viewpoints and consider how they align with your personal values and the ethical frameworks you are using.
- Reflect on the ethical principles: Reflect on the ethical principles relevant to the situation, such as autonomy, beneficence, non-maleficence, and justice. Consider how these principles align with your personal values and the ethical frameworks you are applying.
- Integrate personal values and ethical frameworks: Integrate your personal values and the ethical frameworks you are using to make a decision. Consider how your values and the ethical principles can guide you toward the most ethical and morally justifiable course of action.
- Reflect on the decision: After making a decision, take time to reflect on the process and outcome. Consider whether your decision was consistent with your personal values and the ethical frameworks you applied. Reflect on any lessons learned and areas for improvement in your decision-making process.

Personal values and ethical frameworks are not static. They may evolve over time as you gain more experience and encounter new ethical dilemmas. Regular self-reflection and ongoing learning will help you refine your decision-making process and ensure that your actions align with your values and ethical principles.

Seeking Guidance and Engaging in Ethical Discussions with Colleagues and Mentors
Seeking guidance and engaging in ethical discussions with colleagues and mentors are an important step in navigating ethical dilemmas. Here's how new graduate nurses can effectively seek guidance and engage in ethical discussions:

- Identify trusted colleagues and mentors: Identify colleagues and mentors who have experience and expertise in ethics and ethical decision-making. Look for individuals who are knowledgeable, approachable, and willing to engage in discussions.
- Approach them with respect and openness: When seeking guidance or initiating an ethical discussion, approach your colleagues and mentors with respect and openness. Express your willingness to learn from their insights and perspectives.
- Share the details of the ethical dilemma: Clearly and objectively explain the details of the ethical dilemma you are facing. Provide relevant information about

the situation, including any conflicting values, principles, or professional responsibilities involved.

- Listen actively: Actively listen to the insights and perspectives shared by your colleagues and mentors. Pay attention to their reasoning, experiences, and suggestions. Be open to different viewpoints and consider how they may inform your decision-making process.
- Ask probing questions: Ask thoughtful and probing questions to deepen the discussion. Seek clarification on any points that are unclear or require further exploration. Encourage your colleagues and mentors to elaborate on their perspectives and reasoning.
- Discuss ethical principles and frameworks: Engage in discussions about the ethical principles and frameworks that are relevant to the ethical dilemma. Explore how these principles and frameworks can guide decision-making and address the conflicting values or responsibilities.
- Consider real-life examples and case studies: Discuss real-life examples or case studies that are similar to the ethical dilemma you are facing. Analyze these examples together and explore the ethical considerations, decision-making processes, and outcomes.
- Reflect on the insights gained: After the discussion, take time to reflect on the insights gained from your colleagues and mentors. Consider how their perspectives align or differ from your own. Reflect on how their insights may inform your decision-making process.
- Apply the insights to your decision-making: Integrate the insights gained from the ethical discussions into your decision-making process. Consider how the different perspectives and ethical considerations can help you make a well-informed and ethically sound decision.

Ethical discussions with colleagues and mentors are meant to be collaborative and educational. Be open to learning from others and be willing to challenge your own assumptions. Engaging in these discussions can broaden your understanding of ethical dilemmas and enhance your ethical decision-making skills.

3.5   Conclusion

In conclusion, building a foundation for clinical competence is a crucial aspect of the professional development of new graduate nurses. Self-reflection and personal development are integral to the growth and success of new graduate nurses. By embracing self-reflection as a tool for continuous improvement, setting personal and professional goals, engaging in ongoing learning and development, nurturing emotional intelligence, prioritizing self-care, and applying reflective practice in ethical decision-making, new graduate nurses can enhance their practice, well-being, and overall professional journey.

Review Questions

- Why is self-reflection important for new graduate nurses in their professional development?
- How can self-awareness contribute to a nurse's personal and professional growth?
- What are some practical strategies for engaging in self-reflection as a new graduate nurse?
- How can ongoing learning and professional development benefit new graduate nurses in their careers?
- What are some effective ways for new graduate nurses to stay updated with the latest research and best practices in healthcare?
- Why is goal-setting important for personal and professional development? How can new graduate nurses create SMART goals?
- How can new graduate nurses overcome challenges and obstacles in their personal and professional lives?
- What are some strategies for managing stress and maintaining work-life balance as a new graduate nurse?
- How can mentorship and support from colleagues and loved ones contribute to a nurse's personal and professional growth?
- What are some self-care practices that new graduate nurses should prioritize for their physical, mental, and emotional well-being?
- How can reflective exercises and prompts help new graduate nurses in their self-reflection and personal development journey?
- What additional resources and references are available for further exploration of self-reflection and personal development for new graduate nurses?

References

Falon SL, Kangas M, Crane MF (2021) The coping insights involved in strengthening resilience: the Self-Reflection and Coping Insight Framework. Anxiety Stress Coping 34(6):734–750. https://doi.org/10.1080/10615806.2021.1910676

Gibbs G (1988) Learning by doing: a guide to teaching and learning methods. Further Education Unit, Oxford Polytechnic, Oxford

Jebur AA, Saleh MK, Idan AK (2024) The role of self-awareness in avoiding unethical behavior in the workplace. Business 8:34–47. https://techniumscience.com/index.php/business/article/view/11318

Raghubir AE (2018) Emotional intelligence in professional nursing practice: a concept review using Rodgers's evolutionary analysis approach. Int J Nurs Sci 5(2):126–130. https://doi.org/10.1016/j.ijnss.2018.03.004

Reljić NM, Pajnkihar M, Fekonja Z (2019) Self-reflection during first clinical practice: the experiences of nursing students. Nurse Educ Today 72:61–66. https://doi.org/10.1016/j.nedt.2018.10.019

Shahzad SK, Sarwat S, Ramzan I (2023) Examining the relationship between empathy and English language proficiency in BS English students at KFUEIT. JARH 3(3):30–34. https://jar.bwo-researches.com/index.php/jarh/article/view/176

Slemon A, Jenkins EK, Bailey E (2021) Enhancing conceptual clarity of self-care for nursing students: a scoping review. Nurse Educ Pract 55:103178. https://doi.org/10.1016/j.nepr.2021.103178

Zaga CJ, Freeman-Sanderson A, Happ MB, Hoit JD, McGrath BA, Pandian V, Quraishi-Akhtar T, Rose L, Sutt AL, Tuinman PR, Wallace S (2023) Defining effective communication for critically ill patients with an artificial airway: an international multi-professional consensus. Intensive Crit Care Nurs 76:103393. https://doi.org/10.1016/j.iccn.2023.103393

Part II

Clinical Skills

In this section, we delve into the clinical skills that new graduate nurses need to effectively communicate, provide patient-centered care, manage complex situations, and demonstrate cultural competence. These skills are crucial for building strong relationships with patients, delivering high-quality care, and promoting positive health outcomes. The section begins by providing a comprehensive guide that focuses on the specific skills and competencies needed (Chap. 4). It continues emphasizing the significance of communication and interpersonal skills in healthcare (Chap. 5). It explores the various components of effective communication, such as active listening, empathy, and clear and concise verbal and nonverbal communication. By mastering these skills, new graduate nurses can establish trust, foster collaboration, and ensure accurate information exchange with patients, their families, and the healthcare team. Next, the section focuses on patient-centered care skills (Chap. 6). It highlights the importance of understanding and respecting patients' values, preferences, and needs. It explores the principles of shared decision-making, patient empowerment, and individualized care planning. By adopting a patient-centered approach, new graduate nurses can enhance patient satisfaction, engagement, and overall health outcomes. Furthermore, the section addresses the challenges of managing complex situations in healthcare (Chap. 7). It explores strategies for critical thinking, problem-solving, and decision-making in high-pressure and rapidly changing environments. It emphasizes the importance of remaining calm, organized, and adaptable when faced with complex clinical scenarios. By developing these skills, new graduate nurses can effectively navigate challenging situations and provide optimal care to their patients. Lastly, the section highlights the significance of cultural competence skills in delivering culturally sensitive and inclusive care (Chap. 8). It explores the importance of understanding and respecting diverse cultural beliefs, practices, and values. It discusses strategies for effective cross-cultural communication, addressing health disparities, and promoting cultural humility. By developing cultural competence, new graduate nurses can provide equitable and patient-centered care to individuals from diverse backgrounds. Overall, this section provides valuable insights and guidance for new graduate nurses in developing and honing their communication and interpersonal skills, patient-centered care skills, skill for managing complex situations, and cultural competence skills. By mastering these skills, new graduate nurses can establish strong relationships with patients, deliver high-quality care, navigate complex clinical scenarios, and provide culturally sensitive and inclusive care. Ultimately, these skills contribute to improved patient outcomes, enhanced patient satisfaction, and overall advancement of the nursing profession.

Essential Clinical Skills

4

Contents

> Test your learning and check your understanding of this book's contents: use the "Springer Nature Flashcards" app to access questions using ▶ https://sn.pub/pe441e. To use the app, please follow the instructions in Chap. 1.

4.1   Definition of Essential Clinical Skills

Clinical skills refer to the specific abilities and competencies required to provide direct patient care (Vichittragoonthavon et al. 2020). Clinical skills are usually divided into psychomotor and communication. These skills encompass a wide range of competencies such as history taking, performing physical assessments, administering treatments, and conducting procedures, effective communication, teamwork, and professionalism (Perry et al. 2021). Nurses must also be proficient in basic nursing techniques, including proper hygiene practices, infection control measures, and patient positioning. Additionally, they must possess critical thinking skills to make quick and accurate decisions in high-pressure situations. Overall, essential clinical skills are the foundation of nursing practice and are essential for ensuring the well-being and recovery of patients.

© The Author(s), under exclusive license to Springer Nature Switzerland AG 2024   113
K. Matlhaba, *Enhancing Clinical Competence of Graduate Nurses*,
https://doi.org/10.1007/978-3-031-81407-5_4

4.2   Examples of Essential Clinical Skills Needed for New Graduate Nurse During the Transition Period

4.2.1   Communication Skills

Communication skills refer to the ability to effectively convey and receive information, ideas, and emotions (Stephen 2024). It includes verbal and nonverbal communication, active listening, empathy, and clear expression. Effective communication is crucial in healthcare settings as it plays a vital role in building trust, establishing rapport, and ensuring the delivery of safe and high-quality patient care. Here are the key points to discuss regarding the importance of effective communication with patients, their families, and the healthcare team:

- Building trust and rapport: Effective communication helps build trust and establish a positive rapport with patients and their families. When healthcare professionals communicate clearly and empathetically, patients feel heard, understood, and valued. This fosters a trusting relationship, which is essential for patient satisfaction and engagement in their care.
- Patient-centered care: Effective communication is at the core of patient-centered care. By actively listening to patients, healthcare professionals can understand their unique needs, preferences, and concerns. This enables them to tailor their care plans, accordingly, promoting better patient outcomes and satisfaction.
- Active listening: Active listening is a technique that involves fully focusing on and understanding what the patient is saying. It requires giving undivided attention, maintaining eye contact, and using verbal and nonverbal cues to show interest and understanding. Active listening helps healthcare professionals gather accurate information, identify patient needs, and address any misconceptions or fears.
- Empathy: Empathy is the ability to understand and share the feelings of another person. It is a crucial component of effective communication in healthcare. By demonstrating empathy, healthcare professionals show compassion and understanding toward patients and their families, which can greatly enhance the patient experience and improve patient outcomes.
- Clear verbal communication: Clear and concise verbal communication is essential to ensure that information is accurately conveyed and understood. Healthcare professionals should use simple language, avoid medical jargon, and check for patient comprehension. They should also encourage patients and their families to ask questions and seek clarification when needed.
- Clear written communication: Written communication, such as medical records and discharge instructions, should be clear, accurate, and easily understandable. Healthcare professionals should use plain language, avoid abbreviations, and provide information in a format that is accessible to the patient and their family. This helps prevent misunderstandings and promotes continuity of care.
- Interprofessional collaboration: Effective communication extends beyond the patient-provider relationship and includes communication within the healthcare

team. Clear and timely communication among healthcare professionals ensures coordinated and safe patient care. This involves sharing relevant patient information, discussing treatment plans, and addressing any concerns or changes in the patient's condition.

By emphasizing the importance of effective communication and providing training on active listening, empathy, and clear verbal and written communication, healthcare organizations can enhance patient satisfaction, improve patient outcomes, and create a positive and collaborative healthcare environment.

4.2.2   Patient Assessment

Patient assessment refers to the systematic collection and analysis of patient data to evaluate their health status, identify problems, and develop appropriate care plans (Jarvis 2023). It includes techniques such as physical examination, medical history taking, and diagnostic tests. Conducting a comprehensive patient assessment is a critical step in providing quality healthcare. It involves gathering information about the patient's health status, identifying potential health issues, and establishing a baseline for monitoring changes in their condition. The process typically includes assessing vital signs, performing a physical examination, and gathering relevant medical history. Thorough and accurate documentation of the assessment findings is essential for effective communication, continuity of care, and legal purposes. Here's a breakdown of the process:

1. *Vital signs assessment*
   (a) Measure and record the patient's temperature, pulse rate, respiratory rate, and blood pressure. These vital signs provide important indicators of the patient's overall health and can help identify any abnormalities or changes in their condition.
   (b) Assess the patient's oxygen saturation level using a pulse oximeter. This measurement helps determine the adequacy of oxygenation.
   (c) Document the vital signs accurately, including the date, time, and any relevant contextual information (e.g., activity level, pain level, medication administration).
2. *Physical examination*
   (a) Begin with a general survey of the patient, observing their appearance, behavior, and overall condition.
   (b) Systematically assess each body system, including the head and neck, chest and lungs, heart and cardiovascular system, abdomen, musculoskeletal system, and neurological system.
   (c) Use appropriate assessment techniques such as inspection, palpation, percussion, and auscultation to gather information about the patient's physical health.

(d) Document the findings of the physical examination in a clear and organized manner, including any abnormalities or significant findings.

3. *Medical history*

(a) Gather relevant medical history information, including the patient's past medical conditions, surgeries, allergies, current medications, and family medical history.

(b) Ask about the patient's chief complaint or reason for seeking healthcare, as well as any associated symptoms or concerns.

(c) Inquire about the patient's social history, including lifestyle factors, occupation, and habits (e.g., smoking, alcohol consumption).

(d) Obtain a thorough review of systems by asking about symptoms related to each body system.

(e) Document the medical history information accurately and comprehensively, ensuring that it is organized and easily accessible for future reference.

Importance of Thorough and Accurate Documentation

Thorough and accurate documentation of the patient assessment is crucial for several reasons:

- Communication: Documentation serves as a means of communication among healthcare providers. It ensures that important information about the patient's health status, assessment findings, and interventions is shared accurately and effectively.
- Continuity of care: Accurate documentation allows for continuity of care, ensuring that healthcare providers have access to the patient's complete and up-to-date health information. This is particularly important during care transitions or when multiple healthcare professionals are involved in the patient's treatment.
- Legal and regulatory compliance: Documentation serves as a legal record of the care provided. Accurate and comprehensive documentation helps protect healthcare providers in case of legal disputes and ensures compliance with regulatory requirements.
- Monitoring and evaluation: Thorough documentation enables healthcare providers to monitor the patient's progress, track changes in their condition, and evaluate the effectiveness of interventions. It provides a baseline for comparison and helps identify trends or patterns that may require further assessment or intervention.
- Research and quality improvement: Documentation contributes to research and quality improvement efforts by providing data for analysis and identifying areas for improvement in patient care.

Conducting a comprehensive patient assessment involves assessing vital signs, performing a physical examination, and gathering relevant medical history. Thorough and accurate documentation of the assessment findings is essential for effective communication, continuity of care, and legal purposes. New graduate nurses should prioritize documentation to ensure the provision of safe and high-quality patient care.

4.2.3   Medication Administration

Medication administration involves the safe and accurate delivery of medications to patients (NCSBN 2018). Safe medication administration is vital process that ensures patients' safety and quality of life (Jafaru and Abubakar 2022). Therefore, it includes processes such as medication verification, dosage calculation, and proper administration techniques. Here are the key principles of safe medication administration, including dosage calculations, medication reconciliation, proper documentation, common medication errors, and strategies to prevent them:

1. *Dosage calculations*
   (a) Accurate dosage calculations are essential to administer the correct amount of medication to patients. Nurses should have a solid understanding of basic math calculations and be familiar with different measurement systems (e.g., metric, household).
   (b) Double-check all calculations and use reliable references or tools (e.g., medication calculation formulas, dosage calculation apps) to ensure accuracy.
   (c) Verify calculations with another qualified healthcare professional when necessary, especially for high-risk medications or complex dosage regimens.
2. *Medication reconciliation*
   (a) Medication reconciliation is the process of comparing a patient's current medication regimen with any new medications prescribed during transitions of care (e.g., admission, transfer, discharge).
   (b) Obtain a comprehensive medication history, including prescription medications, over-the-counter drugs, herbal supplements, and allergies.
   (c) Compare the medication orders with the patient's current medications, resolve any discrepancies, and communicate changes to the healthcare team.
   (d) Medication reconciliation helps prevent medication errors, adverse drug events, and drug interactions.
3. *Proper documentation*
   (a) Accurate and timely documentation is crucial for safe medication administration.
   (b) Document medication administration immediately after giving the medication, including the medication name, dosage, route, time, and any relevant observations or patient responses.
   (c) Use clear and standardized documentation practices, following institutional policies and procedures.
   (d) Document any medication refusals, missed doses, or medication errors according to the facility's guidelines.

4. ***Common medication errors***
   (a) Medication errors can occur at various stages, including prescribing, transcribing, dispensing, and administering medications.
   (b) Common medication errors include administering the wrong medication, incorrect dosage, wrong route, administering medication to the wrong patient, or administering medication at the wrong time.
   (c) Other errors may involve medication allergies, drug interactions, or failure to recognize contraindications.
   (d) Communication breakdowns, distractions, fatigue, and lack of knowledge or training contribute to medication errors.
5. ***Strategies to prevent medication errors***
   (a) Use technology, such as barcode scanning systems and electronic medication administration records (eMARs), to verify medication orders and ensure accuracy.
   (b) Follow the "Five Rights" of medication administration: right patient, right medication, right dose, right route, and right time.
   (c) Implement a double-check system for high-risk medications or complex dosage calculations.
   (d) Practice effective communication and collaboration with the healthcare team, including clarifying unclear orders and seeking clarification when needed.
   (e) Stay updated with medication information, including indications, contraindications, side effects, and administration guidelines.
   (f) Adhere to medication administration policies and procedures, including proper hand hygiene, medication storage, and disposal practices.

Safe medication administration involves principles such as accurate dosage calculations, medication reconciliation, and proper documentation. It is essential to be aware of common medication errors and strategies to prevent them. By following these principles and implementing preventive strategies, nurses can significantly reduce medication errors, enhance patient safety, and improve overall healthcare outcomes.

4.2.4   Infection Control

Infection control refers to the measures and practices implemented to prevent the spread of infections in healthcare settings (CDC 2020). It includes techniques such as hand hygiene, proper use of personal protective equipment, and adherence to infection control protocols. Infection control practices are crucial in healthcare settings to prevent the spread of infections and protect both patients and healthcare providers. Here are the key points highlighting the importance of infection control practices, including hand hygiene, personal protective equipment (PPE) usage, and proper disposal of contaminated materials. Additionally, strategies to prevent healthcare-associated infections (HAIs) are discussed:

1. *Hand hygiene*
   (a) Hand hygiene is the single most important practice in preventing the transmission of healthcare-associated infections.
   (b) Healthcare providers should perform hand hygiene using soap and water or an alcohol-based hand sanitizer before and after every patient contact, after touching potentially contaminated surfaces, and before invasive procedures.
   (c) Proper hand hygiene reduces the risk of transmitting pathogens from one patient to another and helps prevent the spread of multidrug-resistant organisms.
2. *Personal protective equipment (PPE) usage*
   (a) PPE, such as gloves, gowns, masks, and eye protection, acts as a barrier between healthcare providers and infectious agents.
   (b) Healthcare providers should use appropriate PPE based on the type of anticipated exposure to infectious materials (e.g., contact, droplet, airborne precautions).
   (c) Proper donning (putting on) and doffing (taking off) techniques should be followed to prevent self-contamination.
   (d) PPE usage is particularly important during procedures that generate splashes, sprays, or aerosols, as well as when caring for patients with known or suspected infectious diseases.
3. *Proper disposal of contaminated materials*
   (a) Contaminated materials, such as used gloves, masks, and other disposable items, should be disposed of properly to prevent the spread of infections.
   (b) Healthcare providers should follow the facility's guidelines for waste segregation, disposal, and handling of sharps.
   (c) Properly labeled and sealed containers should be used for the disposal of biohazardous waste.

Strategies to Prevent Healthcare-Associated Infections (HAIs)

1. *Adherence to standard precautions*
   (a) Standard precautions should be followed consistently for all patients to prevent the transmission of infectious agents.
   (b) These precautions include hand hygiene, proper use of PPE, safe injection practices, respiratory hygiene/cough etiquette, and safe handling of contaminated equipment.
2. *Environmental cleaning and disinfection*
   (a) Regular cleaning and disinfection of patient care areas, surfaces, and equipment help reduce the risk of healthcare-associated infections.
   (b) Use appropriate disinfectants and follow recommended contact times for effective disinfection.
   (c) Pay special attention to high-touch surfaces and equipment.

3. *Antimicrobial stewardship*
   (a) Implement antimicrobial stewardship programs to promote the appropriate and judicious use of antibiotics.
   (b) This helps prevent the development of antibiotic resistance and reduces the risk of healthcare-associated infections, such as *Clostridium difficile* infection.
4. *Vaccination*
   (a) Ensure healthcare providers are up to date with their immunizations, including influenza, hepatitis B, and other recommended vaccines.
   (b) Encourage patients to receive recommended vaccinations to prevent vaccine-preventable infections.
5. *Education and training*
   (a) Provide regular education and training to healthcare providers on infection control practices, including hand hygiene, PPE usage, and proper disposal of contaminated materials.
   (b) Promote a culture of infection prevention and empower healthcare providers to be vigilant in their infection control practices.
6. *Surveillance and monitoring*
   (a) Implement surveillance systems to monitor healthcare-associated infections and identify trends or outbreaks.
   (b) Regularly review and analyze infection data to identify areas for improvement and implement targeted interventions.
   By emphasizing the importance of infection control practices, implementing preventive strategies, and fostering a culture of infection prevention, healthcare facilities can significantly reduce the risk of healthcare-associated infections and ensure the safety of patients and healthcare providers.

4.2.5 Wound Care

Wound care involves the assessment, treatment, and management of wounds to promote healing and prevent complications (Saifullah and Sharma 2024). It includes techniques such as cleaning, dressing, and protecting the wound. Wound assessment, wound dressing techniques, and wound care management are essential components of nursing practice to promote optimal wound healing and prevent complications. Here is an overview of these topics, including information on different types of wounds, wound healing stages, and infection prevention:

1. *Wound assessment*
   (a) Wound assessment involves a systematic evaluation of the wound's characteristics, including its location, size, depth, appearance, and surrounding tissue.
   (b) Assess the wound for signs of infection (e.g., redness, swelling, warmth, pus), presence of necrotic tissue, amount of exudate (drainage), and any underlying structures (e.g., bones, tendons) exposed.

(c) Assess the patient's pain level, sensation, and circulation in the affected area.

(d) Document the findings accurately and regularly to monitor wound progress and guide appropriate interventions.

2. *Types of wounds*

There are various types of wounds, including the following:

(a) Surgical wounds: Incisions made during surgical procedures.

(b) Traumatic wounds: Caused by accidents, injuries, or burns.

(c) Pressure ulcers: Develop due to prolonged pressure on the skin, commonly seen in immobile or bedridden patients.

(d) Diabetic foot ulcers: Occur in individuals with diabetes due to poor circulation and neuropathy.

(e) Venous and arterial ulcers: Result from venous insufficiency or arterial occlusion, respectively.

(f) Chronic wounds: Wounds that fail to heal within the expected timeframe (e.g., pressure ulcers, diabetic foot ulcers).

3. *Wound healing stages*

Wound healing typically progresses through four stages:

(a) Hemostasis: The initial stage involves blood clotting and vasoconstriction to control bleeding.

(b) Inflammatory phase: Inflammation occurs, leading to the removal of debris and the release of growth factors.

(c) Proliferative phase: New tissue forms, including granulation tissue and the development of new blood vessels.

(d) Maturation phase: Collagen fibers reorganize, and the wound gradually strengthens and remodels.

4. *Wound dressing techniques*

(a) Wound dressing techniques aim to create an optimal environment for wound healing, protect the wound, and manage exudate.

(b) Dressing selection depends on the wound characteristics, such as the amount of exudate, presence of infection, and need for moisture balance.

(c) Common types of wound dressings include the following:

- Transparent films: Used for superficial wounds with minimal exudate.
- Hydrocolloids: Provide a moist environment and are suitable for partial-thickness wounds.
- Hydrogels: Maintain moisture and promote autolytic debridement.
- Alginate dressings: Absorb exudate and are useful for moderate to heavily exuding wounds.
- Foam dressings: Absorb exudate and provide cushioning and protection.
- Antimicrobial dressings: Contain agents to help prevent or treat wound infections.

5. *Wound care management*

(a) Wound care management involves a holistic approach to promote wound healing and prevent complications.

(b) Cleanse the wound using a gentle, nontoxic solution (e.g., normal saline) to remove debris and bacteria.

    (c) Debridement may be necessary to remove necrotic tissue or foreign material from the wound bed.

    (d) Use appropriate techniques for wound closure, such as sutures, staples, or adhesive strips, depending on the wound type and healthcare provider's preference.

    (e) Provide appropriate pain management during wound care procedures.

    (f) Educate the patient and caregivers on proper wound care techniques, signs of infection, and the importance of adherence to the treatment plan.

    (g) Monitor the wound regularly for signs of healing, infection, or complications and adjust the treatment plan as needed.

6. **Infection prevention**

    (a) Infection prevention is crucial in wound care to minimize the risk of wound infections.

    (b) Follow strict hand hygiene practices before and after wound care procedures.

    (c) Use appropriate personal protective equipment (PPE) to prevent cross contamination.

    (d) Ensure a clean and sterile environment during wound care procedures.

    (e) Administer prophylactic antibiotics as prescribed for high-risk wounds or patients.

    (f) Monitor for signs of wound infection, such as increased redness, swelling, warmth, pain, or purulent drainage, and promptly report any concerns to the healthcare provider.

By conducting thorough wound assessments, employing appropriate wound dressing techniques, and implementing effective wound care management, new graduate nurses can facilitate optimal wound healing, prevent complications, and promote the overall well-being of patients. Additionally, adherence to infection prevention practices is crucial to minimize the risk of wound infections and promote successful wound healing.

4.2.6 Basic Life Support

Basic life support (BLS) refers to the immediate care provided to individuals experiencing cardiac arrest, respiratory distress, or other life-threatening emergencies. It includes techniques such as cardiopulmonary resuscitation (CPR) and the use of automated external defibrillators (AEDs). Basic life support (BLS) skills are essential for nurses and other healthcare professionals in emergency situations to provide immediate care and potentially save lives (American Heart Association, 2020). Here are the essential skills required for basic life support, including cardiopulmonary resuscitation (CPR), use of automated external defibrillators (AEDs), and recognition of common life-threatening emergencies:

1. **Cardiopulmonary resuscitation (CPR)**

    (a) CPR is a critical skill used to maintain blood flow and oxygenation to vital organs during cardiac arrest or respiratory arrest.

(b) Key skills for CPR include the following:
- Recognition of cardiac arrest: Identifying the absence of responsiveness, absence of normal breathing, and absence of a pulse.
- Activating the emergency response system: Calling for help and activating the emergency medical services (EMS).
- Chest compressions: Performing high-quality chest compressions by placing the heel of one hand on the center of the chest (lower half of the sternum) and interlocking the other hand on top. Compressions should be at least 2 in. deep and delivered at a rate of 100–120 compressions per minute.
- Rescue breaths: Providing rescue breaths by tilting the head back, lifting the chin, and delivering two breaths into the person's mouth while ensuring a proper seal.
- Continuous cycles of compressions and breaths until help arrives or an AED is available.

2. *Use of automated external defibrillators (AEDs):*
   (a) AEDs are portable devices that deliver an electric shock to restore normal heart rhythm in cases of sudden cardiac arrest.
   (b) Key skills for using AEDs include the following:
   - Recognizing the need for defibrillation: Identifying the absence of responsiveness, absence of normal breathing, and absence of a pulse.
   - Activating the emergency response system: Calling for help and activating the EMS.
   - Applying the AED pads: Placing the pads on the person's bare chest as indicated by the AED's visual or audio prompts.
   - Clearing the area and analyzing the heart rhythm: Ensuring no one is touching the person and allowing the AED to analyze the heart rhythm.
   - Delivering a shock: If the AED advises a shock, ensuring everyone is clear and pressing the shock button as instructed.
   - Continuing CPR cycles as directed by the AED until help arrives.

3. *Recognition of common life-threatening emergencies*
   (a) Recognizing life-threatening emergencies is crucial for initiating appropriate interventions and seeking immediate medical assistance.
   (b) Key skills for recognition include the following:
   - Identifying signs of cardiac arrest: Absence of responsiveness, absence of normal breathing, and absence of a pulse.
   - Recognizing respiratory distress or failure: Difficulty breathing, gasping for breath, or complete cessation of breathing.
   - Identifying severe allergic reactions: Swelling of the face, lips, or tongue; difficulty breathing; and signs of anaphylaxis.
   - Recognizing choking: Inability to speak, cough, or breathe and the universal choking sign (hands clutching the throat).
   - Identifying signs of stroke: Sudden weakness or numbness on one side of the body, slurred speech, and facial drooping.

- Recognizing severe bleeding: Profuse bleeding that is difficult to control and may lead to shock.

In addition to these skills, it is important to maintain composure, communicate effectively with bystanders and emergency medical services, and provide reassurance and support to the person in need.

Regular training and practice in BLS skills, including CPR, AED use, and recognition of life-threatening emergencies, are crucial to maintain proficiency and confidence in responding to critical situations. Certification courses, such as basic life support (BLS) courses offered by recognized organizations, can provide comprehensive training and hands-on practice in these essential skills.

4.2.7 Patient Safety

Patient safety refers to the prevention of harm to patients during the provision of healthcare services (National Department of Health 2022). According to WHO (2021), patient safety involves identifying and reducing risks, implementing safety measures, and promoting a culture of safety. Patient safety is a fundamental aspect of clinical practice that aims to prevent harm to patients and ensure their well-being. It involves implementing strategies and protocols to minimize the occurrence of adverse events, such as falls and medication errors. Nurses play a crucial role in promoting a culture of safety and actively contributing to patient safety initiatives. Here are the key points regarding the importance of patient safety and strategies to prevent falls, medication errors, and other adverse events, along with the nurse's role in promoting a culture of safety:

1. *Importance of patient safety*
   (a) Patient safety is essential to prevent harm, improve patient outcomes, and enhance the overall quality of healthcare delivery.
   (b) Adverse events, such as falls, medication errors, healthcare-associated infections, and procedural complications, can lead to patient harm, prolonged hospital stays, increased healthcare costs, and even mortality.
   (c) Prioritizing patient safety helps build trust between healthcare providers and patients, fosters a culture of accountability, and promotes a positive healthcare environment.
2. *Strategies to prevent falls*
   Falls are a common cause of patient harm, especially among older adults and individuals with mobility issues. Preventive strategies include the following:
   (a) Conducting fall risk assessments upon admission and regularly throughout the patient's stay.
   (b) Implementing appropriate interventions based on the patient's risk level, such as bed alarms, nonslip footwear, and assistance with ambulation.
   (c) Ensuring a safe environment by keeping walkways clear, providing adequate lighting, and using handrails and grab bars.

(d) Educating patients and their families about fall prevention measures and encouraging their active participation.

3. ***Strategies to prevent medication errors***

Medication errors can have serious consequences for patient safety. Strategies to prevent medication errors include the following:

(a) Implementing medication reconciliation processes to ensure accurate and up-to-date medication lists.

(b) Using technology, such as barcode scanning and electronic prescribing systems, to reduce errors in medication administration.

(c) Double-checking medication orders, dosages, and patient allergies before administration.

(d) Providing education and training to healthcare providers on medication safety practices.

(e) Encouraging open communication and reporting of medication errors to facilitate learning and system improvement.

4. ***Strategies to prevent other adverse events***

In addition to falls and medication errors, other adverse events can occur in healthcare settings. Strategies to prevent these events include the following:

(a) Implementing infection prevention and control measures, such as hand hygiene, proper sterilization techniques, and adherence to standard precautions.

(b) Ensuring proper patient identification and verification processes to prevent errors in procedures, surgeries, and transfusions.

(c) Using checklists and protocols to enhance communication and teamwork during high-risk procedures.

(d) Promoting a culture of reporting and learning from near misses and adverse events to identify system weaknesses and implement improvements.

5. ***Role of the nurse in promoting a culture of safety***

Nurses play a vital role in promoting a culture of safety within healthcare organizations. Their responsibilities include the following:

(a) Adhering to evidence-based practice guidelines and safety protocols.

(b) Advocating for patient safety and actively participating in safety committees and initiatives.

(c) Engaging in ongoing education and training to enhance knowledge and skills related to patient safety.

(d) Encouraging open communication and reporting of safety concerns or incidents.

(e) Collaborating with interdisciplinary teams to identify and implement safety improvements.

(f) Educating patients and their families about safety measures and empowering them to actively participate in their care.

By prioritizing patient safety, implementing preventive strategies, and actively engaging in safety initiatives, nurses can contribute significantly to creating a culture of safety and improving patient outcomes. Collaboration among healthcare providers, patients, and organizations is essential to ensure a safe and reliable healthcare system.

4.2.8   Documentation and Recordkeeping

Documentation refers to the process of recording information related to patient care, including assessments, interventions, and outcomes. Recordkeeping involves maintaining accurate and complete records of patient information (Demsash et al. 2023). Accurate and timely documentation in patient care is of utmost importance as it serves several crucial purposes in healthcare. It involves recording relevant patient information, interventions, assessments, and outcomes in a systematic and organized manner. Here are the key points regarding the significance of accurate and timely documentation in patient care and the importance of maintaining patient confidentiality:

1. *Continuity of care*
   (a) Accurate and timely documentation ensures the continuity of care by providing a comprehensive and up-to-date record of the patient's medical history, diagnoses, treatments, and outcomes.
   (b) It allows healthcare providers to have a complete understanding of the patient's condition, facilitating effective communication and collaboration among the care team.
2. *Communication and coordination*
   (a) Documentation serves as a means of communication among healthcare providers involved in the patient's care, ensuring that important information is shared accurately and efficiently.
   (b) It helps prevent miscommunication, errors, and omissions, enabling seamless coordination of care across different healthcare settings and transitions of care.
3. *Legal and regulatory requirements*
   (a) Accurate and timely documentation is essential for meeting legal and regulatory requirements in healthcare.
   (b) It provides a legal record of the care provided, including informed consent, treatment plans, medication administration, and any adverse events or complications.
   (c) Documentation also supports billing and reimbursement processes, ensuring compliance with healthcare regulations and standards.
4. *Clinical decision-making and patient safety*
   (a) Documentation plays a crucial role in clinical decision-making by providing healthcare providers with the necessary information to make informed judgments about patient care.
   (b) Accurate documentation of assessments, interventions, and outcomes helps identify trends, monitor progress, and evaluate the effectiveness of treatments.

(c) It contributes to patient safety by reducing the risk of errors, facilitating accurate medication reconciliation, and ensuring the timely identification and response to changes in the patient's condition.

5. *Importance of maintaining patient confidentiality*
    (a) Patient confidentiality is a fundamental ethical and legal principle in healthcare.
    (b) Accurate and timely documentation must be accompanied by strict adherence to patient confidentiality and privacy regulations, such as the Health Insurance Portability and Accountability Act (HIPAA).
    (c) Healthcare providers must ensure that patient information is securely stored, accessed only by authorized individuals, and shared only for legitimate purposes.

Maintaining accurate and timely documentation, whether in paper or electronic form, is essential for effective patient care, communication, legal compliance, and clinical decision-making. It is crucial for new graduate nurses to understand the significance of documentation and the importance of maintaining patient confidentiality to ensure the highest standards of care and protect patient rights.

4.2.9 Time Management and Prioritization

Effective time management and prioritization of nursing tasks are essential skills for nurses to ensure efficient and quality patient care. Delegation and collaboration with the healthcare team also play a crucial role in optimizing workflow and achieving positive patient outcomes. Here are strategies for effective time management, prioritization of nursing tasks, and the importance of delegation and collaboration:

1. *Prioritization of nursing tasks*
    (a) Assess the urgency and importance of each task: Prioritize tasks based on their urgency and impact on patient safety and well-being. Identify critical tasks that require immediate attention.
    (b) Use a systematic approach: Develop a systematic approach, such as the ABCDE method (airway, breathing, circulation, disability, exposure), to prioritize tasks based on the patient's condition and needs.
    (c) Consider patient acuity and complexity: Take into account the acuity and complexity of patients' conditions when prioritizing tasks. Allocate more time and resources to patients with higher acuity levels.
    (d) Communicate with the healthcare team: Collaborate with the healthcare team to gain insights into the overall patient care plan and prioritize tasks accordingly.
    (e) Reevaluate and adjust priorities: Continuously reevaluate and adjust priorities as the patient's condition changes or new tasks arise.

2. **Effective time management**
   (a) Plan and organize: Create a daily or shift schedule, outlining the tasks and responsibilities for each patient. Organize supplies and equipment in advance to minimize time wastage.
   (b) Set realistic goals: Set achievable goals for each task and allocate appropriate time for completion. Avoid overcommitting or taking on more tasks than can be realistically accomplished.
   (c) Avoid multitasking: Focus on one task at a time to maintain concentration and prevent errors. Multitasking can lead to decreased efficiency and increased risk of mistakes.
   (d) Minimize distractions: Minimize interruptions and distractions during critical tasks. Communicate with colleagues and ask for privacy when necessary.
   (e) Utilize technology: Take advantage of technology tools, such as electronic health records (EHRs), mobile apps, and alarms, to streamline documentation, reminders, and task management.
3. **Delegation**
   (a) Assess the need for delegation: Evaluate the workload and complexity of tasks to determine if delegation is appropriate. Delegate tasks that can be safely and effectively performed by other members of the healthcare team.
   (b) Select the right person: Delegate tasks to individuals with the appropriate knowledge, skills, and competence. Consider their workload and availability when assigning tasks.
   (c) Provide clear instructions: Clearly communicate the task, expectations, and any specific instructions or precautions to the person to whom the task is delegated. Ensure they understand and have the necessary resources to complete the task.
   (d) Monitor and provide feedback: Regularly check on the progress of delegated tasks and provide feedback and support as needed. Maintain open communication to address any concerns or questions.
4. **Collaboration with the multidisciplinary team**
   (a) Effective communication: Maintain open and effective communication with the multidisciplinary team to ensure a shared understanding of patient care goals, priorities, and responsibilities.
   (b) Interprofessional collaboration: Collaborate with other healthcare professionals, such as physicians, pharmacists, and therapists, to coordinate care, share information, and optimize patient outcomes.
   (c) Team huddles and rounds: Participate in team huddles and rounds to discuss patient care plans, identify priorities, and address any concerns or changes in the patient's condition.
   (d) Shared decision-making: Engage in shared decision-making processes with the healthcare team to determine the most appropriate interventions and prioritize tasks based on the patient's needs and goals.

Effective time management, prioritization of tasks, delegation, and collaboration with the multidisciplinary team are essential for new graduate nurses to provide safe and efficient patient care. By implementing these strategies, nurses can optimize their workflow, enhance patient outcomes, and promote a positive and collaborative healthcare environment.

4.2.10 Professionalism and Ethical Practice

Professionalism refers to the conduct, behavior, and attitudes expected of professionals in a particular field. Ethical practice involves adhering to ethical principles and standards in professional decision-making and behavior (ANA 2015). Professionalism, ethical decision-making, and maintaining professional boundaries are critical aspects of nursing practice. They ensure the delivery of safe, compassionate, and ethical care to patients. The nursing code of ethics and legal responsibilities provide guidance and standards for nurses to uphold these principles. Here is an emphasis on the importance of professionalism, ethical decision-making, maintaining professional boundaries, and an overview of the nursing code of ethics and legal responsibilities:

1. *Importance of professionalism*
   (a) Professionalism in nursing encompasses a set of behaviors, attitudes, and values that reflect a commitment to the highest standards of patient care, integrity, and ethical conduct.
   (b) Professionalism fosters trust and confidence in the nursing profession and promotes positive relationships with patients, families, and the healthcare team.
   (c) It involves maintaining a professional appearance; demonstrating respect, empathy, and cultural sensitivity; and adhering to ethical and legal standards.
2. *Ethical decision-making*
   (a) Ethical decision-making in nursing involves considering the ethical principles and values that guide nursing practice, such as autonomy, beneficence, non-maleficence, and justice.
   (b) Nurses must assess ethical dilemmas, weigh the potential benefits and harms, and make decisions that prioritize the best interests and well-being of the patient.
   (c) Ethical decision-making requires critical thinking, effective communication, collaboration with the healthcare team, and a commitment to upholding ethical standards.
3. *Maintaining professional boundaries*
   (a) Professional boundaries in nursing refer to the limits and appropriate relationships between nurses and patients, colleagues, and other individuals involved in patient care.
   (b) Maintaining professional boundaries ensures the preservation of trust, confidentiality, and the therapeutic nurse-patient relationship.
   (c) Nurses must establish clear boundaries, avoid dual relationships, maintain objectivity, and refrain from engaging in personal, social, or romantic relationships with patients.

4. *Nursing code of ethics*

ICN provides ethical guidance in relation to nurses' roles, duties, responsibilities, behaviors, professional judgement, and relationships with patients, other people who are receiving nursing care or services, coworkers, and allied professionals (ICN 2021). SANC defined this code of ethics as the foundation of ethical decision-making and is aimed at informing nursing (SANC 2021). In their statement on code of ethics for nurses, the American Nursing Association (2024) (ANA) stated that nurses should demonstrate values of the profession which includes respect, justice, empathy, responsiveness, caring, compassion, trustworthiness, and integrity.

(a) The nursing code of ethics is a set of principles and standards that guide the ethical practice of nursing. It provides a framework for ethical decision-making and professional conduct.

(b) The code of ethics is widely recognized and followed by nurses globally. It includes provisions that address the nurse's responsibilities to patients, the profession, society, and oneself.

(c) The code emphasizes the importance of respecting the dignity and rights of patients, advocating for their well-being, maintaining confidentiality, and engaging in lifelong learning and professional development.

5. *Legal responsibilities*

(a) Nurses have legal responsibilities to ensure compliance with laws, regulations, and standards related to nursing practice.

(b) Legal responsibilities include maintaining patient confidentiality, obtaining informed consent, documenting accurately and timely, administering medications safely, and reporting any incidents or errors.

(c) Nurses must also be aware of their state's nurse practice act, which outlines the scope of nursing practice, licensure requirements, and legal obligations.

By upholding professionalism and ethical decision-making and maintaining professional boundaries, nurses demonstrate their commitment to providing high-quality care, protecting patient rights, and promoting the integrity of the nursing profession. Adhering to the nursing code of ethics and legal responsibilities ensures that nurses practice within the boundaries of the law and ethical standards, ultimately benefiting both patients and the healthcare system as a whole.

Tips to Help New Nurses Develop and Refine Their Clinical Skills

Here are some tips to help new nurses develop and refine their clinical skills:

- Seek mentorship: Find experienced nurses or preceptors who can serve as mentors and provide guidance. They can offer valuable insights, share their expertise, and provide constructive feedback to help you improve your clinical skills.
- Continuously learn and stay updated: Stay current with evidence-based practice guidelines, research, and advancements in healthcare. Attend workshops, conferences, and seminars to enhance your knowledge and skills. Engage in lifelong learning to stay abreast of new developments in your field.

- Practice critical thinking: Develop your critical thinking skills to effectively analyze situations, make sound clinical judgments, and prioritize patient care. Consider different perspectives, gather relevant information, and apply critical thinking frameworks to solve problems and make decisions.
- Take advantage of simulation and skills labs: Utilize simulation and skills labs to practice and refine your clinical skills in a controlled environment. These settings allow you to gain confidence, receive feedback, and make mistakes without compromising patient safety.
- Embrace opportunities for hands-on experience: Actively seek opportunities to gain hands-on experience in various clinical settings. Volunteer for procedures, assist with complex cases, and take on challenging patient assignments to expand your skill set and build confidence.
- Reflect on experiences: Reflect on your clinical experiences to identify areas for improvement and growth. Consider what went well, what could have been done differently, and how you can enhance your skills moving forward. Regular self-reflection promotes self-awareness and continuous improvement.
- Seek feedback and constructive criticism: Request feedback from colleagues, preceptors, and supervisors. Be open to constructive criticism and use it as an opportunity to learn and grow. Actively seek feedback on specific skills or areas you want to improve.
- Utilize clinical resources: Familiarize yourself with clinical resources such as textbooks, practice guidelines, and online databases. These resources can provide valuable information and serve as references when encountering unfamiliar situations or procedures.
- Collaborate with interdisciplinary team members: Engage in effective communication and collaboration with other healthcare professionals. Collaborating with physicians, pharmacists, therapists, and other team members can enhance your clinical skills and promote holistic patient care.
- Practice time management: Develop strong time management skills to prioritize tasks, organize your workload, and ensure timely and efficient patient care. Effective time management allows you to allocate sufficient time for skill development and continuous learning.
- Embrace feedback and learn from mistakes: Embrace a growth mindset and view mistakes as learning opportunities. Learn from your errors, seek guidance on how to improve, and implement strategies to prevent similar mistakes in the future.
- Take care of yourself: Prioritize self-care to maintain physical and emotional well-being. Adequate rest, nutrition, exercise, and stress management are essential for optimal performance and skill development.

Developing clinical skills is a continuous process that takes time and practice. Be patient with yourself, stay motivated, and embrace opportunities for growth and learning.

The Importance of Mastering Essential Clinical Skills as a Foundation for Safe and Effective Patient Care

Mastering essential clinical skills is crucial for ensuring safe and effective patient care. These skills form the foundation of a healthcare provider's ability to properly assess, diagnose, and treat patients. Without a solid understanding of these skills, healthcare professionals may put patients at risk of harm through misdiagnosis or improper treatment. By mastering essential clinical skills, healthcare providers can confidently and accurately care for their patients, leading to better outcomes and improved overall quality of care. Additionally, having a strong foundation in clinical skills allows healthcare providers to adapt to new and emerging healthcare practices, ultimately enhancing their ability to provide comprehensive and patient-centered care. In short, mastering essential clinical skills is essential for ensuring the safety and well-being of patients in any healthcare setting.

Importance of Critical Thinking, Clinical Judgment, and Evidence-Based Practice

Critical thinking, clinical judgment, and evidence-based practice are crucial skills for new graduate nurses as they transition into their professional roles. These skills allow nurses to effectively analyze situations, make sound decisions, and provide the best quality of care to their patients. Critical thinking enables nurses to think creatively, problem-solve, and consider all aspects of a situation before making a decision. Clinical judgment helps nurses to prioritize and anticipate potential complications, ensuring timely and effective interventions. Evidence-based practice is essential for new graduate nurses to stay up to date with the latest research and best practices in healthcare, ultimately leading to better patient outcomes. By cultivating and honing these skills, new graduate nurses can navigate the challenges of the healthcare setting with confidence and competence.

The Need for Ongoing Practice and Self-Reflection to Enhance Clinical Skills

Continuous practice and self-reflection are essential components for enhancing clinical skills. As healthcare professionals, it is crucial to constantly hone our skills and stay up to date with the latest advancements in medicine. Regular practice allows us to refine our techniques and improve our ability to provide quality care to patients. Self-reflection, on the other hand, helps us to identify areas of improvement and learn from our mistakes. By taking the time to reflect on our experiences, we can develop a deeper understanding of our strengths and weaknesses as clinicians. Ultimately, ongoing practice and self-reflection are key to becoming more competent and confident healthcare providers.

4.3   Conclusion

In conclusion, this chapter has provided valuable information on the basic competencies required to excel in the healthcare field. From mastering vital signs to performing sterile procedures, these skills are crucial for ensuring safe and effective patient care. As new nurses, it is essential to continuously practice and refine these skills through hands-on experience and ongoing education. By building a strong foundation of clinical skills, new graduate nurses can feel confident and competent in their ability to provide high-quality care to their patients. This chapter serves as a guide for new nurses entering the profession, equipping them with the knowledge and tools necessary to succeed in their roles.

Review Questions
- What are the key reasons why mastering essential clinical skills is crucial for new graduate nurses?
- Describe the importance of accurate vital signs assessment in patient care. What are the common vital signs and how should they be measured?
- Discuss the principles of safe medication administration and the steps involved in ensuring medication safety.
- Explain the importance of thorough patient assessments and the components of a comprehensive physical assessment.
- What are the fundamental nursing procedures that new graduate nurses should be proficient in? Provide step-by-step instructions for one of these procedures.
- Discuss the principles of infection control and the specific measures that should be taken during wound care.
- Describe the skills required for effective patient monitoring and the significance of timely and accurate monitoring.
- How can new graduate nurses develop and enhance their communication and interpersonal skills in the clinical setting?
- Explain the importance of critical thinking, clinical judgment, and evidence-based practice in the context of essential clinical skills.
- What are some strategies and resources available for new graduate nurses to continue practicing and refining their clinical skills beyond their initial orientation period?

References

American Heart Association (2020) Basic life support (BLS) provider manual. https://shopcpr.heart.org/bls-provider-manual. Accessed 22 Aug 2024

American Nurses Association (2015) Code of ethics for nurses with interpretive statements. https://www.nursingworld.org/coe-view-only. Accessed on 22 Aug 2024

American Nurses Association (ANA) (2024) Code of ethics for nurses. https://www.nursingworld.org/practice-policy/nursing-excellence/ethics/code-of-ethics-for-nurses/. Accessed 22 Aug 2024

Centers for Disease Control and Prevention (2020) Infection control. https://www.cdc.gov/infectioncontrol/index.html. Accessed 22 Aug 2024

Demsash AW, Kassie SY, Dubale AT, Chereka AA, Ngusie HS, Hunde MK, Emanu MD, Shibabaw AA, Walle AD (2023) Health professionals' routine practice documentation and its associated factors in a resource-limited setting: a cross-sectional study. BMJ Health Care Informatics 30(1):e100699. https://doi.org/10.1136/bmjhci-2022-100699

International Council of Nurses (ICN) (2021) THE ICN CODE OF ETHICS FOR NURSES. https://www.icn.ch/sites/default/files/2023-06/ICN_Code-of-Ethics_EN_Web.pdf. Accessed on 22 Aug 2024

Jafaru Y, Abubakar D (2022) Medication administration safety practices and perceived barriers among nurses: a cross-sectional study in northern Nigeria. Glob J Qual Saf Healthc 5(1):10–17. https://doi.org/10.36401/JQSH-21-11

Jarvis C (2023) Physical examination and health assessment-Canadian E-book. Elsevier Health Sciences. https://books.google.com/books?hl=en&lr=&id=IWy1EAAAQBAJ&oi=fnd&pg=PP1&dq=Physical+Examination+and+Health+Assessment&ots=7FTZ2op4e9&sig=qMrZQyMRLFXfePUq9WunTMnylBs. Accessed 22 Aug 2024

National Council of State Boards of Nursing. United States (2018) Medication administration. https://www.ncsbn.org/medication-administration.htm. Accessed 23 Aug 2024

National Department of Health (2022) South Africa. National guideline for patient safety incident reporting and learning in the health sector of South Africa. https://www.ncbi.nlm.nih.gov/pmc/articles/PMC9339949/. Accessed 22 Aug 2024

Perry AG, Potter PA, Ostendorf WR, Laplante N (2021) Clinical nursing skills and techniques-E-book. Elsevier Health Sciences. https://books.google.com/books?hl=en&lr=&id=6UciEAAAQBAJ&oi=fnd&pg=PR1&dq=clinical+skills+involves+history+taking,+performing+physical+assessments,+administering+treatments,+and+conducting+procedures,+effective+communication,+team+work+and+professionalism+&ots=r7ez1iOfk0&sig=9Ni8bdPddcDyNFD_iw39SGrhlYM. Accessed 22 Aug 2024

Saifullah Q, Sharma A (2024) Current trends on innovative technologies in topical wound care for advanced healing and management. Curr Drug Res Rev 16(3):319–332

South African Nursing Council (SANC) (2021) Code of ethics. https://www.sanc.co.za/wp-content/uploads/2021/04/Code-of-Ethics-for-Nursing-in-South-Africa.pdf. Accessed 22 Aug 2024

Stephen JS (2024) Skills and strategies for communication. In: Academic success in online programs: a resource for college students. Springer Nature Switzerland, Cham, pp 157–172. https://doi.org/10.1007/978-3-031-54439-2_11

Vichittragoonthavon S, Klunklin A, Wichaikhum OA, Viseskul N, Turale S (2020) Essential clinical skill components of new graduate nurses: a qualitative study. Nurse Educ Pract 44:102778. https://doi.org/10.1016/j.nepr.2020.102778

World Health Organization (2021) Patient safety. https://www.who.int/health-topics/patient-safety#tab=tab_1. Accessed 4 Aug 2024

Communication and Interpersonal Skills

5

Contents

> Test your learning and check your understanding of this book's contents: use the "Springer Nature Flashcards" app to access questions using ▶ https://sn.pub/pe441e. To use the app, please follow the instructions in Chap. 1.

5.1   Effective Communication

Communication refers to the exchange of information, ideas, and emotions between individuals or groups through verbal, nonverbal, and written means (Aji et al. 2023). Effective communication is essential in healthcare for accurate and collaborative patient care (Sharkiya 2023). Effective communication in nursing is essential for providing quality patient care and ensuring positive outcomes. Nurses must be able to clearly and accurately communicate with patients, their families, and other healthcare team members. This includes using active listening skills, asking clarifying questions, and providing information in a way that is easily understood. Good communication can help build trust, reduce stress, and improve patient satisfaction. Nurses who are effective communicators can also prevent misunderstandings, errors, and complications, leading to better overall patient outcomes. It is crucial for nurses to continuously work on improving their communication skills in order to be successful in their roles and provide optimal care for their patients.

© The Author(s), under exclusive license to Springer Nature Switzerland AG 2024   135
K. Matlhaba, *Enhancing Clinical Competence of Graduate Nurses*,
https://doi.org/10.1007/978-3-031-81407-5_5

Effective Communication Strategies in a Professional Setting
Effective communication is crucial for success as a new graduate nurse in a professional setting. Here are some strategies to enhance your communication skills:

- Active listening: Practice active listening by giving your full attention to the person speaking. Maintain eye contact, nod to show understanding, and avoid interrupting. Clarify and paraphrase information to ensure accurate understanding. Active listening helps build rapport, shows respect, and improves the quality of communication.
- Clear and concise communication: Use clear and concise language when communicating with patients, colleagues, and other healthcare professionals. Avoid using jargon or technical terms that everyone may not understand. Break down complex information into simpler terms and provide explanations as needed.
- Therapeutic communication: Develop skills in therapeutic communication to establish trust and build rapport with patients. Use empathy, compassion, and active listening to create a supportive and caring environment. Practice open-ended questions and reflective responses to encourage patients to express their concerns and feelings.
- Effective handover communication: Handover communication is critical for patient safety and continuity of care. Develop a structured approach to handover communication, such as using the SBAR (situation, background, assessment, recommendation) format. Clearly communicate important patient information, including changes in condition, medications, and upcoming procedures.
- Nonverbal communication: Pay attention to your nonverbal cues, such as body language, facial expressions, and tone of voice. Maintain a professional and approachable demeanor, and be aware of how your nonverbal cues may impact the communication process. Nonverbal communication can convey empathy, confidence, and professionalism.
- Collaborative communication: Nursing is a collaborative profession, and effective communication with the healthcare team is essential. Practice assertive communication by expressing your thoughts, concerns, and ideas in a respectful and confident manner. Seek clarification when needed and actively participate in interdisciplinary discussions and meetings.
- Written communication: Develop strong written communication skills for documentation, reports, and patient education materials. Use clear and concise language and proper grammar and spelling, and organize information in a logical manner. Proofread your written communication to ensure accuracy and clarity.
- Cultural sensitivity: Recognize and respect cultural differences in communication styles. Be mindful of cultural norms, values, and beliefs influencing communication preferences. Adapt your communication approach to meet the needs of diverse patients and colleagues.
- Feedback and reflection: Seek colleagues, supervisors, and patients' feedback to improve your communication skills. Reflect on your communication experiences and identify areas for improvement. Actively work on enhancing your communication skills based on the feedback you received.

Effective communication is a continuous learning process. Be open to feedback, actively seek opportunities to practice and refine your communication skills, and be mindful of the impact your communication has on patient care and professional relationships. By developing strong communication skills, you can enhance patient outcomes, collaborate effectively with the healthcare team, and establish yourself as a competent and trusted nurse.

5.2 The Key Reasons Why Effective Communication Skills Are Essential

1. *Patient outcomes*
   - Effective communication plays a vital role in improving patient outcomes. When nurses communicate clearly and effectively with patients, they can gather accurate information about their health conditions, symptoms, and concerns. This information is essential for making accurate diagnoses, developing appropriate care plans, and delivering personalized care.
   - Clear communication also helps patients understand their treatment options, medications, and self-care instructions, leading to better adherence to treatment plans and improved health outcomes.
2. *Teamwork and collaboration*
   - Effective communication is essential for fostering teamwork and collaboration among healthcare professionals. Nurses need to communicate effectively with physicians, other nurses, therapists, and support staff to ensure coordinated and comprehensive patient care.
   - Clear and timely communication helps prevent errors, reduces misunderstandings, and promotes efficient workflow. It enables healthcare teams to work together seamlessly, share critical information, and make informed decisions for the benefit of the patient.
3. *Patient satisfaction*
   - Effective communication is a key driver of patient satisfaction. When nurses communicate empathetically, actively listen to patients' concerns, and provide clear explanations, patients feel valued, respected, and involved in their care.
   - Good communication helps build trust and rapport between nurses and patients, leading to increased patient satisfaction. Patients who feel heard and understood are more likely to have a positive perception of their healthcare experience.
4. *Trust and patient safety*
   - Communication is fundamental in establishing trust between nurses and patients. When nurses communicate openly, honestly, and respectfully, patients feel confident in their care and are more likely to trust the healthcare team.
   - Effective communication also plays a critical role in patient safety. Clear and accurate communication helps prevent errors, such as medication mistakes or

misinterpretation of orders. It ensures that important information, such as allergies, medical history, and changes in condition, is properly communicated and understood by the entire healthcare team.

5. *Accurate information exchange*
   – Accurate information exchange is essential for safe and effective patient care. Nurses need to communicate patient information, assessments, and care plans accurately and efficiently to ensure continuity of care.
   – Effective communication ensures that important details are not overlooked or misinterpreted, reducing the risk of adverse events and improving patient outcomes.

Effective communication skills are vital in nursing practice as they contribute to improved patient outcomes, promote teamwork and collaboration, enhance patient satisfaction, establish trust, ensure patient safety, and facilitate accurate information exchange. By honing their communication skills, nurses can provide high-quality, patient-centered care and contribute to positive healthcare experiences for patients and their families.

5.3   Verbal and Nonverbal Communication

Verbal communication is a fundamental aspect of nursing practice, and clear and concise verbal communication is essential for effective patient care. Here's a closer look at the importance of clear and concise verbal communication, examples of effective verbal communication techniques, and the challenges of communicating with diverse patient populations:

Importance of Clear and Concise Verbal Communication

- Patient understanding: Clear and concise verbal communication ensures that patients understand their health conditions, treatment plans, and instructions for self-care. It helps prevent misunderstandings and promotes patient compliance with prescribed treatments.
- Collaboration: Effective verbal communication facilitates collaboration among healthcare professionals. It allows nurses to convey important patient information, discuss care plans, and seek input from colleagues, leading to coordinated and comprehensive care.
- Safety: Clear communication is crucial for patient safety. It helps prevent errors, such as medication mistakes or misinterpretation of orders, by ensuring accurate information exchange and understanding among the healthcare team.
- Trust and rapport: Clear and concise verbal communication builds trust and rapport between nurses and patients. It shows that nurses are attentive, respectful, and invested in the patient's well-being, leading to improved patient satisfaction and engagement in their care.

Examples of Effective Verbal Communication Techniques

- Active listening: Actively listening to patients and colleagues demonstrates respect and empathy. It involves giving full attention, maintaining eye contact, and providing verbal and nonverbal cues to show understanding and engagement.
- Appropriate tone and language: Using a calm and reassuring tone of voice, along with simple and jargon-free language, helps patients understand and feel at ease. Adjusting the tone and language based on the patient's cultural background and level of understanding is important.
- Clear instructions: Providing clear and concise instructions to patients and colleagues ensures that information is understood and followed accurately. Breaking down complex information into smaller, manageable parts and using visual aids or written materials can enhance comprehension.

Challenges of Communicating with Diverse Patient Populations

- Language barriers: Language differences can hinder effective communication. Nurses should use professional interpreters or translation services to ensure accurate understanding and avoid miscommunication. Using simple and nontechnical language can also help overcome language barriers.
- Cognitive impairments: Communicating with patients who have cognitive impairments, such as dementia or intellectual disabilities, requires patience and adaptability. Nurses may need to use visual cues, repetition, and simplified language to facilitate understanding.
- Cultural differences: Cultural differences can affect communication styles and expectations. Nurses should be aware of cultural norms, beliefs, and communication preferences to ensure respectful and effective communication. Seeking cultural consultation or involving cultural mediators can be helpful.

Clear and concise verbal communication is vital in nursing practice. It promotes patient understanding, collaboration, safety, and trust. Examples of effective verbal communication techniques include active listening, using appropriate tone and language, and providing clear instructions. Nurses should also be aware of the challenges of communicating with diverse patient populations, such as language barriers and cognitive impairments, and employ strategies to overcome these challenges for effective communication and patient-centered care.

Nonverbal communication, which includes body language, facial expressions, and gestures, plays a crucial role in nursing practice. Here's an explanation of the role of nonverbal communication; how nonverbal cues convey empathy, understanding, and reassurance to patients; and the importance of being aware of one's own nonverbal communication in patient interactions:

Role of Nonverbal Communication

- Enhancing communication: Nonverbal cues complement and reinforce verbal communication, adding depth and meaning to the message being conveyed. They provide additional information and context that words alone may not express.
- Conveying emotions and feelings: Nonverbal communication allows nurses to express empathy, compassion, and understanding without using words. It helps create a supportive and comforting environment for patients.
- Establishing rapport: Nonverbal cues help establish rapport and build trust with patients. They can convey openness, attentiveness, and genuine interest, which are essential for developing a therapeutic nurse-patient relationship.
- Assessing patient's emotional state: Nonverbal cues can provide valuable insights into a patient's emotional state, helping nurses assess their well-being and respond appropriately. They can indicate pain, discomfort, anxiety, or other emotions that may not be explicitly expressed verbally.

Conveying Empathy, Understanding, and Reassurance

- Facial expressions: Smiling, maintaining a warm and friendly facial expression, and using appropriate eye contact can convey empathy, understanding, and reassurance to patients. It helps them feel valued, heard, and supported.
- Body language: Open and relaxed body posture, leaning slightly toward the patient, and nodding to show active listening can communicate empathy and understanding. It signals that the nurse is fully present and engaged in the interaction.
- Touch: Appropriate and gentle touch, such as holding a patient's hand or providing a comforting pat on the shoulder, can convey empathy and reassurance. It can help alleviate anxiety and provide a sense of connection and support.

Importance of Being Aware of One's Own Nonverbal Communication

- Impact on patient interactions: Nurses' nonverbal communication can significantly impact patient interactions. Patients are sensitive to nonverbal cues and can pick up on subtle signals. Being aware of one's own nonverbal communication helps ensure that the intended message aligns with the verbal communication and promotes positive patient experiences.
- Self-reflection: Being conscious of one's own nonverbal communication allows nurses to reflect on their own attitudes, biases, and emotions that may influence patient interactions. It helps them identify areas for improvement and develop self-awareness to provide patient-centered care.
- Cultural sensitivity: Different cultures may have varying interpretations of nonverbal cues. Being aware of cultural differences and adapting nonverbal

communication accordingly are essential to avoid misunderstandings and promote effective communication with patients from diverse backgrounds.

Nonverbal communication, including body language, facial expressions, and gestures, plays a vital role in nursing practice. Nonverbal cues convey empathy, understanding, and reassurance to patients, enhancing communication and building rapport. Nurses should be aware of their own nonverbal communication and its impact on patient interactions to ensure effective and patient-centered care.

Therapeutic Communication

Therapeutic communication is a fundamental concept in nursing practice that focuses on establishing a therapeutic relationship between the nurse and the patient. It involves using effective communication techniques to promote trust, understanding, and collaboration, ultimately enhancing patient outcomes and satisfaction.

Application in Nursing Practice

- Establishing rapport and trust: Therapeutic communication techniques help nurses build rapport and trust with patients. By actively listening, showing empathy, and using open-ended questions, nurses create a safe and supportive environment where patients feel comfortable expressing their concerns and sharing important information.
- Enhancing patient understanding: Through therapeutic communication, nurses can ensure that patients understand their health conditions, treatment options, and self-care instructions. By using clear and concise language, providing explanations, and checking for understanding, nurses empower patients to actively participate in their care.
- Emotional support: Therapeutic communication techniques, such as active listening and reflection, allow nurses to provide emotional support to patients. By acknowledging and validating their feelings, nurses help patients cope with their emotions and promote their overall well-being.
- Collaboration and shared decision-making: Effective therapeutic communication fosters collaboration and shared decision-making between nurses and patients. By involving patients in their care, considering their preferences and values, and providing information to support informed choices, nurses promote patient-centered care.

Techniques for Therapeutic Communication

- Active listening: Actively listening to patients involves giving full attention, maintaining eye contact, and providing verbal and nonverbal cues to show understanding and engagement. It demonstrates respect and empathy, allowing patients to feel heard and valued.

- Empathy: Showing empathy involves understanding and sharing the feelings and experiences of patients. By expressing empathy through verbal and nonverbal cues, nurses create a supportive and compassionate environment.
- Open-ended questions: Using open-ended questions encourages patients to provide more detailed and meaningful responses. It promotes conversation, allows patients to express their thoughts and concerns, and provides nurses with valuable information.
- Reflection: Reflecting on patients' statements or emotions helps nurses validate their feelings and demonstrate understanding. Reflective responses can include summarizing, paraphrasing, or clarifying what the patient has expressed.

Importance of Effective Communication in Sensitive Situations

In sensitive situations, such as delivering bad news or discussing end-of-life care, effective communication is crucial. It helps nurses convey information with sensitivity, compassion, and clarity. By using appropriate language, providing emotional support, and allowing patients and their families to express their emotions and concerns, nurses can navigate these difficult conversations while maintaining trust and respect.

Therapeutic communication is a vital aspect of nursing practice. It involves using effective communication techniques to establish rapport, trust, and collaboration with patients. Techniques such as active listening, empathy, open-ended questioning, and reflection are essential for building therapeutic relationships. Effective communication is particularly important in sensitive situations, as it allows nurses to deliver information with compassion and support. By continuously improving their communication skills, nurses can provide patient-centered care and enhance patient outcomes.

Technology has revolutionized communication in healthcare settings, including nursing practice. Here's an exploration of the role of technology in communication; the benefits and challenges of using electronic health records (EHRs), telehealth, and other communication technologies; and the importance of maintaining privacy, confidentiality, and professionalism when using technology for communication:

Role of Technology in Communication

- Efficient information exchange: Technology enables quick and efficient exchange of patient information among healthcare professionals. It allows nurses to access and share patient data, test results, and treatment plans in real time, facilitating coordinated and collaborative care.
- Remote communication: Telehealth and telecommunication technologies enable nurses to communicate with patients and other healthcare providers remotely. This is particularly valuable for patients in remote areas or those with limited mobility, as it improves access to care and reduces barriers to communication.

- Enhanced documentation: Electronic health records (EHRs) streamline documentation processes, making patient information readily available and easily accessible. Nurses can input and retrieve data efficiently, improving accuracy, continuity of care, and communication among healthcare team members.
- Patient education: Technology provides various platforms for delivering educational materials to patients. Nurses can use multimedia resources, online portals, and mobile applications to educate patients about their health conditions, medications, and self-care instructions.

Benefits and Challenges of Using Technology in Communication

1. *Benefits*
   - Improved efficiency: Technology streamlines communication processes, reducing the time and effort required for information exchange.
   - Enhanced collaboration: Communication technologies facilitate collaboration among healthcare professionals, promoting coordinated and patient-centered care.
   - Increased access to care: Telehealth and remote communication technologies improve access to healthcare services, especially for underserved populations.
   - Better documentation: EHRs improve documentation accuracy, accessibility, and legibility, ensuring comprehensive and up-to-date patient records.
2. *Challenges*
   - Technical issues: Technology can be prone to technical glitches, such as system failures or connectivity issues, which may disrupt communication and workflow.
   - Learning curve: Nurses need to acquire the necessary skills and knowledge to effectively use communication technologies, which may require training and ongoing support.
   - Privacy and security concerns: The use of technology for communication raises concerns about patient privacy and data security. Nurses must adhere to strict protocols and safeguards to protect patient information.
   - Potential for misinterpretation: Communication technologies lack nonverbal cues and nuances present in face-to-face interactions, which may lead to misinterpretation or misunderstanding of messages.

Importance of Privacy, Confidentiality, and Professionalism

When using technology for communication, nurses must prioritize privacy, confidentiality, and professionalism:

- Privacy: Nurses should ensure that patient information is shared securely and only with authorized individuals. They must follow privacy regulations and use encrypted communication platforms when transmitting sensitive data.

- Confidentiality: Nurses must maintain patient confidentiality by not disclosing patient information to unauthorized individuals or discussing patient cases in public or unsecured digital platforms.
- Professionalism: Nurses should communicate professionally and respectfully, adhering to ethical standards and guidelines. They should use appropriate language, tone, and behavior when communicating electronically.

Technology plays a significant role in communication in nursing practice. It improves information exchange, enables remote communication, enhances documentation, and facilitates patient education. While there are benefits to using technology, challenges such as technical issues and privacy concerns must be addressed. Nurses must prioritize privacy, confidentiality, and professionalism when using technology for communication to ensure patient safety and trust.

Self-reflection and continuous improvement are essential for new graduate nurses to enhance their communication skills and develop strong interpersonal abilities. Here's a discussion on encouraging self-reflection, seeking feedback, engaging in self-assessment, and pursuing ongoing professional development:

Encouraging Self-Reflection

- Importance of self-reflection: Self-reflection allows new graduate nurses to assess their communication skills, identify strengths and areas for improvement, and gain self-awareness. It helps them understand how their communication style and behaviors impact patient outcomes and relationships.
- Promoting self-reflection: Encourage new graduate nurses to set aside time for self-reflection regularly. They can journal their experiences, review interactions with patients and colleagues, and analyze their communication effectiveness. This process helps them recognize patterns, challenges, and opportunities for growth.

Seeking Feedback

- Importance of feedback: Feedback from patients, colleagues, and mentors provides valuable insights into a nurse's communication skills. It helps identify blind spots, validates strengths, and offers suggestions for improvement.
- Creating a feedback culture: Encourage new graduate nurses to actively seek feedback from patients, colleagues, and supervisors. They can request specific feedback on their communication skills and behaviors and use it as a learning opportunity to enhance their practice.

Engaging in Self-assessment

1. Self-assessment tools: New graduate nurses can use self-assessment tools, such as communication competency frameworks or checklists, to evaluate their communication skills objectively. These tools provide a structured approach to identify areas of strength and areas that require improvement.
2. Reflective questions: New graduate nurses are encouraged to ask themselves reflective questions such as the following:
   – How effectively do I listen to patients and colleagues?
   – How well do I convey empathy and understanding?
   – Am I able to adapt my communication style to meet the needs of diverse patients?
   – How do I handle difficult conversations or conflicts?
   – Do I effectively communicate information to patients and their families?

Pursuing Ongoing Professional Development

- Continuing education: Encourage new graduate nurses to participate in workshops, seminars, and courses focused on communication and interpersonal skills. These opportunities provide knowledge, strategies, and techniques to enhance their communication abilities.
- Mentoring and coaching: Pair new graduate nurses with experienced mentors or coaches who can provide guidance, support, and feedback on their communication skills. Mentors can share their expertise and help new nurses navigate challenging communication situations.
- Peer learning: Encourage new graduate nurses to engage in peer learning activities, such as case discussions or role-playing exercises, to practice and refine their communication skills. Peer feedback and collaboration can foster growth and improvement.

Self-reflection and continuous improvement are crucial for new graduate nurses to enhance their communication skills. Encouraging self-reflection, seeking feedback, engaging in self-assessment, and pursuing ongoing professional development are key strategies to develop strong communication and interpersonal abilities. By actively working on their communication skills, new graduate nurses can provide patient-centered care, build therapeutic relationships, and contribute to positive patient outcomes.

5.4   Collaboration and Teamwork

Collaboration and teamwork are essential components of nursing practice. In order to provide the best possible care for patients, nurses must work together effectively with other healthcare professionals. This includes communication, sharing knowledge, and supporting each other in decision-making processes. By collaborating and working as a team, nurses can ensure that the needs of their patients are met in a timely and efficient manner. This can lead to improved patient outcomes, increased job satisfaction, and a stronger sense of unity among the healthcare team. Overall, collaboration and teamwork in nursing are crucial for delivering high-quality care and promoting a positive working environment.

5.4.1   Collaborating with Colleagues and Stakeholders to Achieve Goals

As a new graduate nurse, collaborating with colleagues and stakeholders is essential for achieving goals and providing quality patient care. Here are some tips to help you collaborate effectively:

- Build relationships: Take the time to get to know your colleagues and stakeholders. Building positive relationships based on trust and respect will make collaboration easier.
- Communicate effectively: Clear and open communication is key to successful collaboration. Be an active listener, ask questions, and provide feedback. Use both verbal and written communication methods to ensure everyone is on the same page.
- Understand roles and responsibilities: Familiarize yourself with your colleagues' and stakeholders' roles and responsibilities. This will help you understand how to collaborate effectively and utilize each person's expertise.
- Share information: Share relevant information with your colleagues and stakeholders. This includes patient information, research findings, and updates on care plans. Effective information sharing promotes collaboration and ensures everyone is working toward the same goals.
- Seek input and feedback: Value your colleagues' and stakeholders' input and feedback. Encourage them to share their ideas and perspectives. This will foster a collaborative environment where everyone feels heard and valued.
- Be flexible and adaptable: Collaboration often requires compromise and flexibility. Be open to different ideas and approaches and be willing to adapt your plans if necessary. This will help create a collaborative culture where everyone feels comfortable contributing.
- Resolve conflicts constructively: Conflicts may arise during collaboration. It's important to address conflicts in a constructive manner, focusing on finding solutions rather than placing blame. Use effective communication and problem-solving skills to resolve conflicts and maintain positive working relationships.

Collaboration is a continuous process that requires ongoing effort and commitment. You can work together to achieve your goals as a new graduate nurse by actively engaging with your colleagues and stakeholders.

5.4.2 Developing Strong Interpersonal Skills for Effective Teamwork

Developing strong interpersonal skills is crucial for effective teamwork as a new graduate nurse. Here are some tips to help you enhance your interpersonal skills:

- Active listening: Practice active listening by giving your full attention to others when they are speaking. This shows respect and helps you understand their perspectives and concerns.
- Empathy: Cultivate empathy by putting yourself in the shoes of your colleagues and patients. Try to understand their emotions and experiences, which will help you build stronger connections and provide better care.
- Effective communication: Develop clear and concise communication skills. Use appropriate language, tone, and nonverbal cues to convey your message effectively. Be open to feedback and ask for clarification when needed.
- Conflict resolution: Learn how to manage conflicts in a constructive manner. Practice active problem-solving, compromise, and negotiation skills to find resolutions that benefit everyone involved.
- Collaboration: Foster a collaborative mindset by actively seeking input and involving others in decision-making processes. Value the contributions of your team members and encourage a sense of shared responsibility.
- Emotional intelligence: Develop emotional intelligence by recognizing and managing your own emotions, as well as understanding and responding to the emotions of others. This skill helps build trust and rapport within the team.
- Flexibility and adaptability: Be open to change and willing to adapt your approach when necessary. Flexibility allows you to work effectively with different personalities and adapt to evolving situations.
- Respect and professionalism: Treat your colleagues, patients, and stakeholders with respect and professionalism. Show appreciation for their expertise and contributions and maintain a positive and supportive work environment.
- Time management: Develop strong time management skills to prioritize tasks, meet deadlines, and contribute to the team's overall efficiency. Being organized and reliable helps build trust and credibility.
- Reflect and learn: Continuously reflect on your interpersonal skills and seek opportunities for improvement. Actively seek feedback from colleagues and supervisors to identify areas for growth.
- Remember, developing strong interpersonal skills is an ongoing process. By actively working on these skills, you can enhance your ability to work effectively as part of a team and provide quality care as a new graduate nurse.

5.5   Conclusion

This chapter highlights the importance of effective communication and interpersonal skills in the nursing profession. As new graduate nurses enter the field, they must prioritize building strong relationships with patients, colleagues, and other healthcare professionals. By developing active listening skills, showing empathy, and practicing clear and concise communication, nurses can enhance patient outcomes and create a positive work environment. It is essential for new nurses to continuously work on honing their communication skills through education, training, and self-reflection to provide high-quality patient care. Overall, this chapter emphasizes the vital role that communication and interpersonal skills play in nursing practice and the impact they have on overall patient satisfaction and well-being.

Review Questions
- What are the key components of effective communication in the healthcare setting?
- How can new graduate nurses improve their verbal communication skills when interacting with patients, families, and healthcare team members?
- What are some strategies for enhancing nonverbal communication skills as a new graduate nurse?
- How can active listening contribute to building therapeutic relationships with patients and promoting patient-centered care?
- What is the role of empathy in effective communication and how can new graduate nurses develop and demonstrate empathy in their interactions?
- How can new graduate nurses effectively communicate and collaborate within interdisciplinary healthcare teams?
- What are some common challenges in communication within healthcare teams and how can they be addressed?
- How does cultural diversity impact communication in healthcare and what strategies can new graduate nurses employ to ensure culturally sensitive and inclusive care?
- What are the ethical considerations related to communication and interpersonal skills for new graduate nurses?
- How can new graduate nurses utilize technology effectively to enhance communication while maintaining professionalism and patient confidentiality?

References

Aji R, Aji SR, Noorma N, Suratman S (2023) Interpersonal communication. Lambert Academic Publishing. http://repository.poltekkesbengkulu.ac.id/id/eprint/3041
Sharkiya SH (2023) Quality communication can improve patient-centred health outcomes among older patients: a rapid review. BMC Health Serv Res 23(1):886. https://doi.org/10.1186/s12913-023-09869-8

Patient-Centered Care

6

Contents

> Test your learning and check your understanding of this book's contents: use the "Springer Nature Flashcards" app to access questions using ▶ https://sn.pub/pe441e. To use the app, please follow the instructions in Chap. 1.

6.1   Definition of Patient-Centered Care

Patient-centered care is an approach that puts the individual patient at the center of the care process, and it consists of holistic, collaborative, and responsive care components (Baek et al. 2023). Patient-centered care skills involve providing care that is respectful, compassionate, and responsive to the individual needs, values, and preferences of patients (Kwame and Petrucka 2021). It emphasizes shared decision-making and collaboration between healthcare providers and patients. Patient-centered care seeks to empower patients to be active participants in their own healthcare journey, ultimately leading to better health outcomes and increased patient satisfaction. This approach also emphasizes the importance of building strong and trusting relationships between healthcare providers and patients, as well as considering the unique sociocultural and emotional factors that may impact a patient's overall well-being. In essence, patient-centered care places the patient at the center of their healthcare experience, ensuring that their voice is heard and their needs are met with compassion and respect.

Significance in Promoting Positive Patient Outcomes and Experiences
Promoting positive patient outcomes and experiences is of great significance in healthcare. Here are some reasons why:

- Improved health outcomes: When patients have positive experiences and feel supported in their healthcare journey, they are more likely to actively participate in their treatment plans and follow medical advice. This can lead to better health outcomes and improved overall well-being.
- Increased patient satisfaction: Positive patient experiences contribute to higher levels of patient satisfaction. When patients feel heard, respected, and involved in their care, they are more likely to have a positive perception of the healthcare system and the quality of care they receive.
- Enhanced trust and communication: Positive patient experiences help build trust between patients and healthcare providers. Trust is essential for effective communication, as patients are more likely to openly share their concerns, symptoms, and medical history when they feel comfortable and supported. This, in turn, enables healthcare providers to make accurate diagnoses and develop appropriate treatment plans.
- Better adherence to treatment plans: Patients who have positive experiences are more likely to adhere to their treatment plans, including taking medications as prescribed, attending follow-up appointments, and making necessary lifestyle changes. This improves the effectiveness of the treatment and reduces the risk of complications or relapses.
- Increased engagement and empowerment: Positive patient experiences promote patient engagement and empowerment. When patients are actively involved in their care, they become partners in decision-making and take ownership of their health. This can lead to better self-management of chronic conditions and improved overall health outcomes.
- Positive reputation and referrals: Healthcare organizations that prioritize positive patient experiences often develop a strong reputation for quality care. Satisfied patients are more likely to recommend the healthcare facility or provider to others, leading to increased referrals and a larger patient base.

Promoting positive patient outcomes and experiences is crucial for delivering patient-centered care, improving health outcomes, and building strong relationships between patients and healthcare providers.

The Shift from a Provider-Focused Approach to One That Prioritizes the Unique Needs, Values, and Goals of Each Patient
The shift from a provider-focused approach to a patient-centered approach is essential in healthcare, especially for new graduate nurses. Here's why prioritizing the unique needs, values, and goals of each patient is important:

- Individualized care: Every patient is unique, with different needs, values, and goals. By adopting a patient-centered approach, new graduate nurses can tailor their care plans to meet the specific requirements of each patient. This individualized care improves patient outcomes and enhances their overall experience.
- Respect for autonomy: Patient-centered care respects the autonomy and decision-making capabilities of patients. It recognizes that patients have the right to be involved in their care and make informed choices about their health. New graduate nurses can empower patients by providing them with information, involving them in care decisions, and respecting their preferences.
- Improved communication: Prioritizing the unique needs, values, and goals of each patient promotes effective communication between new graduate nurses and their patients. It encourages active listening, empathy, and understanding. This open and honest communication fosters trust and enhances the nurse-patient relationship and improves patient satisfaction.
- Enhanced patient engagement: Patient-centered care encourages active participation and engagement from patients in their healthcare journey. New graduate nurses can involve patients in setting goals, developing care plans, and monitoring progress. This engagement promotes patient empowerment, responsibility, and accountability for their health.
- Cultural sensitivity: Each patient comes from a unique cultural background with specific values, beliefs, and practices. By prioritizing the unique needs of each patient, new graduate nurses can provide culturally sensitive care. This includes respecting cultural traditions, beliefs, and preferences, which leads to improved patient trust, satisfaction, and outcomes.
- Holistic approach: Patient-centered care takes into account the physical, emotional, social, and spiritual aspects of a patient's well-being. New graduate nurses can adopt a holistic approach by considering all these dimensions and addressing them in their care plans. This comprehensive approach promotes better patient outcomes and a higher quality of life.
- Continuity of care: Prioritizing the unique needs, values, and goals of each patient helps in establishing continuity of care. New graduate nurses can ensure that care is consistent, coordinated, and personalized across different healthcare settings. This continuity improves patient safety, reduces errors, and enhances the overall patient experience.

Shifting from a provider-focused approach to a patient-centered approach is crucial for new graduate nurses. By prioritizing the unique needs, values, and goals of each patient, they can deliver individualized care, respect patient autonomy, improve communication, enhance patient engagement, provide culturally sensitive care, adopt a holistic approach, and ensure continuity of care. This shift ultimately leads to better patient outcomes and experiences.

6.2 Key Components of Patient-Centered Care

- Respect for patients' values, preferences, and needs: Healthcare providers should respect and consider the individual values, preferences, and needs of each patient. This involves actively listening to patients, involving them in decision-making, and tailoring care to their specific circumstances.
- Effective communication: Clear and open communication between healthcare providers and patients is essential for patient-centered care. This includes providing information in a way that patients can understand, listening to their concerns, and addressing any questions or uncertainties they may have.
- Shared decision-making: Patient-centered care involves involving patients in the decision-making process regarding their healthcare. Healthcare providers should provide patients with information about their condition, treatment options, and potential risks and benefits and work together with patients to make decisions that align with their values and preferences.
- Empathy and compassion: Healthcare providers should demonstrate empathy and compassion toward their patients. This involves understanding and acknowledging patients' emotions, providing emotional support, and showing genuine care and concern for their well-being.
- Continuity of care: Patient-centered care involves providing continuous and coordinated care throughout a patient's healthcare journey. This includes ensuring smooth transitions between different healthcare settings, effective communication between healthcare providers, and ongoing support and follow-up.
- Accessible and equitable care: Patient-centered care should be accessible and equitable for all patients, regardless of their background, socioeconomic status, or other factors. This involves addressing barriers to access, promoting health equity, and ensuring that all patients receive the same level of care and attention.
- Patient and family engagement: Patient-centered care recognizes the importance of involving patients and their families in their healthcare. This includes actively engaging patients in their own care, encouraging their participation in decision-making, and involving family members or caregivers in the care process when appropriate.

These components work together to ensure that healthcare is centered around the needs and preferences of the individual patient, promoting better outcomes and patient satisfaction.

6.3 The Essential Skills and Principles Required for the New Graduate Nurses to Provide Patient-Centered Care in the Healthcare Setting

To provide patient-centered care in the healthcare setting, new graduate nurses should possess the following essential skills and principles:

- Clinical competence: It is essential for nurses to have a strong foundation of clinical knowledge and skills. They should be proficient in performing nursing procedures, administering medications, and monitoring patient conditions.
- Communication skills: Effective communication is crucial for building trust and understanding with patients. Nurses should be able to listen actively, communicate clearly, and provide information in a compassionate and empathetic manner.
- Empathy and compassion: Nurses should have the ability to understand and share the feelings of their patients. They should demonstrate empathy and compassion to provide emotional support and create a caring environment.
- Critical thinking: New graduate nurses should be able to analyze complex situations, make sound judgments, and prioritize patient needs. Critical thinking skills help in problem-solving, decision-making, and providing safe and effective care.
- Cultural competence: Nurses should respect and value the diversity of patients' cultural backgrounds, beliefs, and practices. Cultural competence helps in providing individualized care that is sensitive to the unique needs of each patient.
- Teamwork and collaboration: Nurses work as part of a multidisciplinary team, and effective teamwork is essential for providing coordinated and holistic care. New graduate nurses should be able to collaborate with other healthcare professionals and communicate effectively within the team.
- Ethical practice: Nurses should adhere to ethical principles and professional standards in their practice. They should respect patient autonomy, maintain confidentiality, and advocate for the rights and well-being of their patients.
- Continuous learning: Healthcare is constantly evolving, and new graduate nurses should have a commitment to lifelong learning. They should stay updated with the latest evidence-based practices, advancements in technology, and healthcare policies.

By developing these skills and principles, new graduate nurses can provide patient-centered care that focuses on the individual needs, preferences, and goals of each patient.

6.4   Strategies for Building Rapport, Establishing Trust, and Engaging Patients

Building rapport, establishing trust, and engaging patients are crucial skills for new graduate nurses. Here are some strategies to achieve these goals:

- Introduce yourself and establish a personal connection: Begin by introducing yourself to the patient and their family members. Use a warm and friendly tone, maintain eye contact, and address them by their preferred name. Take a moment to engage in small talk and show genuine interest in their well-being.
- Active listening: Practice active listening skills by giving your full attention to the patient. Maintain eye contact, nod, and use verbal and nonverbal cues to show that you are actively listening. Encourage patients to express their concerns,

fears, and questions, and provide them with ample time to speak without interruption.

- Empathy and compassion: Show empathy and compassion toward patients by acknowledging their emotions and validating their experiences. Use empathetic statements such as "I understand this must be difficult for you" or "I'm here to support you." Be sensitive to their needs and emotions and offer emotional support when appropriate.
- Clear and effective communication: Use clear and simple language when communicating with patients to ensure they understand the information you provide. Avoid medical jargon and explain medical terms in a way that patients can comprehend. Encourage patients to ask questions and clarify any doubts they may have.
- Respect patient autonomy: Respect patients' autonomy by involving them in their care decisions. Provide them with information about their condition, treatment options, and potential risks and benefits. Encourage patients to express their preferences and involve them in the decision-making process.
- Be reliable and trustworthy: Build trust with patients by being reliable and trustworthy. Follow through on your commitments, such as returning with requested information or following up on their concerns. Be honest and transparent in your communication, and admit when you don't know something, but assure them that you will find the information they need.
- Personalize care: Tailor your care to meet the individual needs and preferences of each patient. Take the time to understand their values, cultural background, and personal preferences. Incorporate these factors into their care plan to make them feel heard and respected.
- Involve family members and caregivers: Engage family members and caregivers in the care process, when appropriate. Keep them informed about the patient's condition, involve them in decision-making, and provide them with support and resources as needed.
- Follow-up and continuity of care: Demonstrate your commitment to patient care by following up with patients after procedures or treatments. Ensure smooth transitions between different healthcare settings, and provide clear instructions for follow-up care. This shows patients that you are invested in their well-being beyond their immediate hospital stay.

By implementing these strategies, new graduate nurses can build rapport, establish trust, and engage patients effectively, leading to better patient outcomes and satisfaction.

6.5   Guidance to Actively Participate as a Member of Multiple Disciplinary Team

As a new graduate nurse, it is important to actively participate as a member of multiple disciplinary teams in order to provide the best possible care for patients. This can be achieved by communicating effectively with other team members, sharing knowledge and expertise, and being open to learning from others. It is important to understand and respect the role that each member of the team plays in the overall care of patients and to contribute in a positive and collaborative manner. By actively participating as a member of multiple disciplinary teams, new graduate nurses can not only enhance their own skills and knowledge but also contribute to improved patient outcomes and experiences.

Interdisciplinary Rounds and Care Conferences
New graduate nurses can actively participate in interdisciplinary rounds and care conferences by following these strategies:

- Prepare in advance: Before the rounds or conference, review the patient's medical history, care plan, and any relevant documentation. Familiarize yourself with the patient's condition, medications, and treatment goals.
- Be proactive: Take the initiative to contribute to the discussion. Share your observations, concerns, and suggestions regarding the patient's care. Offer insights based on your nursing knowledge and experience.
- Listen actively: Pay attention to what other healthcare professionals are saying during the rounds or conference. Listen to their perspectives, recommendations, and questions. This will help you understand the holistic approach to patient care.
- Ask questions: Do not hesitate to ask questions if you need clarification or want to learn more about a particular aspect of the patient's care. This shows your engagement and willingness to learn from other team members.
- Collaborate with other disciplines: Interdisciplinary rounds and care conferences are opportunities to collaborate with professionals from different disciplines. Engage in discussions, share information, and seek input from doctors, therapists, social workers, and other team members.
- Advocate for the patient: As a nurse, you play a crucial role in advocating for your patients. Speak up if you notice any discrepancies or potential risks or if you believe a different approach may be beneficial for the patient's well-being.
- Document and follow-up: Take notes during the rounds or conference to ensure accurate documentation of the discussed care plan. Follow up on any assigned tasks or responsibilities promptly to ensure continuity of care.

Remember, active participation in interdisciplinary rounds and care conferences not only enhances patient care but also promotes professional growth and collaboration within the healthcare team.

Care Planning to Promote Holistic and Patient-Centered Approaches

New graduate nurses can actively participate in care planning to promote holistic and patient-centered approaches by following these strategies:

- Develop a comprehensive understanding of the patient: Take the time to gather information about the patient's medical history, current condition, and personal preferences. This includes reviewing medical records, conducting assessments, and engaging in therapeutic communication with the patient and their family.
- Collaborate with the healthcare team: Actively engage with other healthcare professionals involved in the patient's care, such as doctors, therapists, social workers, and pharmacists. Share your nursing perspective, and contribute to the development of a holistic care plan that addresses the physical, emotional, social, and spiritual needs of the patient.
- Advocate for the patient's preferences and values: Ensure that the patient's preferences, values, and cultural beliefs are considered in the care planning process. Act as a liaison between the patient and the healthcare team, ensuring that their voice is heard and respected.
- Incorporate evidence-based practice: Stay up to date with current research and evidence-based guidelines relevant to the patient's condition. Use this knowledge to contribute to the development of a care plan that is based on the best available evidence.
- Prioritize patient education: Recognize the importance of patient education in promoting holistic care. Take the time to educate the patient and their family about their condition, treatment options, and self-care strategies. Empower them to actively participate in their own care.
- Continuously reassess and modify the care plan: Regularly reassess the patient's condition and evaluate the effectiveness of the care plan. Collaborate with the healthcare team to make necessary modifications and adjustments to ensure that the care plan remains patient-centered and holistic.
- Emphasize interdisciplinary collaboration: Actively seek opportunities to collaborate with professionals from different disciplines. Engage in interdisciplinary rounds, care conferences, and team meetings to share insights, exchange information, and contribute to the development of a comprehensive care plan.

By actively participating in care planning, new graduate nurses can contribute to the promotion of holistic and patient-centered approaches, ultimately enhancing the overall quality of care provided to patients.

6.6   Ethical Considerations Related to Patient-Centered Care

Patient-centered care is a fundamental aspect of healthcare that aims to prioritize the needs and preferences of patients. However, in order to provide truly patient-centered care, it is important to also consider the ethical implications of taking a patient-centered approach. One ethical consideration is the principle of autonomy, which emphasizes the importance of respecting a patient's right to make their own healthcare decisions. This means healthcare providers must ensure patients are fully informed and can make decisions based on their values and beliefs. Another ethical consideration is the principle of beneficence, which requires healthcare providers to act in the best interest of their patients. In a patient-centered approach, this may involve collaborating with patients to develop treatment plans that align with their goals and values. Ultimately, by integrating ethical considerations into patient-centered care, healthcare providers can ensure that they are truly serving the best interests of their patients.

The Principles of Beneficence, Non-maleficence, and Respect for Autonomy
In patient care, the principles of beneficence, non-maleficence, and respect for autonomy are essential in guiding healthcare professionals in their decision-making (Cheraghi et al. 2023; Varkey 2021). Beneficence requires healthcare providers to act in the best interest of the patient, striving to promote their well-being and improve their health outcomes. Non-maleficence, on the other hand, emphasizes the importance of avoiding harm and minimizing risks to the patient. Finally, respect for autonomy acknowledges the patient's right to make informed decisions about their own healthcare, ensuring that they are informed of all available options and their consequences. By adhering to these principles, healthcare professionals can ensure that they are providing ethical and patient-centered care that respects the dignity and autonomy of each individual.

Examples of Ethical Dilemmas That New Graduate Nurses May Encounter
The principles of beneficence, non-maleficence, and respect for autonomy are fundamental ethical principles in healthcare. Here are brief explanations of each principle and examples of ethical dilemmas that new graduate nurses may encounter:

- Beneficence: This principle emphasizes the duty to do good and promote the well-being of patients. It involves taking actions that benefit the patient and improve their health outcomes.
- Example ethical dilemma: A new graduate nurse is assigned to care for a patient who refuses a lifesaving treatment due to personal beliefs. The nurse must balance the patient's autonomy with the duty to promote their well-being.
- Non-maleficence: This principle focuses on the duty to do no harm and prevent harm to patients. It involves avoiding actions that may cause harm or worsen the patient's condition.
- Example ethical dilemma: A new graduate nurse administers a medication to a patient without double-checking the dosage, resulting in an adverse reaction. The nurse must address the harm caused and take steps to prevent similar incidents in the future.
- Respect for autonomy: This principle recognizes the right of patients to make their own decisions about their healthcare. It involves respecting the patient's choices, values, and preferences.

Example ethical dilemma: A new graduate nurse is caring for an elderly patient with a terminal illness who expresses a desire to discontinue treatment and opt for palliative care. The nurse must respect the patient's autonomy while providing support and ensuring they have all the necessary information to make an informed decision.

These principles often intersect, and nurses must navigate complex ethical dilemmas while upholding these principles in their practice. It is important for new graduate nurses to seek guidance from experienced colleagues and adhere to the ethical standards set by their profession.

The Need for Ethical Decision-Making and Advocacy

Ethical decision-making is a logical process which involves making the best moral decisions through systematic reasoning in a situation that brings about conflicting choices (Sari et al. 2018). Patient advocacy refers to the ethical obligation to ensure that the needs of the patient and family and medical decisions are made in line with their wishes (Kurt and Gurdogan 2023). New graduate nurses play a crucial role in applying ethical decision-making and advocacy to ensure the best interests of the patient are upheld. Here are some reasons why this is important:

- Ethical decision-making and advocacy help new graduate nurses prioritize the needs and preferences of the patient. By considering the patient's values, beliefs, and goals, nurses can provide individualized care that respects their autonomy and promotes their well-being.
- New graduate nurses often encounter ethical dilemmas in their practice. These dilemmas may involve conflicting values, limited resources, or complex treatment decisions. Applying ethical decision-making frameworks, such as the principles of beneficence, non-maleficence, and respect for autonomy, helps nurses navigate these dilemmas and make informed choices that prioritize the patient's best interests.
- Advocacy is essential for ensuring patient safety. New graduate nurses must be vigilant in identifying and addressing potential risks or errors in patient care. By advocating for necessary resources, following evidence-based practices, and speaking up about concerns, nurses can help prevent harm and promote a safe healthcare environment.
- Ethical decision-making and advocacy involve effective communication and collaboration with the healthcare team. New graduate nurses need to actively participate in interdisciplinary discussions, share their perspectives, and advocate for the patient's needs. By working together, healthcare professionals can make well-informed decisions that align with ethical principles and promote optimal patient outcomes.
- Applying ethical decision-making and advocacy skills allows new graduate nurses to develop professionally. By actively engaging in ethical discussions, seeking guidance from experienced colleagues, and staying updated on ethical guidelines and standards, nurses can enhance their critical thinking abilities and

ethical reasoning. This, in turn, contributes to their overall competence and growth as healthcare professionals.

New graduate nurses must apply ethical decision-making and advocacy to ensure the best interests of the patient are upheld. By prioritizing patient-centered care, navigating ethical dilemmas, promoting patient safety, collaborating with the healthcare team, and fostering professional growth, nurses can make a positive impact on patient outcomes and the overall quality of care.

6.7 Conclusion

Chapter 6 on patient-centered care emphasizes the importance of prioritizing the needs and preferences of patients in the healthcare setting. By actively involving patients in their care decisions, healthcare providers can enhance satisfaction, improve outcomes, and promote a stronger patient-provider relationship. Patient-centered care also encourages a holistic approach to healthcare that considers the physical, emotional, and psychological well-being of patients. Moving forward, it is crucial for healthcare professionals to continue implementing patient-centered practices to ensure that all individuals receive high-quality and personalized care that meets their unique needs. By embracing patient-centered care principles, healthcare providers can truly make a positive difference in the lives of their patients.

Review Questions
- What is patient-centered care and why is it important in nursing practice?
- How can new graduate nurses effectively communicate with patients to establish rapport and build trust?
- What are some strategies for actively listening to patients and demonstrating empathy in patient interactions?
- How can new graduate nurses involve patients in shared decision-making and respect their autonomy?
- What role does cultural competence play in providing patient-centered care, and how can new graduate nurses develop cultural sensitivity?
- How can interdisciplinary collaboration contribute to patient-centered care, and what are some ways new graduate nurses can actively participate in interdisciplinary teams?
- What ethical considerations should new graduate nurses be aware of when providing patient-centered care?
- How can new graduate nurses advocate for patients and ensure their needs and preferences are respected in the healthcare setting?
- What are the benefits and challenges of utilizing technology in patient-centered care, and how can new graduate nurses navigate these challenges?
- How can new graduate nurses evaluate the effectiveness of their patient-centered care practices and continuously improve their skills in this area?

References

Baek H, Han K, Cho H, Ju J (2023) Nursing teamwork is essential in promoting patient-centered care: a cross-sectional study. BMC Nurs 22(1):433. https://doi.org/10.1186/s12912-023-01592-3

Cheraghi R, Valizadeh L, Zamanzadeh V, Hassankhani H, Jafarzadeh A (2023) Clarification of ethical principle of the beneficence in nursing care: an integrative review. BMC Nurs 22(1):89. https://doi.org/10.1186/s12912-023-01246-4

Kurt D, Gurdogan EP (2023) Professional autonomy and patient advocacy in nurses. Collegian 30(2):327–334. https://doi.org/10.1016/j.colegn.2022.09.015

Kwame A, Petrucka PM (2021) A literature-based study of patient-centered care and communication in nurse-patient interactions: barriers, facilitators, and the way forward. BMC Nurs 20(1):158. https://doi.org/10.1186/s12912-021-00684-2

Sari D, Baysal E, Celik GG, Eser I (2018) Ethical decision-making levels of nursing students. Pak J Med Sci 34(3):724. https://doi.org/10.12669/pjms.343.14922

Varkey B (2021) Principles of clinical ethics and their application to practice. Med Princ Pract 30(1):17–28. https://doi.org/10.1159/000509119

Managing Complex Situations

7

Contents

> Test your learning and check your understanding of this book's contents: use the "Springer Nature Flashcards" app to access questions using ▶ https://sn.pub/pe441e. To use the app, please follow the instructions in Chap. 1.

7.1 Definition of Complex Situation in Healthcare Facilities

Complex situation is defined as challenging and multifaceted situations that require critical thinking, problem-solving, and decision-making skills (Ahmady and Shahbazi 2020; Kim et al. 2021; Silva et al. 2024). These situations often involve uncertainty, ambiguity, and the need to consider multiple factors (Khan et al. 2018). In healthcare, complex situations can involve patients with multiple comorbidities, ethical dilemmas, or situations that require coordination with various healthcare professionals.

The Importance of Critical Thinking and Problem-Solving Skills in Managing Complex Situations
Critical thinking and problem-solving skills are essential for nurses in managing complex situations in nursing. Here are the key reasons why these skills are crucial:

- Clinical decision-making: Critical thinking and problem-solving skills enable nurses to make sound clinical decisions based on evidence, patient assessment, and critical analysis. They help nurses gather relevant information, identify patterns, and evaluate the best course of action to provide safe and effective care.

- Patient safety: Complex situations in nursing often involve high-stakes decisions that can impact patient safety. Critical thinking skills allow nurses to assess risks, anticipate potential complications, and implement appropriate interventions to prevent harm to patients.
- Prioritization and time management: Nurses frequently face situations where multiple tasks and priorities compete for attention. Critical thinking skills help nurses analyze the urgency and importance of each task, make informed decisions about prioritization, and manage their time effectively to ensure optimal patient care.
- Collaboration and interdisciplinary communication: Complex situations often require collaboration with other healthcare professionals. Critical thinking skills enable nurses to effectively communicate their assessments, concerns, and recommendations to the interdisciplinary team. They also facilitate active participation in collaborative problem-solving and decision-making processes.
- Adaptability and flexibility: Nursing is a dynamic field, and complex situations can arise unexpectedly. Critical thinking skills help nurses adapt to changing circumstances, think on their feet, and make quick and effective decisions in high-pressure situations.
- Identifying and managing complications: Complex situations in nursing often involve complications or unexpected outcomes. Critical thinking skills enable nurses to recognize and assess these complications, analyze the underlying causes, and implement appropriate interventions to manage them effectively.
- Ethical decision-making: Complex situations may present ethical dilemmas that require careful consideration and ethical decision-making. Critical thinking skills help nurses analyze ethical principles, consider the perspectives of all stakeholders, and make decisions that uphold patient autonomy, beneficence, and justice.
- Continuous improvement and quality improvement: Critical thinking skills encourage nurses to reflect on their practice, identify areas for improvement, and seek evidence-based solutions to enhance patient outcomes. They also facilitate active participation in quality improvement initiatives to address complex issues and promote best practices.

To develop and enhance critical thinking and problem-solving skills in nursing, nurses can engage in activities such as case studies, simulation exercises, reflective practice, and ongoing education. Seeking mentorship from experienced nurses and participating in interdisciplinary discussions can also foster the development of these skills. Ultimately, honing these skills empowers nurses to navigate complex situations, provide high-quality care, and advocate for the best interests of their patients.

Approach to Assess, Analyze, and Prioritize Patient Needs in Complex and Rapidly Changing Environments

Assessing, analyzing, and prioritizing patient needs in complex and rapidly changing environments require a systematic and organized approach. Here is a suggested approach to help nurses effectively manage these situations:

1. *Initial assessment*
   - Begin by conducting a rapid initial assessment of the patient's condition, focusing on the ABCs (airway, breathing, circulation) and any immediate life-threatening issues.
   - Gather essential information such as vital signs, level of consciousness, and chief complaint.
   - Use your clinical judgment and experience to quickly identify any obvious or immediate needs that require immediate attention.

2. *Gather comprehensive data*
   - Conduct a thorough and systematic assessment to gather comprehensive data about the patient's condition.
   - Collect information related to the patient's medical history, current symptoms, medications, allergies, and any recent changes in their condition.
   - Utilize appropriate assessment tools and techniques to gather objective data, such as physical examinations, diagnostic tests, and laboratory results.

3. *Analyze and prioritize*
   - Analyze the collected data to identify patterns, trends, and potential complications.
   - Use critical thinking skills to prioritize patient needs based on the severity of the condition, potential for deterioration, and the patient's overall stability.
   - Consider the patient's physiological, psychological, and social needs when determining priorities.

4. *Consider the context*
   - Take into account the specific context and environment in which the patient is situated.
   - Consider factors such as available resources, staffing levels, and the acuity of other patients in the area.
   - Adapt your approach and priorities based on the unique circumstances of the situation.

5. *Collaborate and communicate*
   - Engage in effective communication and collaboration with the interdisciplinary team, including physicians, other nurses, and allied healthcare professionals.
   - Share relevant information, observations, and concerns to ensure a comprehensive understanding of the patient's needs.
   - Seek input and guidance from experienced colleagues or supervisors when faced with complex or rapidly changing situations.

6. *Reassess and adjust*
   - Continuously reassess the patient's condition and response to interventions.

- Modify the plan of care as needed based on new information or changes in the patient's condition.
- Prioritize ongoing monitoring and reassessment to identify any emerging needs or complications.

7. *Document and evaluate*
   - Document all assessments, interventions, and changes in the patient's condition accurately and in a timely manner.
   - Evaluate the effectiveness of interventions and the patient's response to treatment.
   - Reflect on the outcomes and identify areas for improvement in managing complex and rapidly changing situations.

Practice and experience play a significant role in developing proficiency in assessing, analyzing, and prioritizing patient needs in complex and rapidly changing environments. Continuously seek opportunities for learning, engage in reflective practice, and seek feedback from experienced colleagues to enhance your skills in managing these situations effectively.

7.2   Key Components of Managing Complex Situations

- Approach to assess, analyze, and prioritize patient needs in complex and rapidly changing environments.
- Importance of interdisciplinary collaboration in coordinating care and seeking input from experts in complex cases.
- The importance of maintaining calmness, prioritizing tasks, and following established protocols in high-stress situations.
- Effectively delegating responsibilities, mobilizing resources, and providing timely interventions to ensure patient safety and positive outcomes.
- The decision-making process, including the consideration of evidence-based practice, ethical principles, and patient preferences.

7.3   Management of Emergencies and Crises

Importance of Maintaining Calmness, Prioritizing Tasks, and Following Established Protocols in High-Stress Situations
Maintaining calmness, prioritizing tasks, and following established protocols are crucial in high-stress situations in healthcare. Here's why these practices are important:

1. *Maintaining calmness*
   - High-stress situations can be chaotic and overwhelming. Maintaining calmness allows healthcare professionals to think clearly, make rational decisions, and provide effective care.

- Calmness helps to create a sense of stability and reassurance for patients and their families, promoting trust and confidence in the healthcare team.
- It enables healthcare professionals to effectively communicate and collaborate with the interdisciplinary team, ensuring coordinated and efficient care.

2. *Prioritizing tasks*
   - High-stress situations often involve multiple tasks and competing priorities. Prioritizing tasks helps healthcare professionals focus on the most critical and time-sensitive actions.
   - Prioritization ensures that urgent and life-threatening needs are addressed promptly, minimizing the risk of adverse outcomes.
   - It helps prevent task overload and allows for efficient use of time and resources, optimizing patient care delivery.

3. *Following established protocols*
   - Established protocols and guidelines are developed based on evidence-based practice and best available evidence. Following these protocols ensures standardized and consistent care delivery.
   - Protocols provide a structured approach to managing specific situations, reducing the risk of errors and improving patient outcomes.
   - They serve as a reference point during high-stress situations, providing guidance and support to healthcare professionals when making critical decisions.

4. *Enhancing patient safety*
   - Maintaining calmness, prioritizing tasks, and following established protocols contribute to patient safety in high-stress situations.
   - Calmness reduces the likelihood of errors and promotes a safe and controlled environment for patient care.
   - Prioritizing tasks ensures that urgent needs are addressed promptly, minimizing the risk of harm to patients.
   - Following established protocols helps healthcare professionals adhere to evidence-based practices, reducing the risk of adverse events and improving patient outcomes.

5. *Promoting teamwork and collaboration*
   - In high-stress situations, effective teamwork and collaboration are essential. Maintaining calmness fosters a positive and collaborative environment, promoting effective communication and cooperation among team members.
   - Prioritizing tasks helps allocate responsibilities and resources efficiently, ensuring that all team members are working toward a common goal.
   - Following established protocols facilitates standardized communication and decision-making, enhancing teamwork and coordination among healthcare professionals.

6. *Reducing stress and burnout*
   - High-stress situations can take a toll on healthcare professionals' well-being. Maintaining calmness, prioritizing tasks, and following established protocols help reduce stress and prevent burnout.
   - Calmness allows healthcare professionals to manage their own stress levels and cope effectively with challenging situations.

– Prioritizing tasks and following protocols provide a structured approach, reducing the feeling of being overwhelmed and increasing confidence in managing high-stress situations.

Maintaining calmness, prioritizing tasks, and following established protocols are essential practices in high-stress situations in healthcare. These practices contribute to patient safety, enhance teamwork and collaboration, and reduce stress for healthcare professionals. By incorporating these practices into their approach, healthcare professionals can effectively navigate high-stress situations and provide optimal care to their patients.

Guidance on How to Effectively Delegate Responsibilities, Mobilize Resources, and Provide Timely Interventions to Ensure Patient Safety and Positive Outcomes

For new graduate nurses, effectively delegating responsibilities, mobilizing resources, and providing timely interventions are critical skills to ensure patient safety and positive outcomes. Here is some guidance to help you in these areas:

1. *Delegating responsibilities*
   – Understand your scope of practice and the scope of practice of other healthcare team members. Delegate tasks that are within their scope and appropriate for their level of expertise.
   – Clearly communicate the task, expectations, and any specific instructions or considerations to the person you are delegating to.
   – Provide necessary information, such as patient background, current condition, and any relevant updates, to ensure the delegated task is performed safely and effectively.
   – Follow up and provide support as needed while also allowing the person you delegated to work independently and take ownership of the task.
2. *Mobilizing resources*
   – Familiarize yourself with the available resources in your healthcare setting, such as equipment, supplies, and support services.
   – Assess the needs of the patient and the situation, and determine which resources are required to provide appropriate care.
   – Communicate effectively with the interdisciplinary team to mobilize the necessary resources. Clearly articulate the patient's needs, the urgency of the situation, and any specific requirements.
   – Advocate for the patient by ensuring that the required resources are obtained in a timely manner.
3. *Providing timely interventions*
   – Stay vigilant and continuously assess the patient's condition. Recognize any changes or deterioration promptly.
   – Prioritize interventions based on the urgency and severity of the patient's condition. Address immediate life-threatening issues first.

- Act quickly and decisively, following established protocols and evidence-based practices.
- Communicate effectively with the interdisciplinary team to coordinate interventions and ensure a timely response.
- Document all interventions and their outcomes accurately and in a timely manner.

4. *Prioritizing patient safety*
   - Make patient safety your top priority in all aspects of care. Be aware of potential risks and take proactive measures to prevent harm.
   - Follow infection control protocols and adhere to patient safety guidelines.
   - Communicate effectively with the patient and their family, providing clear instructions and addressing any concerns or questions they may have.
   - Continuously monitor the patient for any signs of deterioration or complications, and take appropriate action to ensure their safety.

5. *Seek guidance and support*
   - Recognize that as a new graduate nurse, you may encounter situations that require guidance and support.
   - Don't hesitate to ask for help or clarification from experienced colleagues, supervisors, or other healthcare professionals.
   - Engage in ongoing learning and professional development to enhance your knowledge and skills in delegation, resource mobilization, and timely interventions.

Developing these skills takes time and experience. Be open to learning from your experiences, reflect on your practice, and seek feedback to continuously improve. By effectively delegating responsibilities, mobilizing resources, and providing timely interventions, you can contribute to patient safety and positive outcomes as a new graduate nurse.

The Role of Self-Care and Resilience in Managing Complex Situations

Resilience is of utmost importance in nursing due to the demanding and challenging nature of the profession. Here are some key reasons why resilience is crucial for nurses:

1. *Coping with stress and adversity*
   - Nursing can be highly stressful, with long hours, heavy workloads, and exposure to emotionally and physically demanding situations. Resilience helps nurses cope with these stressors and bounce back from adversity.
   - Resilient nurses are better equipped to manage the emotional toll of caring for patients in difficult circumstances, such as dealing with loss, trauma, or challenging patient interactions.
   - By developing resilience, nurses can maintain their well-being and prevent burnout, ensuring they can continue to provide high-quality care.

2. *Adapting to change*
   - The healthcare industry is constantly evolving, with new technologies, treatments, and protocols emerging. Resilience enables nurses to adapt to these changes and embrace new ways of delivering care.
   - Resilient nurses are open to learning and growth, willing to acquire new skills and knowledge to keep up with advancements in healthcare.
   - They can navigate through organizational changes, such as restructuring or policy updates, and remain flexible in their approach to care delivery.
3. *Enhancing problem-solving skills*
   - Resilience fosters strong problem-solving skills, allowing nurses to effectively address challenges and find solutions.
   - Resilient nurses can think critically and creatively, finding innovative ways to overcome obstacles and provide optimal care to their patients.
   - They are able to remain calm and focused during crises, making sound decisions under pressure.
4. *Building strong relationships and communication*
   - Resilience promotes effective communication and the ability to build strong relationships with patients, families, and colleagues.
   - Resilient nurses can effectively communicate with empathy, actively listen, and provide emotional support to patients and their families.
   - They can collaborate and work well within interdisciplinary teams, fostering a positive and supportive work environment.
5. *Improving patient outcomes*
   - Resilient nurses are better equipped to handle the challenges and complexities of patient care, leading to improved patient outcomes.
   - They can maintain a high level of professionalism and provide consistent, safe, and compassionate care even in difficult situations.
   - Resilient nurses are more likely to engage in continuous learning and quality improvement initiatives, contributing to better patient care and outcomes.
6. *Personal growth and self-care*
   - Resilience allows nurses to prioritize their own well-being and engage in self-care practices.
   - Resilient nurses recognize the importance of maintaining their physical, emotional, and mental health to sustain their ability to care for others.
   - They actively seek support, engage in stress-reducing activities, and set boundaries to prevent burnout and promote work-life balance.

Resilience is essential in nursing to cope with stress, adapt to change, enhance problem-solving skills, build relationships, improve patient outcomes, and promote personal growth. By developing resilience, nurses can thrive in their profession and provide the best possible care to their patients.

Self-care and resilience play crucial roles in managing complex situations effectively. Here's how they contribute to navigating and coping with complexity:

1. *Self-care for emotional well-being*
   - Complex situations can be emotionally challenging and draining. Practicing self-care helps maintain emotional well-being, allowing individuals to better manage their emotions and reactions.
   - Engaging in activities that promote relaxation, stress reduction, and emotional balance, such as exercise, mindfulness, hobbies, or spending time with loved ones, can help individuals recharge and maintain resilience.
   - Self-care also involves setting boundaries, recognizing personal limits, and seeking support when needed. Taking care of one's own emotional needs enables individuals to approach complex situations with a clear and balanced mindset.

2. *Resilience for problem-solving*
   - Resilience is the ability to bounce back from adversity and adapt to challenging circumstances. It enables individuals to approach complex situations with a problem-solving mindset.
   - Resilient individuals are more likely to view challenges as opportunities for growth and learning. They can identify potential solutions, think creatively, and adapt their approach as needed.
   - Resilience helps individuals maintain a positive attitude, persistence, and determination in the face of complexity. It allows them to stay focused on finding solutions rather than becoming overwhelmed by the challenges.

3. *Self-care for physical well-being*
   - Complex situations often require individuals to invest significant physical and mental energy. Prioritizing self-care for physical well-being is essential to sustain energy levels and overall health.
   - Adequate sleep, proper nutrition, regular exercise, and taking breaks during demanding situations are all important aspects of self-care. These practices help individuals maintain physical stamina and mental clarity, enabling them to navigate complex situations more effectively.
   - Neglecting physical well-being can lead to fatigue, decreased cognitive function, and increased vulnerability to stress, hindering the ability to manage complexity.

4. *Resilience for adaptability*
   - Complex situations often involve uncertainty, ambiguity, and unexpected changes. Resilience allows individuals to adapt and adjust their strategies and plans as needed.
   - Resilient individuals are open to new information, feedback, and alternative perspectives. They can quickly assess the situation, make necessary adjustments, and remain flexible in their approach.
   - Resilience helps individuals embrace change and view it as an opportunity for growth rather than a threat. This adaptability is crucial in managing complex situations that may require shifting priorities or strategies.

5. *Self-care for reflection and learning*
   - Self-care practices, such as journaling, reflection, and seeking feedback, provide opportunities for individuals to process complex situations and learn from their experiences.
   - Taking time for self-reflection allows individuals to gain insights into their strengths, areas for improvement, and personal triggers in complex situations. This self-awareness contributes to better decision-making and problem-solving skills.
   - Engaging in continuous learning and professional development also falls under self-care. It helps individuals stay updated with new knowledge and skills relevant to managing complexity.

Self-care and resilience are intertwined and essential in managing complex situations. Self-care promotes emotional and physical well-being, enabling individuals to approach complexity with a clear mindset. Resilience allows individuals to adapt, problem-solve, and remain flexible in the face of challenges. By prioritizing self-care and developing resilience, individuals can effectively navigate complex situations and maintain their well-being.

7.4   Conclusion

Navigating and managing complex situations is a crucial skill for new graduate nurses to develop in order to provide optimal patient care. By utilizing critical thinking, effective communication, and teamwork and seeking guidance from experienced nurses and mentors, new graduates can confidently handle challenging situations that may arise in the healthcare setting. It is important for new nurses to continuously learn and grow in their practice, as encountering and managing complex situations will ultimately lead to their growth and success in the nursing profession. Remember, with perseverance, dedication, and a willingness to learn, new graduate nurses can navigate and manage any situation that comes their way.

Applied Practical Exercises
- Case study analysis: Provide new graduate nurses with complex patient case studies and ask them to analyze the situation, identify potential challenges, and develop a plan of action. Encourage them to consider factors such as patient acuity, interdisciplinary collaboration, ethical considerations, and communication strategies.
- Simulation scenarios: Conduct simulation exercises that simulate complex situations, such as a deteriorating patient, a medication error, or a conflict within the healthcare team. Allow new graduate nurses to practice their critical thinking, decision-making, and communication skills in a

controlled environment. Provide debriefing sessions to discuss their actions, strengths, and areas for improvement.

- Team-based problem-solving: Divide new graduate nurses into small groups and present them with a complex situation. Assign each group member a specific role within the healthcare team (e.g., nurse, physician, pharmacist), and ask them to collaborate and develop a comprehensive plan to address the situation. Encourage them to consider different perspectives, communicate effectively, and make decisions collectively.

- Ethical dilemma discussions: Present new graduate nurses with ethical dilemmas commonly encountered in healthcare settings. Facilitate group discussions where they can explore different viewpoints, analyze the ethical principles involved, and propose solutions. Encourage them to consider the potential consequences of their decisions and reflect on the impact on patient care.

- Emergency response drills: Organize emergency response drills where new graduate nurses can practice their skills in managing critical situations, such as cardiac arrest or respiratory distress. Provide them with scenarios, equipment, and simulated patients, and assess their ability to prioritize tasks, communicate effectively, and provide appropriate interventions under pressure.

- Reflection and self-assessment: Assign new graduate nurses to keep a reflective journal where they document complex situations they have encountered during their clinical practice. Encourage them to reflect on their actions, emotions, and lessons learned. Provide guidance on self-assessment tools that can help them identify areas for improvement, and set goals for professional development.

- Role-playing exercises: Assign new graduate nurse's different roles within a complex situation, such as a patient's family member, a healthcare team leader, or a nurse facing a challenging ethical dilemma. Ask them to role-play these scenarios, allowing them to practice their communication, negotiation, and conflict resolution skills in a safe and supportive environment.

- Critical thinking exercises: Provide new graduate nurses with critical thinking exercises that require them to analyze complex situations, identify potential risks, and propose strategies to mitigate those risks. Encourage them to consider evidence-based practice, patient safety principles, and interdisciplinary collaboration in their decision-making process.

- These applied practical exercises provide new graduate nurses with opportunities to apply their knowledge and skills in managing complex situations. They promote critical thinking, decision-making, effective communication, and collaboration, helping new nurses develop the confidence and competence needed to navigate challenging healthcare scenarios.

References

Ahmady S, Shahbazi S (2020) Impact of social problem-solving training on critical think-ing and decision making of nursing students. BMC Nurs 19(1):94. https://doi.org/10.1186/s12912-020-00487-x

Khan S, Vandermorris A, Shepherd J, Begun JW, Lanham HJ, Uhl-Bien M, Berta W (2018) Embracing uncertainty, managing complexity: applying complexity thinking principles to transformation efforts in healthcare systems. BMC Health Serv Res 18:1–8. https://doi.org/10.1186/s12913-018-2994-0

Kim YH, Kang YA, Ok JH, Choe K (2021) Expert nurses' coping strategies in ethically chal-lenging situations: a qualitative study. BMC Nurs 20:1–8. https://doi.org/10.1186/s12912-021-00709-w

Silva, A., Dupuis, K.L., Dhanani, S., James, L., Lotherington, K. e Silva VS (2024) Coping strate-gies used by registered nurses in acute and critical care settings: a scoping review protocol. Crit Care Nurs 11. https://cjccn.ca/wp-content/uploads/2024/06/CJCCN-2024-Spring-final.pdf#page=11

Cultural Competence Skills

8

Contents

> Test your learning and check your understanding of this book's contents: use the "Springer Nature Flashcards" app to access questions using ▶ https://sn.pub/pe441e. To use the app, please follow the instructions in Chap. 1.

8.1   Definition of Cultural Competence

Cultural competence skill refers to the ability to effectively work with individuals from diverse cultural backgrounds and provide care that is sensitive to their cultural beliefs, values, and practices (DiBiasio et al. 2023; Schouten et al. 2023). Cultural competence involves understanding and respecting cultural differences, addressing health disparities, and promoting equitable care.

The Significance of Cultural Competence in Nursing Practice

Cultural competence in nursing practice is of utmost importance as it allows nurses to effectively care for patients from diverse backgrounds. By being culturally competent, nurses can better understand their patients' beliefs, values, and practices, leading to improved communication and trust between the nurse and patient. This ultimately results in better health outcomes as patients are more likely to adhere to treatment plans and feel supported in their healthcare journey. Additionally, cultural competence helps to reduce disparities in healthcare and promotes a more inclusive and respectful healthcare environment for all individuals. In today's globalized world, cultural competence is essential for nurses to provide high-quality and patient-centered care to a diverse population.

Cultural Competence as a Lifelong Journey

Cultural competence is not something that can be achieved overnight; rather, it is a lifelong journey that requires ongoing learning and reflection. As individuals interact with people from different cultures, they must continuously educate themselves about different customs, beliefs, and perspectives in order to build understanding and empathy. This journey involves stepping out of one's comfort zone, challenging assumptions, and actively seeking out opportunities to engage with diverse communities. By committing to this ongoing process of self-improvement, individuals can continue to grow and evolve in their ability to navigate and appreciate the rich tapestry of human diversity. Ultimately, cultural competence is not a destination, but a continuous path toward greater awareness and inclusivity.

Core Skills and Strategies to Develop and Enhance Their Cultural Competence

Developing and enhancing cultural competence is essential for individuals to effectively navigate diverse cultural contexts. Here are some core skills and strategies to develop and enhance cultural competence:

- Self-awareness: Start by reflecting on your own cultural background, biases, and assumptions. Understand how your own cultural experiences shape your perspectives and behaviors.
- Open-mindedness: Cultivate an open and nonjudgmental attitude toward different cultures. Be willing to learn and appreciate diverse perspectives, values, and practices.
- Cultural knowledge: Educate yourself about different cultures, including their history, traditions, customs, and social norms. Read books, watch documentaries, and engage in conversations with people from different cultural backgrounds.
- Active listening: Practice active listening when interacting with individuals from different cultures. Pay attention to their verbal and nonverbal cues, and try to understand their perspectives without imposing your own biases.
- Empathy and respect: Cultivate empathy and respect for individuals from different cultures. Recognize and value their unique experiences, beliefs, and values.
- Flexibility and adaptability: Be open to adapting your behavior and communication style to accommodate cultural differences. Recognize that what may be considered appropriate in one culture may not be in another.
- Cross-cultural communication: Develop effective cross-cultural communication skills. This includes being mindful of language barriers, using clear and concise language, and being sensitive to cultural nuances in verbal and nonverbal communication.
- Building relationships: Actively seek opportunities to build relationships with individuals from different cultures. Engage in meaningful conversations,

participate in cultural events, and collaborate on projects that promote cultural understanding and inclusivity.

- Continuous learning: Cultivate a mindset of continuous learning and improvement. Stay updated on current cultural trends, global issues, and intercultural communication strategies.
- Seek feedback: Regularly seek feedback from individuals from different cultures to understand how your actions and behaviors are perceived. Use this feedback to make necessary adjustments and improve your cultural competence.

Developing cultural competence is an ongoing process that requires self-reflection, learning, and practice. By actively engaging with diverse cultures and embracing cultural differences, you can enhance your cultural competence and become more effective in multicultural settings.

Importance of Effective Communication in Cultural Competence

Effective communication plays a crucial role in cultural competence in nursing. As healthcare providers, nurses must be able to understand and respect the diverse cultural backgrounds of their patients in order to provide optimal care. Culturally competent communication involves not only speaking the same language as the patient but also being sensitive to their beliefs, customs, and values. By effectively communicating with patients from different cultures, nurses can build trust, establish rapport, and ensure that the patient's needs and preferences are understood and addressed. This can ultimately lead to better health outcomes and a more positive healthcare experience for all parties involved. Therefore, developing strong communication skills is essential for nurses to uphold cultural competence and provide quality care to a diverse patient population.

Effective communication is crucial in fostering cultural competence within any organization or community. When individuals are able to effectively communicate with people from different cultures, they are better able to understand and appreciate those cultural differences. This leads to a more inclusive and diverse environment where everyone feels respected and valued. Effective communication also helps to avoid misunderstandings and conflicts that can arise from cultural differences. By being able to communicate clearly and respectfully with people from diverse backgrounds, individuals can work together more harmoniously and create a more cohesive and supportive community. In essence, effective communication is the key to building cultural competence and promoting diversity and inclusivity.

8.2   Cultural Assessment in Nursing Practice

Cultural assessment in nursing practice is the process of evaluating a patient's cultural beliefs, values, practices, and preferences in order to provide culturally competent care. This assessment helps nurses understand how a patient's cultural background may influence their health beliefs, treatment decisions, and overall health outcomes. By being aware of and sensitive to cultural differences, nurses can better tailor their care to meet the unique needs and preferences of each individual patient. Cultural assessment includes asking open-ended questions, actively listening to patients, and recognizing the importance of cultural considerations in providing effective and holistic care. Ultimately, cultural assessment plays a crucial role in promoting patient-centered care and addressing health disparities among diverse populations.

The Significance of Cultural Assessment in Nursing Practice
Cultural assessment plays a crucial role in nursing practice as it allows healthcare professionals to provide more effective and culturally competent care to their patients. By understanding a patient's cultural background, beliefs, values, and practices, nurses can tailor their care to meet the individual needs and preferences of each patient. This can help improve communication between nurses and patients, increase patient satisfaction, and ultimately lead to better health outcomes. Additionally, cultural assessment helps nurses to identify and address any cultural barriers that may impact a patient's healthcare experience. Overall, incorporating cultural assessment into nursing practice is essential for providing high-quality, patient-centered care.

Guidance on Conducting Culturally Sensitive Assessments
Conducting culturally sensitive assessments is essential for new graduate nurses to provide quality and patient-centered care to individuals from diverse cultural backgrounds. Here are some guidance and tips for new graduate nurses on conducting culturally sensitive assessments:

- Develop cultural awareness: Start by developing cultural awareness and understanding your own biases and assumptions. Recognize that cultural beliefs, values, and practices may influence a patient's health beliefs and behaviors.
- Respect and dignity: Treat every patient with respect, dignity, and sensitivity. Be mindful of cultural norms regarding personal space, eye contact, and touch. Use appropriate titles and honorifics based on cultural preferences.
- Build rapport and trust: Take the time to build rapport and establish trust with the patient. Use active listening skills, show empathy, and validate their experiences. This can help create a safe and open environment for the patient to share their health concerns.
- Use open-ended questions: Ask open-ended questions that allow patients to share their health beliefs, practices, and concerns in their own words. Avoid assumptions and stereotypes. Encourage patients to express their thoughts and feelings without judgment.
- Use culturally appropriate language: Use language that is culturally appropriate and easily understood by the patient. Avoid medical jargon and complex terminology. Consider using professional interpreters or language services if needed.
- Understand health beliefs and practices: Learn about the cultural beliefs, values, and practices that may influence a patient's health. This includes understanding

concepts of health and illness, traditional healing practices, and dietary preferences.

- Assess social determinants of health: Consider the social determinants of health that may impact the patient's well-being, such as socioeconomic status, education, housing, and access to healthcare. These factors can influence health outcomes and treatment plans.
- Incorporate family and community: Recognize the importance of family and community in the patient's healthcare decision-making process. Involve family members or trusted individuals in discussions with the patient, if appropriate and with their consent.
- Be mindful of nonverbal communication: Be aware of nonverbal communication cues that may vary across cultures. Facial expressions, body language, and gestures may have different meanings in different cultures. Be sensitive to these differences.
- Seek cultural consultation: If you encounter a patient from a cultural background that you are unfamiliar with, seek cultural consultation from colleagues, cultural liaisons, or community resources. They can provide valuable insights and guidance.
- Document cultural considerations: Document any cultural considerations or preferences discussed during the assessment. This information can help inform the patient's plan of care and ensure continuity of culturally sensitive care.

Cultural competence is an ongoing process of learning and growth. Continuously educate yourself, seek feedback, and reflect on your own practice to improve your cultural sensitivity and provide the best possible care to your patients from diverse cultural backgrounds.

The Need for New Graduate Nurses to Approach Cultural Assessment with Humility, Respect, and Sensitivity
As new graduate nurses enter the workforce, it is crucial for them to approach cultural assessment with humility, respect, and sensitivity. Understanding and respecting the diverse cultures and beliefs of their patients is essential in providing effective and patient-centered care. Without approaching cultural assessment with these qualities, there is a risk of unintentionally causing harm or perpetuating stereotypes. By approaching cultural assessment with humility, new graduate nurses can acknowledge that they may not have all the answers and are open to learning from their patients. Respect allows them to honor the values and beliefs of their patients, fostering trust and cooperation. Lastly, sensitivity enables them to communicate effectively and empathize with their patients, ultimately leading to better outcomes and improved patient satisfaction. In today's ever-evolving healthcare landscape, it is more important than ever for new graduate nurses to prioritize cultural competence in their practice.

The Challenges and Barriers That New Graduate Nurses May Encounter When Striving to Become Culturally Competent

New graduate nurses may encounter several challenges and barriers when striving to become culturally competent. These challenges can arise from various factors, including personal, organizational, and systemic barriers. Here are some common challenges and barriers that new graduate nurses may face:

- Limited cultural knowledge: New graduate nurses may have limited knowledge and understanding of different cultures, including their beliefs, values, and healthcare practices. This lack of knowledge can hinder their ability to provide culturally competent care.
- Time constraints: New graduate nurses often face time constraints in their clinical practice. This can make it challenging to spend sufficient time with patients to understand their cultural backgrounds and provide individualized care.
- Language barriers: Language barriers can pose a significant challenge in providing culturally competent care. New graduate nurses may struggle to communicate effectively with patients who have limited English proficiency, leading to misunderstandings and potential gaps in care.
- Bias and stereotypes: Unconscious biases and stereotypes can influence the perceptions and interactions of new graduate nurses with patients from different cultural backgrounds. These biases can hinder the development of cultural competence and lead to disparities in care.
- Lack of cultural awareness training: Some healthcare organizations may not provide adequate cultural awareness training for new graduate nurses. Without proper training, nurses may not have the necessary skills and knowledge to navigate cultural differences and provide culturally competent care.
- Organizational culture: The organizational culture within healthcare settings can either support or hinder the development of cultural competence. If the organizational culture does not prioritize diversity, inclusion, and cultural competence, new graduate nurses may face barriers in their efforts to become culturally competent.
- Limited resources: Limited access to resources, such as interpreters, cultural competency guides, and educational materials, can impede new graduate nurses' ability to provide culturally competent care. Lack of resources can make it challenging to address the unique needs of patients from diverse cultural backgrounds.
- Ethical dilemmas: New graduate nurses may encounter ethical dilemmas when providing care to patients from different cultural backgrounds. Balancing cultural beliefs and practices with evidence-based care can be challenging and require careful consideration.
- Resistance to change: Resistance to change within healthcare systems and among colleagues can be a barrier to developing cultural competence. Some healthcare professionals may be resistant to adopting new practices or approaches that promote cultural competence.
- Lack of support and mentorship: New graduate nurses may lack support and mentorship from experienced nurses who can guide them in their journey toward

cultural competence. Without proper support, it can be challenging to navigate the complexities of providing culturally competent care.

It is important for healthcare organizations to recognize and address these challenges and barriers by providing ongoing education, training, and support for new graduate nurses. By addressing these barriers, healthcare organizations can create an environment that promotes cultural competence and improves the quality of care for patients from diverse cultural backgrounds.

Strategies for Overcoming These Barriers
To overcome the barriers and challenges that new graduate nurses may face in their journey towards cultural competence, several strategies can be implemented. Here are some strategies to consider:

- Cultural competence training: Provide comprehensive cultural competence training programs for new graduate nurses. These programs should focus on increasing cultural awareness, knowledge, and skills. Include topics such as cultural beliefs, practices, healthcare disparities, and effective communication strategies.
- Mentorship and preceptorship programs: Establish mentorship and preceptorship programs that pair new graduate nurses with experienced nurses who have a strong understanding of cultural competence. Mentors can provide guidance and support and share their experiences to help new nurses navigate cultural challenges.
- Language services: Ensure access to language interpretation services to overcome language barriers. Provide training on how to effectively utilize interpreters and promote the use of professional interpreters to ensure accurate communication with patients who have limited English proficiency.
- Cultural liaisons and resources: Designate cultural liaisons within the healthcare organization who can serve as resources for new graduate nurses. These liaisons can provide guidance, answer questions, and offer cultural insights to support culturally competent care.
- Incorporate cultural competence in orientation programs: Include cultural competence as a core component of the orientation programs for new graduate nurses. This will help set the foundation for understanding the importance of cultural competence and provide them with the necessary tools and resources.
- Encourage self-reflection and awareness: Promote self-reflection and awareness among new graduate nurses regarding their own biases and assumptions. Encourage them to continuously examine their beliefs and attitudes toward different cultures and seek opportunities for personal growth.
- Create a supportive organizational culture: Foster a supportive organizational culture that values diversity, inclusion, and cultural competence. Encourage open discussions about cultural differences, provide opportunities for learning and growth, and recognize and celebrate efforts toward cultural competence.
- Provide access to resources: Ensure that new graduate nurses have access to resources and tools that support their cultural competence journey. This can

include cultural assessment tools, cultural competency guides, and educational materials on specific cultural groups.

- Collaborative approach: Encourage collaboration and teamwork among healthcare professionals from different cultural backgrounds. Foster an environment where knowledge and experiences are shared and where colleagues can learn from each other's cultural perspectives.
- Continuous education and professional development: Offer ongoing education and professional development opportunities that focus on cultural competence. This can include workshops, seminars, webinars, and conferences that explore current research and best practices in culturally competent care.
- Evaluate and provide feedback: Regularly evaluate the cultural competence of new graduate nurses and provide constructive feedback. This feedback can help identify areas for improvement and provide opportunities for growth.

By implementing these strategies, healthcare organizations can help new graduate nurses overcome barriers and challenges in their journey toward cultural competence. This will ultimately enhance the quality of care provided to diverse patient populations and promote health equity.

Support for New Graduate Nurses in Their Journey Toward Cultural Competence

- Support for new graduate nurses in their journey toward cultural competence is crucial for providing quality and equitable healthcare to diverse patient populations. Here are some ways to support new graduate nurses in developing cultural competence:
- Cultural competence training: Provide comprehensive training programs that focus on cultural awareness, sensitivity, and competence. This can include workshops, seminars, and online courses that cover topics such as cultural beliefs, practices, and healthcare disparities.
- Mentorship programs: Pair new graduate nurses with experienced nurses who have a strong understanding of cultural competence. Mentors can provide guidance, share their experiences, and help new nurses navigate challenging situations related to cultural differences.
- Diversity and inclusion initiatives: Create a supportive and inclusive work environment that values diversity. Encourage open discussions about cultural differences, promote cultural celebrations, and provide resources for learning about different cultures.
- Cultural immersion experiences: Offer opportunities for new graduate nurses to immerse themselves in different cultures. This can include clinical rotations in diverse communities, international healthcare experiences, or partnerships with community organizations.
- Ongoing education and professional development: Provide continuous education and professional development opportunities that focus on cultural competence.

This can include conferences, webinars, and journal clubs that explore current research and best practices in culturally competent care.

- Resources and tools: Make resources and tools readily available to new graduate nurses to support their learning and practice. This can include cultural assessment tools, language interpretation services, and cultural competency guides.
- Feedback and evaluation: Regularly provide feedback and evaluation to new graduate nurses on their cultural competence skills. This can help identify areas for improvement and provide opportunities for growth.
- Collaboration and teamwork: Encourage collaboration and teamwork among healthcare professionals from different cultural backgrounds. This can foster a supportive environment where knowledge and experiences are shared, leading to improved cultural competence.
- Community engagement: Encourage new graduate nurses to engage with the local community and build relationships with diverse patient populations. This can include volunteering at community events, participating in cultural awareness initiatives, and partnering with community organizations.
- Continuous support and encouragement: Provide ongoing support and encouragement to new graduate nurses in their journey toward cultural competence. Recognize their efforts, celebrate their successes, and provide resources for self-reflection and personal growth.

By implementing these strategies, healthcare organizations can support new graduate nurses in their journey toward cultural competence, ultimately improving the quality of care provided to diverse patient populations.

The Importance of Cultural Competence in Promoting Health Equity and Reducing Healthcare Disparities
Cultural competence plays a crucial role in promoting health equity and reducing healthcare disparities. By understanding and respecting the cultural beliefs, values, and norms of diverse populations, healthcare providers can better engage with their patients and provide more effective and tailored care. This means addressing language barriers, acknowledging historical traumas, and being sensitive to cultural preferences and practices. When healthcare providers are culturally competent, they can build trust with their patients, improve health outcomes, and ultimately decrease disparities in healthcare access and quality. It is essential for healthcare systems to prioritize cultural competence in order to ensure that all individuals have equal access to quality care and can achieve optimal health outcomes.

Nurses' Role in Advocating for Culturally Appropriate Care and Addressing Systemic Barriers That May Disproportionately Affect Certain Cultural Groups
Nurses play a crucial role in advocating for culturally appropriate care and addressing systemic barriers that may disproportionately affect certain cultural groups. Here are some ways in which nurses can fulfill this role:

- Cultural assessment: Nurses can conduct cultural assessments to understand the beliefs, values, and practices of patients from different cultural backgrounds. This helps in providing individualized care that respects and incorporates the patient's cultural preferences.
- Communication and language: Nurses can bridge the communication gap by using interpreters or language services to ensure effective communication with patients who have limited English proficiency. They can also learn basic phrases in different languages to establish rapport and trust with patients.
- Cultural sensitivity and respect: Nurses should demonstrate cultural sensitivity and respect toward patients' beliefs, values, and practices. This includes avoiding stereotypes, being open-minded, and actively listening to patients' concerns and preferences.
- Advocacy for culturally appropriate care: Nurses can advocate for policies and practices that promote culturally appropriate care within healthcare organizations. This may involve collaborating with interdisciplinary teams, participating in cultural competency training, and providing feedback on policies and procedures.
- Addressing systemic barriers: Nurses can identify and address systemic barriers that may disproportionately affect certain cultural groups. This can include advocating for equitable access to healthcare services, addressing language barriers, and promoting diversity and inclusion within healthcare organizations.
- Health education and promotion: Nurses can provide culturally tailored health education materials and programs to empower patients from different cultural backgrounds. This helps in promoting health literacy and reducing health disparities.
- Collaboration with community resources: Nurses can collaborate with community organizations and resources to ensure that patients have access to culturally appropriate support services. This may involve connecting patients with community health centers, social services, and cultural organizations.

By fulfilling these roles, nurses can contribute to providing culturally appropriate care and addressing systemic barriers, ultimately improving health outcomes for all cultural groups.

8.3   Conclusion

In conclusion, it is imperative for nurses to develop cultural competence skills in their practice in order to provide quality care to patients from diverse backgrounds. By understanding and respecting the beliefs, values, and practices of different cultures, nurses can establish trust and build strong relationships with their patients. This ultimately leads to improved communication, better health outcomes, and a more positive overall experience for both the patient and the healthcare provider. Cultural competence skills also help nurses to navigate potential challenges and barriers that may arise when caring for patients from different cultural backgrounds.

Overall, integrating cultural competence into nursing practice is essential for providing holistic and patient-centered care.

Review Questions
- What is cultural competence and why is it important for new graduate nurses to develop this skill?
- How does effective communication contribute to cultural competence in nursing practice?
- What are some strategies that new graduate nurses can employ to enhance their cultural competence?
- Why is cultural assessment an essential component of nursing practice? What are some key considerations when conducting culturally sensitive assessments?
- What are some common challenges and barriers that new graduate nurses may face when striving to become culturally competent? How can these barriers be overcome?
- How does cultural competence contribute to promoting health equity and reducing healthcare disparities?
- What are some misconceptions, biases, and stereotypes that can hinder effective cross-cultural interactions? How can nurses address and overcome these biases?
- How can new graduate nurses advocate for culturally appropriate care and address systemic barriers that may disproportionately affect certain cultural groups?
- Why is cultural competence considered a lifelong journey? What are some strategies for continuous learning and development in this area?
- How can new graduate nurses embrace cultural diversity and seek opportunities for cultural immersion and education in their practice?

References

DiBiasio PA, Vallabhajosula S, Eigsti HJ (2023) Assessing cultural competence: a comparison of two measures and their utility in global learning experiences within healthcare education. Physiotherapy 118:97–104. https://doi.org/10.1016/j.physio.2022.09.007

Schouten BC, Manthey L, Scarvaglieri C (2023) Teaching intercultural communication skills in healthcare to improve care for culturally and linguistically diverse patients. Patient Educ Couns 115:107890. https://doi.org/10.1016/j.pec.2023.107890

Part III

Mentorship and Support

In this section, we explore the ongoing journey of professional development, lifelong learning, transitioning to specialty areas, and sustaining clinical competence in the healthcare field. As healthcare practices and technologies continue to evolve, it is crucial for new graduate nurses to stay current, adapt to changes, and continuously enhance their skills and knowledge. The section begins by emphasizing the importance of professional development and lifelong learning in the nursing profession (Chap. 9). It explores the various avenues and opportunities available for new graduate nurses to expand their knowledge, acquire new skills, and stay updated with the latest advancements in their field. By engaging in continuous learning, new graduate nurses can provide the best possible care to their patients and contribute to the advancement of their profession. Next, the section focuses on the transition to specialty areas within healthcare (Chap. 10). It discusses the unique challenges and considerations that new graduate nurses may encounter when transitioning from a general practice to a specialized area. It explores strategies for acquiring specialized knowledge, developing specific skills, and adapting to the unique demands of the specialty. By effectively navigating this transition, new graduate nurses can excel in their chosen specialty and provide specialized care to their patients. Furthermore, the section addresses the importance of sustaining clinical competence throughout one's career (Chap. 11). It explores strategies for maintaining and enhancing clinical skills, staying updated with evidence-based practices, and engaging in self-assessment and reflection. It emphasizes the significance of embracing a growth mindset, seeking feedback, and actively participating in professional development activities. By sustaining clinical competence, healthcare professionals can continue to provide high-quality care, adapt to changes in their field, and meet the evolving needs of their patients. The section highlights the role of mentorship and collaboration in professional development and sustaining clinical competence. It discusses the benefits of seeking guidance from experienced professionals, engaging in interdisciplinary collaboration, and participating in professional networks and organizations. By leveraging these resources, new graduate nurses can gain valuable insights, expand their professional network, and foster a culture of continuous learning and improvement. Finally, this section provides valuable insights and guidance for new graduate nurses in their journey of professional development, lifelong learning, transitioning to specialty areas, and sustaining clinical competence. By embracing these principles, healthcare professionals can stay current, adapt to changes, excel in their chosen specialty, and provide the best possible care to their patients throughout their careers. Ultimately, this commitment to ongoing learning and growth contributes to the advancement of the nursing profession as a whole.

Professional Development and Lifelong Learning

9

Contents

> Test your learning and check your understanding of this book's contents: use the "Springer Nature Flashcards" app to access questions using ▶ https:// sn.pub/pe441c. To use the app, please follow the instructions in Chap. 1.

9.1 The Rapidly Evolving Nature of Healthcare

Healthcare is an industry that is continuously evolving at a rapid pace. With advancements in technology, research, and treatments, the landscape of healthcare is constantly changing. From the development of new medications and therapies to the implementation of innovative medical devices and procedures, healthcare professionals are constantly adapting to new methods of care. Additionally, the rise of telemedicine and digital health solutions has revolutionized the way patients can access and receive healthcare services. The ongoing advancements in healthcare are not only improving patient outcomes but also shaping the future of medicine for generations to come.

© The Author(s), under exclusive license to Springer Nature Switzerland AG 2024 187
K. Matlhaba, *Enhancing Clinical Competence of Graduate Nurses*,
https://doi.org/10.1007/978-3-031-81407-5_9

The Need for Healthcare Professionals Especially Nurses to Adapt to New Knowledge, Technologies, and Best Practices

In today's rapidly evolving healthcare landscape, the need for healthcare professionals, especially nurses, to adapt to new knowledge, technologies, and best practices has become more crucial than ever. With advancements in medical research, new treatments, and innovative technologies continually emerging, nurses must stay current with the latest developments to provide the best possible care for their patients. By staying informed and continuously learning, nurses can improve patient outcomes, enhance their own skills, and contribute to the overall advancement of healthcare. Furthermore, adapting to new knowledge and best practices also ensures that nurses are able to effectively address the changing needs and challenges of the healthcare industry, ultimately leading to better patient care and improved healthcare delivery. It is essential for healthcare professionals to embrace lifelong learning and be open to incorporating new ideas and technologies into their practice in order to stay relevant and provide the highest standard of care to their patients.

That Professional Development is Not Limited to Acquiring New Skills or Knowledge But also Encompasses Personal Growth, Self-Reflection, and the Development of a Professional Identity

Professional development refers to the ongoing process of acquiring and enhancing the knowledge, skills, and competencies necessary for professional growth and advancement in a specific field (Van Beveren et al. 2018). Professional development goes beyond just acquiring new skills and knowledge in a particular field. It also includes aspects such as personal growth, self-reflection, and the development of one's professional identity. In order to truly excel in a career, it is important to not only expand our technical expertise but also to cultivate qualities such as emotional intelligence, resilience, and effective communication skills. Self-reflection allows us to identify areas for improvement and to continuously strive toward becoming the best version of ourselves. Furthermore, developing our professional identity involves understanding our values, beliefs, and goals within the context of our chosen profession. By focusing on these aspects of professional development, individuals can enhance their overall success and satisfaction in their careers.

9.2   Professional Development and Lifelong Learning

Lifelong learning refers to the continuous acquisition of knowledge, skills, and competencies throughout one's professional career (Mlambo et al. 2021; Reychav et al. 2023; World Health Organization 2013). It involves staying updated with current evidence, advancements, and best practices in the field. Lifelong learning is a crucial aspect of nursing practice as it allows nurses to continuously improve their knowledge and skills in order to provide the best possible care for their patients. As the field of healthcare is constantly evolving with new technologies, treatments, and best practices, it is important for nurses to stay up to date on the latest developments. Lifelong learning in nursing practice involves ongoing education, training, and professional development opportunities that enable nurses to enhance their clinical abilities, critical thinking skills, and patient care techniques. By committing to lifelong learning, nurses can ensure that they are equipped to deliver high-quality and evidence-based care throughout their careers. This dedication to continuous learning also demonstrates a commitment to professionalism and a willingness to adapt to change in order to meet the needs of patients and the healthcare system.

9.2.1 Benefits of Continuing Education and Lifelong Learning in Nursing

- Enhanced knowledge and skills: Continuing education and lifelong learning help nurses stay updated with the latest evidence-based practices, technologies, and treatments. This enables them to provide the best possible care to their patients.
- Professional growth and advancement: By continuously learning and expanding their knowledge, nurses can enhance their professional competence and open up opportunities for career advancement, such as specialization or leadership roles.
- Improved patient outcomes: Keeping up with the latest advancements in healthcare through continuing education and lifelong learning allows nurses to provide more effective and evidence-based care, leading to better patient outcomes.
- Personal satisfaction: Lifelong learning can contribute to personal and professional fulfilment by allowing nurses to pursue their interests, develop new skills, and stay engaged in their profession.

Continuing education and lifelong learning are vital for nurses to stay current and competent and provide the best possible care to their patients. It is a lifelong commitment to professional growth and development that benefits both nurses and the healthcare system as a whole.

Embracing a Mindset of Continuous Learning and Professional Growth
Embracing a mindset of continuous learning and professional growth as a new graduate nurse is crucial for your success and development in the nursing profession. Here are some tips to help you cultivate this mindset:

- Recognize the importance of lifelong learning: Understand that nursing is a constantly evolving field and new research, technologies, and best practices emerge regularly. Embrace the idea that learning doesn't stop after graduation but continues throughout your career.
- Stay curious and ask questions: Be curious about your patients, their conditions, and the treatments you provide. Ask questions to your colleagues, mentors, and experienced nurses. Seek opportunities to learn from their expertise and experiences.
- Seek out learning opportunities: Take advantage of continuing education programs, workshops, conferences, and seminars. Look for opportunities to expand your knowledge and skills in areas that interest you or align with your career goals.

- Stay updated with evidence-based practice: Stay current with the latest research and evidence-based guidelines in nursing. Regularly read professional journals, attend webinars, and participate in online forums to stay informed about the latest advancements in your field.
- Set goals for professional development: Identify areas where you want to grow and set goals for yourself. This could include obtaining certifications, pursuing advanced degrees, or developing specific skills. Break down your goals into smaller, achievable steps and create a plan to work toward them.
- Seek mentorship and guidance: Find experienced nurses who can serve as mentors and provide guidance in your professional development. They can offer valuable insights, share their experiences, and provide support as you navigate your nursing career.
- Reflect on your experiences: Take time to reflect on your clinical experiences and identify areas for improvement. Reflective practice allows you to learn from your successes and challenges, and it helps you identify areas where you can grow and develop as a nurse.
- Embrace feedback: Be open to receiving feedback from your colleagues, supervisors, and patients. Constructive feedback can help you identify areas for improvement and guide your professional growth.
- Network with other professionals: Connect with other nurses and healthcare professionals through professional associations, online communities, and networking events. Building a network of peers and mentors can provide valuable support, learning opportunities, and career guidance.
- Take care of yourself: Remember to prioritize self-care and maintain a healthy work-life balance. Continuous learning and professional growth are important, but it's equally important to take care of your physical and mental well-being.

By embracing a mindset of continuous learning and professional growth, you will not only enhance your knowledge and skills as a nurse but also contribute to your personal and professional fulfilment. It will enable you to provide the best possible care to your patients and open up opportunities for career advancement and specialization in the future.

Seeking Opportunities for Further Education, Certifications, and Specialization

As a new graduate nurse, seeking opportunities for further education, certifications, and specialization can greatly enhance your knowledge, skills, and career prospects. Here are some avenues you can explore:

- Advanced degree programs: Consider pursuing an advanced degree such as a Master of Science in Nursing (MSN) or a Doctor of Nursing Practice (DNP). These programs can provide you with specialized knowledge and skills in areas such as nursing leadership, education, informatics, or advanced clinical practice.

- Specialty certifications: Investigate specialty certifications that align with your interests and career goals. Certifications are available in various nursing specialties, such as critical care, pediatrics, oncology, gerontology, and more. These certifications demonstrate your expertise and commitment to a specific area of nursing.
- Continuing education courses: Take advantage of continuing education courses offered by nursing organizations, hospitals, and universities. These courses can help you stay updated with the latest evidence-based practices and advancements in nursing. They may cover topics such as pharmacology, patient safety, wound care, or specific disease management.
- Professional development programs: Many healthcare organizations offer professional development programs for their nurses. These programs may include leadership development, mentorship opportunities, and specialized training in areas such as quality improvement, research, or patient advocacy.
- Specialty training programs: Explore specialty training programs that provide in-depth education and hands-on experience in a specific area of nursing. For example, you may find programs focused on critical care, emergency nursing, labor and delivery, or psychiatric nursing. These programs can help you develop specialized skills and knowledge in your chosen field.
- Research opportunities: If you have an interest in research, seek out research opportunities within your healthcare organization or academic institutions. Participating in research projects can deepen your understanding of evidence-based practice and contribute to advancements in nursing knowledge.
- Professional associations and conferences: Join professional nursing associations related to your area of interest. These associations often offer educational resources, networking opportunities, and access to conferences and workshops. Attending conferences and workshops can expose you to the latest research, best practices, and industry trends.
- Preceptorship and mentorship programs: Seek out preceptorship or mentorship programs that pair you with experienced nurses in your desired specialty. These programs provide valuable guidance, support, and opportunities for learning from seasoned professionals.
- Online learning platforms: Explore online learning platforms that offer nursing-specific courses and certifications. Platforms like Coursera, Udemy, and Nurse.com provide a wide range of courses on various nursing topics, allowing you to learn at your own pace and convenience.
- Collaborate with nurse educators: Engage with nurse educators in your workplace or academic institutions. They can provide guidance on educational opportunities, certifications, and specialization options that align with your career goals.

Remember to research and evaluate the credibility and relevance of any educational programs or certifications you consider. It's important to choose opportunities that align with your interests, career goals, and the needs of your patients and healthcare organization. Continuous learning and professional development will not only enhance your nursing practice but also open doors to new opportunities and advancement in your career.

Staying Updated with Current Evidence-Based Practices and Healthcare Advancements

Staying updated with current evidence-based practices and healthcare advancements is essential for all nurses, including new graduate nurses. Here are some strategies to help you stay informed:

- Read professional journals: Subscribe to reputable nursing journals and publications that focus on evidence-based practice and healthcare advancements. Regularly read articles and research studies to stay updated with the latest findings and recommendations in nursing.
- Join professional associations: Join nursing associations and organizations that provide resources, educational opportunities, and updates on current practices. These associations often publish newsletters, host webinars, and organize conferences that cover the latest trends and advancements in nursing.
- Attend continuing education programs: Take advantage of continuing education programs offered by nursing organizations, hospitals, and universities. These programs often cover topics such as new treatment modalities, emerging technologies, and best practices in various nursing specialties.
- Participate in webinars and online courses: Many nursing organizations and educational institutions offer webinars and online courses on specific topics or areas of interest. These virtual learning opportunities allow you to stay updated from the comfort of your own home and at your own pace.
- Engage in professional development activities: Seek out professional development activities within your workplace or community. This can include attending workshops, seminars, or conferences that focus on evidence-based practice and healthcare advancements.
- Utilize online resources: Explore reputable online resources such as nursing websites, research databases, and healthcare organizations' websites. These platforms often provide access to clinical guidelines, research articles, and educational materials that can help you stay updated.
- Network with colleagues: Engage in discussions with your colleagues, both within your workplace and through online nursing communities. Share knowledge, experiences, and resources to stay informed about current practices and advancements.
- Seek mentorship: Find experienced nurses or nurse educators who can serve as mentors. They can provide guidance and share their expertise on evidence-based practices and healthcare advancements. Regular discussions with a mentor can help you stay updated and gain valuable insights.
- Stay active on social media: Follow reputable nursing organizations, healthcare professionals, and nursing influencers on social media platforms. They often share updates, research findings, and educational resources that can keep you informed about current practices.

- Reflect on your practice: Take time to reflect on your own clinical experiences and patient outcomes. Evaluate the effectiveness of your interventions and seek opportunities for improvement. Reflective practice can help you identify areas where you need to stay updated and enhance your knowledge and skills.

Remember, staying updated with evidence-based practices and healthcare advancements is an ongoing process. Embrace a mindset of continuous learning and make it a priority to stay informed. By doing so, you will provide the best possible care to your patients and contribute to the advancement of nursing practice.

9.3   Mentorship and Collaboration in Professional Development

Mentorship is defined as a relationship in which a more experienced and knowledgeable individual (mentor) provides guidance, support, and advice to a less experienced individual (mentee) to facilitate their personal and professional growth (Khunou and Matlhaba 2023; Wang et al. 2024). Mentorship and collaboration play a crucial role in the professional development of nurses in their practice. Having a mentor provides guidance, support, and opportunities for learning and growth. They can help new nurses navigate the complexities of the healthcare environment, develop their clinical skills, and build their confidence. Collaboration with colleagues also enhances knowledge sharing, teamwork, and the delivery of high-quality patient care. By working together and sharing experiences, nurses can challenge each other to improve their practice and stay current on the latest developments in healthcare. Overall, mentorship and collaboration in nursing practice are essential for ongoing professional development and ensuring the best possible outcomes for patients.

9.3.1   Roles of Mentee and Mentor in the Mentorship Partnership

Mentee and mentor roles play a significant role in professional development and growth. Let's explore the responsibilities and benefits of both roles:

Mentee Role

- Active engagement: As a mentee, it is important to actively engage in the mentoring relationship. This includes being open to learning, seeking guidance, and actively participating in discussions and activities.
- Goal setting: Work with your mentor to set clear and achievable goals for your professional development. These goals can be related to communication skills, career advancement, or specific areas of improvement.
- Seeking guidance: Take initiative in seeking guidance and advice from your mentor. Share your challenges, ask questions, and seek feedback on your

performance. Be receptive to constructive criticism and use it as an opportunity for growth.

- Reflecting and applying: Reflect on the guidance and insights provided by your mentor and apply them to your practice. Actively work on improving your communication skills and implementing the strategies discussed with your mentor.
- Accountability: Hold yourself accountable for your own growth and progress. Take responsibility for following through on action plans and commitments made with your mentor.

Mentor Role

- Guidance and support: As a mentor, provide guidance and support to your mentee. Share your knowledge, expertise, and experiences to help them develop their communication skills and achieve their goals.
- Active listening: Listen attentively to your mentee's concerns, challenges, and goals. Create a safe and supportive environment where they feel comfortable sharing their thoughts and seeking advice.
- Providing feedback: Offer constructive feedback to your mentee on their communication skills. Identify areas for improvement and provide specific suggestions for enhancing their abilities. Encourage their strengths and acknowledge their progress.
- Sharing resources: Share relevant resources, such as articles, books, or training opportunities, that can help your mentee further develop their communication skills. Provide them with tools and techniques they can apply in their practice.
- Encouragement and motivation: Encourage and motivate your mentee to take risks, step out of their comfort zone, and continue their professional development journey. Celebrate their successes and provide support during challenging times.

Benefits for the Mentee

- Personal growth: Mentees can gain valuable insights, knowledge, and skills from their mentors, leading to personal and professional growth.
- Networking opportunities: Mentors can introduce mentees to their professional networks, opening doors to new opportunities and connections.
- Increased confidence: Mentees can gain confidence in their communication skills through the guidance and support of their mentors.
- Career advancement: Effective communication skills can contribute to career advancement opportunities for mentees.

Benefits for the Mentor

- Satisfaction: Mentoring allows mentors to make a positive impact on the professional development of their mentees, leading to a sense of fulfilment.

- Skill development: Mentoring provides an opportunity for mentors to enhance their leadership, coaching, and communication skills.
- Knowledge sharing: Mentors can share their expertise and experiences, contributing to the growth and development of the nursing profession.
- Networking: Mentoring relationships can expand mentors' professional networks and create new connections.

The mentee and mentor roles are essential for professional development. As a mentee, actively engage in the mentoring relationship, seek guidance, and apply the insights provided by your mentor. As a mentor, provide guidance, support, and feedback to your mentee, and contribute to their growth and development. Both roles offer numerous benefits, including personal growth, increased confidence, and networking opportunities.

9.3.2   The Role of Mentorship in Professional Development

Mentorship plays a crucial role in the professional development of individuals, as it provides guidance, support, and opportunities for growth and learning. A mentor can offer valuable insights, share their own experiences, and help navigate the challenges and obstacles that one may face in their career. Through mentorship, individuals can receive feedback, advice, and encouragement that can help them develop their skills, expand their knowledge, and make informed decisions about their career path. By fostering a relationship with a mentor, individuals can gain access to new perspectives, expand their network, and ultimately enhance their professional development and achieve their goals.

Seeking Feedback from Preceptors, Mentors, and Colleagues
Seeking feedback from preceptors, mentors, and colleagues is an effective way to gain valuable insights into your performance and areas for improvement. Here are some steps to help you seek feedback effectively:

- Choose the right time and place: Find a suitable time and place to have a conversation with your preceptors, mentors, or colleagues. Ensure that both parties are comfortable and have enough time for a meaningful discussion.
- Be specific about what you want feedback on: Before approaching someone for feedback, be clear about the specific areas or aspects of your work that you would like feedback on. This will help guide the conversation and ensure that you receive targeted feedback.
- Be open and receptive: Approach the feedback conversation with an open mind and a willingness to listen. Be prepared to receive both positive feedback and constructive criticism. Remember that feedback is meant to help you grow and improve.
- Ask open-ended questions: Instead of asking yes or no questions, ask open-ended questions that encourage detailed responses. For example, instead of asking, "Did I do a good job?", ask, "What are some areas where I can improve?".

- Actively listen and take notes: During the feedback conversation, actively listen to what the other person is saying. Take notes to capture important points and suggestions. This will show that you value their feedback and are committed to learning and growth.
- Seek clarification if needed: If you do not fully understand a piece of feedback or need further clarification, do not hesitate to ask for more information. Seek examples or specific instances to help you better understand the feedback.
- Reflect on the feedback: After the conversation, take some time to reflect on the feedback you received. Consider how it aligns with your own self-assessment and identify any patterns or recurring themes.
- Develop an action plan: Based on the feedback you received, develop an action plan to address the areas for improvement. Set specific goals and outline the steps you will take to work toward those goals.
- Follow up and show appreciation: Once you have implemented changes based on the feedback, follow up with the person who provided the feedback. Share your progress and express your appreciation for their guidance and support.

Remember, seeking feedback is an ongoing process. Regularly check in with your preceptors, mentors, and colleagues to continue receiving feedback and refining your skills. Embrace feedback as an opportunity for growth and improvement.

Engaging in Constructive Conversations to Gain Insights and Perspectives
Engaging in constructive conversations is a powerful way to gain insights and perspectives from others. Here are some tips to help you have meaningful and productive conversations:

- Create a safe and respectful environment: Foster an atmosphere of trust and respect where everyone feels comfortable expressing their thoughts and opinions. Encourage open dialog and ensure that everyone has an equal opportunity to contribute.
- Listen actively: Practice active listening by giving your full attention to the person speaking. Avoid interrupting and genuinely try to understand their perspective. Show empathy and validate their feelings and experiences.
- Ask open-ended questions: Use open-ended questions to encourage the other person to share their thoughts in more detail. Avoid leading questions or questions that can be answered with a simple "yes" or "no." Instead, ask questions that invite deeper reflection and discussion.
- Seek clarification: If you do not fully understand something the other person said, ask for clarification. Paraphrase their statements to ensure you have understood correctly. This demonstrates your genuine interest in understanding their perspective.
- Express your own thoughts and opinions respectfully: Share your own thoughts and opinions in a respectful manner. Use "I" statements to express your perspective and avoid making assumptions or generalizations. Be open to the possibility of changing your viewpoint based on new insights.

- Practice empathy and perspective-taking: Try to put yourself in the other person's shoes and understand their point of view. Consider their background, experiences, and beliefs that may shape their perspective. This can help you develop a more comprehensive understanding of the topic at hand.
- Stay focused on the topic: Keep the conversation focused on the specific topic or issue you want insights on. Avoid getting sidetracked or going off on tangents. This will help maintain clarity and ensure that the conversation remains productive.
- Manage emotions and conflicts: Emotions can sometimes run high during discussions. If conflicts arise, remain calm and composed. Use active listening and empathy to de-escalate tensions and find common ground. Remember that the goal is to gain insights and perspectives, not to win an argument.
- Reflect on the conversation: After the conversation, take some time to reflect on the insights and perspectives you gained. Consider how they align with your own thoughts and beliefs. Use this reflection to broaden your understanding and potentially reshape your own perspectives.

Engaging in constructive conversations requires active participation, respect, and a willingness to learn from others. By embracing different viewpoints and seeking diverse perspectives, you can gain valuable insights and broaden your understanding of various topics.

Establishing Mentorship Relationships to Support Personal and Professional Development

Establishing mentorship relationships can be incredibly beneficial for personal and professional development. Here are some steps to help you establish and nurture mentorship relationships:

- Identify your goals and needs: Before seeking a mentor, clarify your goals and needs. Determine what specific areas you want to develop or improve in your personal and professional life. This will help you find a mentor who aligns with your goals and can provide relevant guidance.
- Research potential mentors: Look for individuals who have expertise and experience in the areas you want to focus on. Consider professionals in your field, leaders in your industry, or individuals who have achieved success in areas you aspire to. Research their background, accomplishments, and values to ensure a good fit.
- Reach out and make a connection: Once you have identified potential mentors, reach out to them, and express your interest in establishing a mentorship relationship. Be clear about why you admire their work and how you believe they can support your development. Personalize your message to show genuine interest.
- Be respectful of their time: Understand that mentors are often busy individuals. When reaching out, be respectful of their time and availability. Clearly communicate your expectations for the mentorship relationship, and be open to their input on the frequency and format of interactions.

- Establish clear goals and expectations: Once you have found a mentor, discuss, and establish clear goals and expectations for the mentorship relationship. Define what you hope to achieve and how you envision the mentor supporting your development. This will provide a framework for your interactions.
- Maintain regular communication: Regularly communicate with your mentor to keep the relationship active and productive. Schedule regular meetings or check-ins, either in person or virtually, to discuss progress, seek guidance, and address any challenges you may be facing.
- Be open and receptive to feedback: Embrace feedback from your mentor with an open mind and a willingness to learn and grow. Actively listen to their insights and suggestions and be open to making changes based on their guidance. Remember, their feedback is meant to support your development.
- Take initiative and be proactive: Do not solely rely on your mentor to drive the relationship. Take initiative and be proactive in seeking opportunities for growth and development. Share your progress, ask for specific feedback, and actively pursue learning opportunities.
- Express gratitude and show appreciation: Regularly express your gratitude and appreciation for your mentor's guidance and support. Acknowledge the impact they have had on your personal and professional growth. This will help nurture a positive and mutually beneficial mentorship relationship.

Mentorship is a two-way street. While your mentor provides guidance and support, you also have a responsibility to actively engage and take ownership of your development. Be proactive, receptive, and grateful for the mentorship relationship, and it can have a significant impact on your personal and professional growth.

9.4   Tools and Frameworks for Self-Assessment

The Importance of a Growth Mindset and a Commitment to Lifelong Learning

In the field of nursing, it is essential to adopt a growth mindset and have a commitment to lifelong learning in order to provide the best possible care for patients. Nursing practice is constantly evolving with new technologies, treatments, and research emerging all the time. Nurses who are open to learning and growth are better equipped to adapt to these changes and provide evidence-based care. By continually expanding their knowledge and skills, nurses can stay current with best practices and deliver high-quality care to their patients. A growth mindset also encourages nurses to seek out opportunities for professional development and personal growth, leading to increased job satisfaction and career advancement. In a field as dynamic as healthcare, a commitment to lifelong learning is crucial for nurses to excel in their practice and ultimately improve patient outcomes.

Staying Current, Adapting to Change, and Providing the Best Possible Care to Patients

In the ever-evolving field of healthcare, it is essential for healthcare professionals to stay current with the latest research, technology, and best practices in order to provide the best possible care to their patients. This requires a commitment to lifelong learning and a willingness to adapt to change. By staying up to date with advancements in medicine and healthcare delivery, healthcare providers can ensure they are offering the most effective treatments and interventions for their patients. Additionally, being open to change and continuously seeking ways to improve patient care can lead to better outcomes and satisfaction for both patients and providers. Ultimately, by prioritizing staying current and adapting to change, healthcare professionals can offer the highest quality of care to their patients.

9.5 Conclusion

Building a foundation for clinical competence is a crucial aspect of the professional development of new graduate nurses. By understanding the transition process, focusing on clinical skill development, honing critical thinking and decision-making abilities, fostering effective communication and collaboration, and prioritizing professional growth and self-care, new graduate nurses can establish a strong foundation for clinical competence and embark on a successful nursing career.

Review Questions
- Why is professional development and lifelong learning important in the healthcare profession?
- What are the key components of a personal development plan for professional growth?
- Discuss different strategies and resources available for professional development and lifelong learning in healthcare.
- How can mentorship and collaboration contribute to professional development?
- How can technology, such as online platforms and mobile applications, support lifelong learning in healthcare?
- Explain the role of self-reflection and self-assessment in professional development. How can healthcare professionals effectively assess their strengths and areas for improvement?
- Discuss the benefits and challenges of attending conferences, workshops, and seminars for professional development.
- How can healthcare professionals engage in self-directed learning? Provide examples of self-directed learning activities.
- Explain the concept of a growth mindset and its relevance to lifelong learning in healthcare.

- How can healthcare professionals stay current with the latest advancements and evidence-based practices in their field?
- Discuss the potential of simulation-based training and virtual reality in enhancing clinical skills and decision-making.
- How can healthcare professionals actively engage in peer-to-peer learning and participate in professional networks and communities?
- What role does feedback and constructive criticism play in professional development? How can healthcare professionals seek and utilize feedback effectively?
- Discuss the ethical considerations and challenges in lifelong learning for healthcare professionals.
- How can professional development and lifelong learning contribute to improved patient outcomes and healthcare quality? Provide examples.

References

Khunou SH, Matlhaba KL (2023) Literature review: The support needs of the nurse mentors in their mentoring role. Jurnal Ners dan Kebidanan (Journal of Ners and Midwifery) 10(2):288–301. https://doi.org/10.26699/jnk.v10i2.ART.p288-301

Mlambo M, Silén C, McGrath C (2021) Lifelong learning and nurses' continuing professional development, a metasynthesis of the literature. BMC Nurs 20:1–3. https://doi.org/10.1186/s12912-021-00579-2

Reychav I, Elyakim N, McHaney R (2023) Lifelong learning processes in professional development for online teachers during the Covid era. Front Educ 8:1041800. https://doi.org/10.3389/feduc.2023.1041800

Van Beveren L, Roets G, Buysse A, Rutten K (2018) We all reflect, but why? A systematic review of the purposes of reflection in higher education in social and behavioral sciences. Educ Res Rev 24:1–9. https://doi.org/10.1016/j.edurev.2018.01.002

Wang Y, Hu S, Yao J, Pan Y, Wang J, Wang H (2024) Clinical nursing mentors' motivation, attitude, and practice for mentoring and factors associated with them. BMC Nurs 23(1):76. https://doi.org/10.1186/s12912-024-01757-8

World Health Organization (2013) Transforming and scaling up health professionals' education and training: World Health Organization Guidelines 2013. https://www.who.int/publications/i/item/transforming-and-scaling-up-health-professionals%E2%80%99-education-and-training. Accessed 23 Aug 2024

Transitioning to Specialty Areas

10

Contents

> Test your learning and check your understanding of this book's contents: use the "Springer Nature Flashcards" app to access questions using ▶ https://sn.pub/pe441e. To use the app, please follow the instructions in Chap. 1.

10.1   Specialty Areas in Healthcare

Specialty areas of nursing practice that require additional education, training, and expertise. Examples of specialty areas in nursing include pediatrics, critical care, oncology, mental health, and geriatrics (Giuffrida et al. 2023; Lee and Roh 2023). Healthcare is a vast field with many specialty areas that cater to the diverse needs of patients. Some of these specialty areas include cardiology, oncology, neurology, pediatrics, and emergency medicine. Each specialty area requires specific training and expertise to address the unique health concerns of patients within that particular field. For example, cardiologists focus on heart health and the treatment of cardiovascular diseases, while oncologists specialize in the diagnosis and treatment of cancer. These specialized healthcare professionals play a crucial role in providing quality care and improving outcomes for patients with complex medical conditions. Emphasizing the importance of collaboration and interdisciplinary care, these specialty areas work together to ensure comprehensive and patient-centered healthcare delivery.

The Importance of Specialty Areas in Healthcare

Specialty areas in healthcare play a crucial role in providing specialized care and expertise to patients. Here are some reasons why specialty areas are important:

- These areas allow healthcare professionals to develop in-depth knowledge and expertise in a specific field, which enables them to provide specialized care and stay updated with the latest advancements in their area of specialization.
- Because the specialized healthcare professionals have a deep understanding of specific conditions, diseases, or procedures, this expertise allows them to provide more accurate diagnoses, develop tailored treatment plans, and deliver better patient outcomes.
- By focusing on specific areas, specialty healthcare professionals can optimize the allocation of healthcare resources. They can efficiently utilize equipment, facilities, and personnel to provide specialized care, reducing unnecessary costs and improving overall healthcare efficiency.
- Specialty areas encourage collaboration and teamwork among healthcare professionals. Nurse specialists often closely work together with primary care physicians, therapists, and other specialists to provide comprehensive and coordinated care to patients.
- Specialty areas drive research and innovation in healthcare. Specialists often engage in research activities to advance knowledge and develop new treatment options. This leads to continuous improvement in healthcare practices and the development of new technologies and therapies which can have a great impact on the new graduate nurses' professional growth.
- Specialty areas are essential for addressing complex and challenging medical cases. Certain conditions or diseases require specialized knowledge and skills that can only be provided by healthcare professionals with expertise in a specific field.
- Specialty areas contribute to higher patient satisfaction. Patients feel more confident and reassured when they receive care from healthcare professionals who specialize in their specific condition or medical needs.

Specialty areas in healthcare are vital for delivering high-quality, specialized care, improving patient outcomes, and advancing medical knowledge and innovation.

The Increasing Demand for Specialized Expertise

The demand for specialized expertise in healthcare has been steadily increasing for several reasons:

- Advancements in medical knowledge: The field of medicine is constantly evolving, with new discoveries and advancements being made regularly. This has led to a deeper understanding of diseases, conditions, and treatment options. As a result, there is a growing need for healthcare professionals who have specialized knowledge and expertise in specific areas to provide the best possible care.

- Aging population: The global population is aging, and older adults often have complex healthcare needs. Conditions such as chronic diseases, age-related ailments, and geriatric care require specialized knowledge and skills to manage effectively. Healthcare professionals with expertise in geriatrics, palliative care, and other related fields are in high demand to cater to the needs of the aging population.
- Technological advancements: Technology has revolutionized healthcare in many ways, from advanced diagnostic tools to innovative treatment options. Specialized expertise is required to operate and interpret the results of these technologies effectively. Healthcare professionals with specialized training in areas such as radiology, medical imaging, and robotic surgery are in high demand to utilize these technologies for improved patient care.
- Complex and rare conditions: Some medical conditions are rare or highly complex, requiring specialized expertise for accurate diagnosis and treatment. Examples include rare genetic disorders, rare cancers, and autoimmune diseases. Healthcare professionals with specialized knowledge in these areas are essential to provide appropriate care and improve patient outcomes.
- Personalized medicine: The concept of personalized medicine, which tailors medical treatment to an individual's specific characteristics, is gaining prominence. This approach requires healthcare professionals with specialized expertise in genomics, pharmacogenomics, and precision medicine to analyze genetic data and develop personalized treatment plans.
- Multidisciplinary care: Many healthcare conditions require a multidisciplinary approach, involving collaboration among healthcare professionals from different specialties. For example, cancer treatment often involves a team of oncologists, surgeons, radiologists, and other specialists working together. The demand for specialized expertise in these multidisciplinary teams is increasing to provide comprehensive and coordinated care.
- Patient preferences: Patients are becoming more informed and proactive in managing their healthcare. They often seek out healthcare professionals with specialized expertise in their specific condition or medical needs. This demand for specialized care is driven by the desire for personalized attention and the belief that specialized expertise leads to better outcomes.

The increasing demand for specialized expertise in healthcare is driven by advancements in medical knowledge, an aging population, technological advancements, complex and rare conditions, personalized medicine, the need for multidisciplinary care, and patient preferences. Healthcare professionals with specialized training and expertise are essential to meet these evolving healthcare needs effectively.

10.2 Terminology Related to Specialized Areas in Nursing

The following terms are often used interchangeably, but there are some differences in their roles and responsibilities. Below are their definitions and descriptions.

- Advanced nurse practitioner (ANP): ANP is another term for an APN who has completed advanced education and training in a specific area of nursing practice. ANPs have a broader scope of practice than CNSs and can diagnose and treat illnesses, prescribe medications, and provide primary care services. They often work in primary care settings, such as family practice clinics or community health centers.
- Advanced nurse specialist (ANS): This term is similar to nurse specialist and is used to describe a nurse who has advanced knowledge and skills in a specific area of nursing practice. Like nurse specialists, their scope of practice may vary depending on the specific role and setting.
- Advanced practice nurse (APN): This is a broad term that refers to a registered nurse who has completed advanced education and training in a specific area of nursing practice. APNs have a higher level of knowledge and skills than a registered nurse and are authorized to provide advanced nursing care.
- Clinical nurse specialist (CNS): A CNS is an APN who specializes in a specific clinical area, such as pediatrics, geriatrics, or oncology. They provide direct patient care, but they also have a role in education, research, and consultation. CNSs often work in hospitals, clinics, or other healthcare settings.
- Nurse specialist (NS): This term is sometimes used to refer to a nurse who has specialized knowledge and skills in a specific area of nursing practice. Nurse specialists may have advanced education and training, but their scope of practice may vary depending on the specific role and setting.

It's important to note that the specific roles and responsibilities of these nursing roles can vary depending on the country, state, or healthcare organization. It's always best to refer to the specific regulations and guidelines in your area to understand the exact scope of practice for each role.

In South Africa, nursing specialties are classified into two categories, namely, clinical and nonclinical specialized areas. As stated by the South African Nursing Council, for a nurse to become a nurse specialist, they must undergo training and acquire a postgraduate diploma in that specific specialization and get professional registration as additional qualification (SANC 2005). The table below shows different fields and the descriptions for new graduate nurses to have an understanding and make decisions on their areas of interests.

Clinical Specialized Areas and Their Descriptions (Author's Own)

Clinical specialized areas and their descriptions

Child nursing	Child nursing, also known as pediatric nursing, focuses on providing healthcare to infants, children, and adolescents. Child nurses are trained to assess and manage the unique healthcare needs of children, including physical, emotional, and developmental aspects
Community health nursing	Community health nursing involves providing healthcare services to individuals, families, and communities in various settings outside of hospitals. Community health nurses work to promote health, prevent diseases, and provide education and support to improve the overall Well-being of the community
Critical care nursing (adult)	Critical care nursing in the adult population involves providing specialized care to critically ill patients in intensive care units (ICUs) or other critical care settings. Critical care nurses are trained to monitor and manage patients with life-threatening conditions, such as severe injuries, organ failure, or postsurgical complications
Critical care nursing (child)	Critical care nursing in the pediatric population focuses on providing specialized care to critically ill infants, children, and adolescents in pediatric intensive care units (PICUs) or other critical care settings. Pediatric critical care nurses are trained to assess and manage the unique needs of critically ill children, including respiratory support, medication administration, and monitoring
Emergency nursing	Emergency nursing involves providing immediate and specialized care to patients who require urgent medical attention. Emergency nurses work in emergency departments and are trained to assess and stabilize patients with acute illnesses, injuries, or trauma
Forensic nursing	Forensic nursing combines the fields of nursing and forensic science. Forensic nurses provide care to individuals who have experienced violence, abuse, or trauma. They also collect evidence, document injuries, and collaborate with law enforcement agencies in legal investigations
Infection prevention and control nursing	Infection prevention and control nursing focuses on preventing and controlling the spread of infections in healthcare settings. These nurses develop and implement strategies to minimize the risk of healthcare-associated infections, educate healthcare staff, and monitor compliance with infection control protocols
Mental health nursing	Mental health nursing involves providing care to individuals with mental health disorders or psychiatric conditions. Mental health nurses assess, diagnose, and develop treatment plans for patients experiencing mental health challenges. They may work in psychiatric hospitals, community mental health centers, or other healthcare settings
Midwifery	Midwifery is a specialized area of nursing that focuses on providing care to women during pregnancy, childbirth, and the postpartum period. Midwives support women in their reproductive health journey, provide prenatal care, assist with labor and delivery, and offer postpartum care to both the mother and newborn

Nephrology nursing	Nephrology nursing involves caring for patients with kidney diseases or disorders. Nephrology nurses assist in the management of patients undergoing dialysis and kidney transplantation or those with chronic kidney disease. They monitor patients' kidney function, administer medications, and provide education on kidney health
Occupational health nursing	Occupational health nursing focuses on promoting and maintaining the health and safety of workers in various occupational settings. Occupational health nurses assess workplace hazards, provide health screenings, promote wellness programs, and assist in the management of work-related injuries or illnesses
Oncology and palliative nursing	Oncology and palliative nursing involve caring for patients with cancer and providing support to individuals with life-limiting illnesses. Oncology nurses administer chemotherapy, manage symptoms, provide emotional support, and educate patients and their families about cancer treatments and end-of-life care
Ophthalmic nursing	Ophthalmic nursing specializes in providing care to patients with eye disorders or undergoing eye surgeries. Ophthalmic nurses assist in eye examinations, administer eye medications, educate patients on eye health, and provide postoperative care for patients undergoing eye surgeries
Orthopedic nursing	Orthopedic nursing focuses on providing care to patients with musculoskeletal conditions or injuries or undergoing orthopedic surgeries. Orthopedic nurses assist in the management of fractures, joint replacements, and spinal surgeries. They provide education on mobility, rehabilitation, and assistive devices
Perioperative nursing	Perioperative nursing involves providing care to patients before, during, and after surgical procedures. Perioperative nurses assist in preparing patients for surgery, ensure a sterile environment in the operating room, monitor patients during surgery, and provide postoperative care and education
Primary care nursing	Primary care nursing involves providing comprehensive and continuous healthcare to individuals and families in primary care settings, such as clinics or family practice settings. Primary care nurses assess, diagnose, treat common illnesses, manage chronic conditions, and promote preventive care and health education
Nonclinical specialized areas and their descriptions	
Health services management	Health services management, also known as healthcare administration or healthcare management, involves overseeing and managing the operations of healthcare organizations. Health services managers are responsible for planning, organizing, and coordinating the delivery of healthcare services
Nursing education	Nursing education focuses on preparing and educating future nurses. Nurse educators work in academic institutions, such as nursing schools or colleges, and are responsible for developing and delivering nursing curricula, teaching nursing courses, and supervising clinical experiences for nursing students. They play a crucial role in shaping the knowledge, skills, and competencies of future nurses. Nurse educators may also be involved in conducting research, mentoring students, and providing professional development opportunities for practicing nurses

The main difference between clinical specialized areas and nonclinical specialized areas in nursing lies in the nature of the work and the setting in which it is performed. Here's a breakdown of the key distinctions:

Clinical Specialized Areas in Nursing
- Direct patient care: Clinical specialized areas involve direct patient care, where nurses work directly with patients to assess, diagnose, treat, and manage their healthcare needs. Examples of clinical specialized areas include critical care, emergency nursing, pediatrics, obstetrics, oncology, and psychiatric nursing.
- Hands-on skills: Nurses in clinical specialized areas require specific clinical skills and knowledge related to their specialty. They perform tasks such as administering medications, conducting physical assessments, providing wound care, operating medical equipment, and implementing specialized treatments or interventions.
- Patient interaction: Nurses in clinical specialized areas have frequent and direct interaction with patients and their families. They provide emotional support, education, and counseling to patients and collaborate with the healthcare team to develop and implement care plans.
- Clinical settings: Clinical specialized areas are typically found in hospitals, clinics, long-term care facilities, and other healthcare settings where direct patient care is provided. Nurses in these areas work closely with physicians, other healthcare professionals, and interdisciplinary teams.

Nonclinical Specialized Areas in Nursing
- Indirect patient care: Nonclinical specialized areas involve roles that support patient care indirectly. Nurses in nonclinical roles may work in administration, education, research, informatics, case management, quality improvement, or healthcare policy.
- Analytical and administrative skills: Nurses in nonclinical specialized areas often utilize analytical and administrative skills to support healthcare operations. They may analyze data, develop policies and procedures, manage healthcare programs, coordinate care, or provide education and training to other healthcare professionals.
- Limited direct patient interaction: Nurses in nonclinical specialized areas may have limited direct patient interaction compared to their clinical counterparts. Their focus is on supporting the delivery of care rather than providing hands-on patient care.
- Diverse work settings: Nonclinical specialized areas offer a wide range of work settings, including healthcare organizations, government agencies, research institutions, insurance companies, pharmaceutical companies, and educational institutions. Nurses in these roles may work in offices, classrooms, research labs, or remote settings.

The nonclinical nursing specialized areas provide opportunities for nurses to contribute to the healthcare system in different ways, beyond direct patient care.

They play vital roles in ensuring the smooth operation of healthcare organizations and in educating and training the next generation of nurses.

It's important to note that both clinical and nonclinical specialized areas in nursing are valuable and contribute to the overall healthcare system. Nurses in both areas play critical roles in improving patient outcomes, promoting health, and advancing the nursing profession. The choice between clinical and nonclinical specialization depends on individual interests, skills, and career goals.

10.3   Transitioning and Adapting to the Specialized Areas

Transitioning and adapting to specialized areas in nursing practice can be both exciting and challenging. Nurses who decide to pursue a specialization must undergo additional training and education to ensure they have the skills and knowledge necessary to excel in their chosen field. This transition can be daunting as nurses may need to learn new protocols, procedures, and medical technologies specific to their specialty. However, with dedication, hard work, and a willingness to learn, nurses can successfully adapt to their new role and provide quality care to patients in specialized areas such as critical care, pediatrics, oncology, or labor and delivery. Embracing change and seeking out opportunities for professional growth will help nurses thrive in their specialized practice and make a positive impact on the health and well-being of their patients.

The Transition of New Graduate Nurses to Specialty Areas is of Significant Importance for Several Reasons

- Enhancing clinical competence: Transitioning to a specialty area allows new graduate nurses to develop and enhance their clinical competence in a specific field. Specialty areas often require specialized knowledge and skills that go beyond the general nursing education provided in undergraduate programs. By transitioning to a specialty area, new graduate nurses can gain expertise and proficiency in delivering specialized care to patients.
- Meeting the needs of specialized patient populations: Specialty areas cater to specific patient populations with unique healthcare needs. Transitioning new graduate nurses to these areas ensures that there are enough healthcare professionals with the necessary skills and knowledge to provide specialized care. This is particularly important in areas such as critical care, pediatrics, oncology, and mental health, where patients require specialized interventions and treatments.
- Improving patient outcomes: When new graduate nurses transition to specialty areas, they can contribute to improved patient outcomes. Specialized knowledge and skills acquired during the transition process enable nurses to provide evidence-based care, implement specialized interventions, and effectively manage complex patient conditions. This, in turn, can lead to better patient outcomes, reduced complications, and improved quality of care.
- Addressing workforce needs: Specialty areas often face challenges in recruiting and retaining experienced nurses. By facilitating the transition of new graduate

nurses to these areas, healthcare organizations can address workforce needs and ensure a sustainable supply of skilled nurses in specialty fields. This is particularly crucial as the demand for specialized healthcare services continues to grow.

- Professional growth and career advancement: Transitioning to a specialty area offers new graduate nurses' opportunities for professional growth and career advancement. Specializing in a specific field allows nurses to develop expertise, gain recognition, and pursue advanced roles and certifications. This can lead to increased job satisfaction, higher earning potential, and expanded career opportunities.
- Contributing to healthcare innovation: Specialty areas often serve as hubs for healthcare innovation and research. By transitioning to these areas, new graduate nurses can actively contribute to advancements in patient care, participate in research studies, and contribute to evidence-based practice. This involvement in innovation and research can have a positive impact on the overall healthcare system.

The transition of new graduate nurses to specialty areas is crucial for enhancing clinical competence, meeting the needs of specialized patient populations, improving patient outcomes, addressing workforce needs, facilitating professional growth, and contributing to healthcare innovation. It is an essential process that benefits both the nurses and the patients they serve.

The transition process for new graduate nurses to specialty areas typically involves several stages. Here is an overview of the transition process, along with the common challenges faced by new graduate nurses during each stage:

1. Orientation

   - Orientation is the initial stage of the transition process, where new graduate nurses are introduced to the healthcare organization, its policies, and procedures.
   - Common challenges during orientation include information overload, adapting to a new work environment, and understanding the organization's culture and expectations.

2. Preceptorship

   - Preceptorship is a structured period where new graduate nurses work closely with an experienced nurse (preceptor) who guides and supports them in their transition.
   - Challenges during preceptorship include building a productive relationship with the preceptor, managing the expectations of both the preceptor and the new graduate nurse, and gaining confidence in clinical skills and decision-making.

3. Independent practice

   - Independent practice is the stage where new graduate nurses gradually assume full responsibility for patient care, with decreasing supervision from the preceptor.

– Challenges during independent practice include managing a higher patient load, prioritizing tasks, making independent clinical judgments, and developing time management skills.

Common Challenges Faced by New Graduate Nurses During the Transition Process Include the Following

- Lack of experience: New graduate nurses may feel overwhelmed by the transition to a specialty area due to their limited clinical experience. They may encounter unfamiliar patient conditions, complex treatments, and specialized equipment, which can be challenging to navigate initially.
- Confidence and self-doubt: New graduate nurses may experience self-doubt and lack confidence in their abilities during the transition process. They may question their clinical judgment, worry about making mistakes, and feel anxious about their performance.
- Time management: Balancing multiple patient assignments, documentation, and other responsibilities can be challenging for new graduate nurses. Time management skills may take time to develop, leading to stress and potential difficulties in meeting deadlines and providing timely care.
- Communication and collaboration: Effective communication and collaboration with interdisciplinary healthcare team members are essential in specialty areas. New graduate nurses may face challenges in effectively communicating with physicians, specialists, and other healthcare professionals, leading to potential misunderstandings or delays in patient care.
- Emotional impact: Transitioning to a specialty area can be emotionally demanding for new graduate nurses. They may encounter complex patient situations, end-of-life care, and emotionally charged interactions with patients and their families. Coping with these emotional challenges and maintaining their own well-being can be difficult.
- Adapting to new policies and procedures: Each healthcare organization has its own policies, procedures, and documentation systems. New graduate nurses may find it challenging to adapt to these new protocols and navigate the electronic health record systems used in specialty areas.

Addressing these challenges requires a supportive environment, ongoing education, mentorship, and opportunities for reflection and self-assessment. Providing resources, debriefing sessions, and access to experienced nurses can help new graduate nurses navigate the transition process more effectively and build confidence in their specialty area.

The Need for New Graduate Nurses to Adapt to New Roles, Responsibilities, and Environments When Transitioning into a Specialty Area

When new graduate nurses transition into a specialty area, they often need to adapt to new roles, responsibilities, and environments. Here are some reasons why this adaptation is necessary:

- Specialized knowledge and skills: Transitioning into a specialty area requires new graduate nurses to acquire specialized knowledge and skills specific to that area. They need to learn about the unique aspects of the specialty, including disease processes, treatment modalities, and specialized procedures. Adapting to these new roles and responsibilities involves continuous learning and professional development.

- Expanded scope of practice: Specialty areas often have an expanded scope of practice compared to general nursing. New graduate nurses need to understand and adhere to the specific regulations, protocols, and guidelines of their specialty. They may have additional responsibilities such as medication management, advanced assessments, or specialized interventions. Adapting to these expanded roles requires a thorough understanding of the specialty's scope of practice.
- Collaborative teamwork: Specialty areas often involve working closely with a multidisciplinary team of healthcare professionals. New graduate nurses need to adapt to the collaborative nature of these teams and learn how to effectively communicate and coordinate care with other team members. This may involve understanding the roles and responsibilities of different team members and developing effective teamwork skills.
- Different patient populations: Specialty areas often focus on specific patient populations, such as pediatrics, geriatrics, or critical care. New graduate nurses need to adapt to the unique needs and characteristics of these patient populations. This may involve learning about developmental milestones, age-specific assessments, and specialized care techniques. Adapting to the different patient populations requires flexibility and a willingness to learn and adapt to new approaches.
- Environmental factors: Specialty areas may have different physical environments and resources compared to general nursing units. New graduate nurses need to adapt to the specific equipment, technology, and facilities available in their specialty area. They may also need to become familiar with the workflow, policies, and procedures specific to that area. Adapting to the new environment involves being open to change and actively seeking opportunities to learn and familiarize oneself with the surroundings.
- Emotional and psychological challenges: Some specialty areas, such as oncology or palliative care, may involve dealing with emotionally challenging situations. New graduate nurses need to adapt to the emotional and psychological demands of their specialty area. This may involve developing coping mechanisms, seeking support from colleagues, and engaging in self-care practices to maintain their well-being.
- Professional growth and development: Transitioning into a specialty area provides new graduate nurses with opportunities for professional growth and development. Adapting to new roles, responsibilities, and environments allows them to expand their knowledge, skills, and expertise. It also opens doors for further specialization, advanced practice roles, and leadership opportunities in the future.

New graduate nurses need to adapt to new roles, responsibilities, and environments when transitioning into a specialty area. This adaptation involves acquiring specialized knowledge and skills, understanding the expanded scope of practice, collaborating with multidisciplinary teams, adapting to different patient populations, familiarizing oneself with the environment, addressing emotional challenges, and embracing opportunities for professional growth. With time, experience, and support, new graduate nurses can successfully navigate these transitions and thrive in their chosen specialty area.

The Key Considerations and Steps Involved in Transitioning to a Specialty Area

Transitioning to a specialty area in nursing requires careful consideration and planning. Here are some key considerations and steps involved in the transition process:

- Self-assessment: Start by assessing your own interests, strengths, and career goals. Reflect on why you want to transition to a specialty area and how it aligns with your long-term aspirations. Consider your personal preferences, such as working with specific patient populations or being involved in certain types of care.
- Research and exploration: Conduct thorough research on the specialty area you are interested in. Learn about the scope of practice, required competencies, and the specific skills and knowledge needed. Explore different specialty areas through shadowing experiences, attending conferences or workshops, and talking to nurses already working in those areas. This will help you gain a better understanding of what the transition entails.
- Education and training: Determine if additional education or training is required to transition to the specialty area. Some specialty areas may require certification or advanced degrees. Identify the educational programs or courses available to acquire the necessary knowledge and skills. Consider pursuing certifications or specialty-specific courses to enhance your qualifications.
- Networking and mentorship: Connect with nurses already working in the specialty area you are interested in. Seek out mentors who can provide guidance and support during the transition process. Networking with professionals in the field can provide valuable insights, advice, and potential job opportunities.
- Professional development: Engage in continuous professional development to enhance your knowledge and skills in the specialty area. Attend conferences, workshops, and seminars related to the specialty. Join professional organizations or specialty-specific nursing associations to stay updated with the latest advancements, and connect with other professionals in the field.
- Clinical experience: Gain hands-on clinical experience in the specialty area. Look for opportunities to work or volunteer in settings that offer exposure to the specialty. This could include internships, externships, or part-time positions. Clinical experience will help you develop the necessary skills and confidence in the specialty area.
- Transition plan: Develop a transition plan that outlines the steps and timeline for transitioning to the specialty area. Set specific goals and objectives to guide your progress. Identify any additional certifications or training you need to complete and create a timeline for achieving them. Consider seeking guidance from experienced nurses or nurse educators to help you create a realistic and achievable plan.

- Job search and application: Once you feel prepared, start searching for job opportunities in the specialty area. Update your resume and tailor it to highlight relevant experiences and skills. Prepare for interviews by researching common interview questions and practicing your responses. Be proactive in networking and reaching out to potential employers or nurse recruiters in the specialty area.
- Orientation and mentoring: Once you secure a position in the specialty area, take advantage of the orientation and mentoring programs offered by the organization. These programs will help you acclimate to the new role, responsibilities, and environment. Seek guidance from experienced nurses and mentors to navigate any challenges or uncertainties that may arise during the transition.
- Continuous learning and growth: Transitioning to a specialty area is an ongoing process. Commit to continuous learning and professional growth in the specialty. Stay updated with the latest research, guidelines, and best practices. Seek opportunities for advanced certifications, specialty-specific courses, and professional development activities to further enhance your expertise.

Transitioning to a specialty area requires dedication, perseverance, and a commitment to lifelong learning. By carefully considering these key steps and taking proactive measures, you can successfully transition to a specialty area and thrive in your nursing career.

Support and Resources for New Graduate Nurses into Specialty Areas

1. Role of mentors and preceptors

    – Mentors and preceptors play a crucial role in supporting new graduate nurses during their transition to specialty areas. They provide guidance, share their expertise, and offer emotional support. Mentors and preceptors help new graduates navigate the challenges of their new roles, answer questions, and provide feedback to enhance their learning and development.

2. Orientation programs

    – Orientation programs are designed to provide new graduate nurses with the necessary knowledge and skills to succeed in their specialty areas. These programs typically include classroom education, hands-on training, and shadowing experienced nurses. Effective orientation programs ensure that new graduates receive comprehensive training, understand the expectations of their roles, and have opportunities to practice and apply their skills in a supportive environment.

3. Availability of resources and support systems

    – Hospitals and healthcare organizations recognize the importance of providing resources and support systems for new graduate nurses. These resources may include access to educational materials, online learning platforms, clinical guidelines, and policies specific to the specialty area. Support systems can include nurse residency programs, peer support groups, and access to experienced nurses who can provide guidance and mentorship.

4. Professional organizations and networks

- Professional organizations and networks can be valuable resources for new graduate nurses. These organizations often offer educational opportunities, networking events, and access to research and best practices in specific specialty areas. Joining professional organizations allows new graduates to connect with experienced nurses, gain insights into their specialty area, and stay updated on advancements in their field.
5. Collaboration and interdisciplinary support

- New graduate nurses benefit from collaboration and support from the interdisciplinary team. Working closely with physicians, nurse practitioners, pharmacists, and other healthcare professionals allows new graduates to learn from their expertise, seek guidance, and provide holistic care to patients. Interdisciplinary support systems foster a collaborative environment where new graduates can ask questions, share experiences, and receive valuable input from different perspectives.

  It is essential for healthcare organizations to prioritize the availability of mentors, effective orientation programs, and resources to support new graduate nurses. By providing a supportive environment and access to necessary resources, healthcare organizations can facilitate the successful transition of new graduate nurses into specialty areas.

10.4   Self-Assessment and Reflection in Specialized Areas

Self-assessment and reflection are essential tools for growth and development in any specialized area. By taking the time to honestly evaluate our skills, knowledge, and performance, we can identify areas where we excel and areas where we may need improvement. Reflection allows us to learn from our experiences, both successes and failures, and make necessary adjustments to enhance our abilities. In specialized areas, such as medicine, education, or technology, self-assessment and reflection can help individuals stay current with advancements in their field and continuously strive for excellence. Overall, engaging in self-assessment and reflection is key to personal and professional growth in specialized areas.

The Importance of Self-Assessment and Reflection to Identify Personal Interests, Strengths, and Areas for Development

Self-assessment and reflection are crucial steps in personal and professional development. They play a significant role in identifying personal interests, strengths, and areas for development. Here's why self-assessment and reflection are important:

- Clarifying personal interests: Self-assessment helps individuals gain clarity about their interests and passions. It allows them to explore what truly motivates and excites them. By understanding their interests, individuals can make informed decisions about their career paths and pursue opportunities that align with their passions.

- Identifying strengths: Self-assessment helps individuals recognize their strengths and areas of expertise. It allows them to identify the skills and abilities they excel in. Understanding one's strengths enables individuals to leverage them in their personal and professional lives, leading to increased confidence, satisfaction, and success.
- Recognizing areas for development: Self-assessment also helps individuals identify areas where they may need further development or improvement. It allows them to acknowledge their weaknesses or areas of limited knowledge or skills. Recognizing these areas for development provides individuals with the opportunity to seek learning experiences, training, or mentorship to enhance their capabilities.
- Setting goals: Self-assessment and reflection provide a foundation for setting meaningful and achievable goals. By understanding their interests, strengths, and areas for development, individuals can set goals that align with their aspirations and address their growth areas. Setting goals based on self-assessment helps individuals stay focused, motivated, and committed to their personal and professional development.
- Making informed decisions: Self-assessment enables individuals to make informed decisions about their career choices, educational pursuits, and personal growth. By understanding their interests and strengths, individuals can choose paths that align with their values and goals. It helps them avoid pursuing opportunities that may not be a good fit and instead focus on areas where they can thrive and find fulfillment.
- Enhancing self-awareness: Self-assessment and reflection promote self-awareness, which is essential for personal and professional growth. By reflecting on their experiences, strengths, and areas for development, individuals gain a deeper understanding of themselves. This self-awareness allows individuals to make conscious choices, manage their emotions, and adapt to different situations effectively.
- Promoting continuous learning: Self-assessment encourages individuals to engage in continuous learning and improvement. By identifying areas for development, individuals can seek out learning opportunities, training programs, or mentorship to enhance their knowledge and skills. This commitment to continuous learning fosters personal and professional growth and keeps individuals adaptable and relevant in a rapidly changing world.

Self-assessment and reflection are vital for personal and professional development. They help individuals clarify their interests, identify strengths, recognize areas for development, set meaningful goals, make informed decisions, enhance self-awareness, and promote continuous learning. By engaging in self-assessment and reflection, individuals can navigate their personal and professional journeys with purpose, fulfillment, and success.

Some Common Challenges Faced by New Graduate Nurses in this Transition to Specialized Areas

Transitioning to specialty areas can present unique challenges for new graduate nurses. Some common challenges faced by new graduate nurses in this transition include the following:

- Limited clinical experience: New graduate nurses may have limited exposure to the specific patient population or procedures in the specialty area. This lack of experience can make it challenging to adapt to the specialized care required. They may need to invest extra time and effort in learning and gaining proficiency in the new skills and knowledge needed for the specialty.
- Increased responsibility and autonomy: Specialty areas often come with increased responsibility and autonomy compared to general nursing. New graduate nurses may feel overwhelmed by the higher expectations and decision-making required in their new roles. They may need to develop confidence in their abilities and seek support from experienced colleagues or mentors to navigate these challenges.
- Learning complex procedures and protocols: Specialty areas often involve complex procedures, protocols, and specialized equipment. New graduate nurses may find it challenging to learn and master these procedures, especially if they have not been exposed to them during their education or clinical rotations. They may need additional training, guidance, and practice to become proficient in performing these procedures safely and effectively.
- Adapting to a new team and environment: Transitioning to a specialty area means joining a new team and adapting to a different work environment. New graduate nurses may face challenges in building relationships with colleagues, understanding team dynamics, and integrating into the existing workflow. They may need to actively seek opportunities to collaborate, communicate, and establish rapport with their new team members.
- Managing time and prioritizing care: Specialty areas often involve complex patient care needs and a higher patient acuity level. New graduate nurses may struggle with time management and prioritizing care effectively. They may need to develop strategies for organizing their workload, delegating tasks when appropriate, and seeking assistance when needed to ensure safe and efficient patient care.
- Emotional and psychological demands: Some specialty areas deal with emotionally challenging situations, such as critical care, oncology, or palliative care. New graduate nurses may find it emotionally taxing to witness and manage patients' suffering or end-of-life care. They may need to develop coping mechanisms, seek support from colleagues or counselors, and engage in self-care practices to maintain their emotional well-being.
- Continuous learning and professional development: Specialty areas often require ongoing learning and professional development to stay updated with advancements and best practices. New graduate nurses may face challenges in balancing their learning needs with their clinical responsibilities. They may need to actively seek out educational opportunities, engage in self-study, and participate in

professional development activities to enhance their knowledge and skills in the specialty.

- Navigating the transition period: The transition period itself can be challenging for new graduate nurses. They may experience feelings of uncertainty, self-doubt, and imposter syndrome as they navigate the new roles, responsibilities, and expectations. They may need support from mentors, preceptors, or nurse educators to provide guidance, feedback, and reassurance during this transition phase.

It's important to note that while these challenges may exist, they are not insurmountable. With time, experience, support, and a commitment to continuous learning, new graduate nurses can overcome these challenges and thrive in their chosen specialty areas.

Different Specialty Areas, Research Their Requirements, and Consider Their Compatibility with Their Skills, Values, and Career Goals

When considering transitioning to a specialty area, it is essential to research the requirements of different specialties and evaluate their compatibility with your skills, values, and career goals. Here are some steps to help you in this process:

- Research specialty areas: Start by researching different specialty areas within nursing. Explore the scope of practice, patient population, and specific skills and knowledge required for each specialty. Look for information on professional organizations, certifications, and educational programs associated with each specialty.
- Assess your skills and knowledge: Evaluate your current skills, knowledge, and experience. Identify the areas where you excel and the skills you enjoy utilizing. Consider how these align with the requirements of different specialty areas. Assess any gaps in your skills or knowledge that may need to be addressed through additional education or training.
- Reflect on your values and interests: Consider your personal values and interests. Reflect on the type of work environment, patient population, or healthcare issues that resonate with you. Think about the aspects of nursing that you find most fulfilling and rewarding. This reflection will help you identify specialty areas that align with your values and interests.
- Consider long-term career goals: Think about your long-term career goals and aspirations. Consider how transitioning to a specific specialty area may align with those goals. Evaluate the potential for growth, advancement, and opportunities for professional development within each specialty. This consideration will help you choose a specialty that supports your long-term career trajectory.
- Seek advice and guidance: Reach out to nurses already working in the specialty areas you are interested in. Seek their advice and insights into the requirements, challenges, and rewards of their specialties. Connect with mentors or professionals in the field who can provide guidance and support in your decision-making process.
- Attend specialty-specific events: Attend conferences, workshops, or seminars related to the specialty areas you are considering. These events provide

opportunities to learn more about the specialties, network with professionals in the field, and gain a deeper understanding of the requirements and trends within each specialty.

- Explore educational programs and certifications: Look into educational programs or certifications associated with the specialty areas you are interested in. Determine if additional education or certification is required to transition to those specialties. Research the availability, cost, and time commitment of these programs to assess their feasibility for your career goals.
- Evaluate work-life balance: Consider the work-life balance associated with different specialty areas. Some specialties may require irregular hours, on-call shifts, or high-intensity work environments. Evaluate how these factors align with your personal preferences and lifestyle.
- Shadow or volunteer: If possible, try to shadow or volunteer in different specialty areas to gain firsthand experience. This will provide you with insights into the day-to-day responsibilities, challenges, and rewards of each specialty. It can help you make an informed decision about which specialty area is the best fit for you.
- Review job market and demand: Research the job market and demand for nurses in the specialty areas you are considering. Evaluate the availability of job opportunities and the potential for growth and job security within each specialty. This information can help you make a decision based on the practical aspects of your career.

By thoroughly researching different specialty areas, considering their requirements, and evaluating their compatibility with your skills, values, and career goals, new graduate nurses can make an informed decision about transitioning to a specialty area that aligns with their aspirations and sets up for success in their nursing career.

The Importance of Acquiring Specialized Knowledge and Skills

Acquiring specialized knowledge and skills is of great importance for several reasons:

- Expertise in a specific area: Specialized knowledge and skills allow individuals to become experts in a specific area of their field. This expertise sets them apart from their peers and positions them as valuable resources within their organization or industry. It enables them to provide specialized services, advice, and solutions that others may not be able to offer.
- Enhanced job performance: Acquiring specialized knowledge and skills directly contributes to improved job performance. When individuals have a deep understanding of a specific area, they can perform their tasks more efficiently and effectively. They are better equipped to handle complex challenges, make informed decisions, and deliver high-quality results. This can lead to increased productivity, job satisfaction, and recognition within the workplace.
- Career advancement opportunities: Specialized knowledge and skills open doors to career advancement opportunities. Employers often seek individuals with expertise in specific areas to fill leadership, management, or specialized roles. Acquiring specialized knowledge and skills can make individuals more

competitive in the job market and increase their chances of securing promotions or higher-level positions.

- Increased professional confidence: Acquiring specialized knowledge and skills boosts professional confidence. When individuals have a deep understanding of a specific area, they feel more competent and capable in their work. This confidence translates into better performance, effective decision-making, and the ability to handle challenges with ease. It also enhances their credibility and reputation among colleagues, clients, and stakeholders.
- Adaptability to changing environments: Specialized knowledge and skills enable individuals to adapt to changing environments and industry trends. As industries evolve, new technologies, practices, and challenges emerge. Having specialized knowledge and skills allows individuals to stay ahead of these changes and adapt their approach accordingly. They can quickly learn and apply new concepts, tools, and techniques, ensuring their continued relevance and success in their field.
- Contribution to innovation and advancement: Specialized knowledge and skills are essential for driving innovation and advancement in a particular field. Individuals with specialized expertise are often at the forefront of research, development, and problem-solving. They can identify gaps, propose innovative solutions, and contribute to the advancement of their field. Their specialized knowledge and skills enable them to push boundaries, challenge existing practices, and drive positive change.
- Collaboration and interdisciplinary work: Specialized knowledge and skills facilitate collaboration and interdisciplinary work. When individuals have expertise in a specific area, they can effectively communicate and collaborate with professionals from different disciplines. They can contribute unique insights, perspectives, and solutions to interdisciplinary projects or teams. This collaboration leads to more comprehensive and innovative outcomes.
- Personal and professional growth: Acquiring specialized knowledge and skills is a continuous learning process that promotes personal and professional growth. It expands individuals' intellectual horizons, challenges them to think critically, and encourages lifelong learning. Specialized knowledge and skills also provide individuals with a sense of accomplishment and fulfillment, contributing to their overall personal and professional satisfaction.

Acquiring specialized knowledge and skills is crucial for becoming an expert in a specific area, enhancing job performance, accessing career advancement opportunities, increasing professional confidence, adapting to changing environments, contributing to innovation, facilitating collaboration, and promoting personal and professional growth. By investing in specialized knowledge and skills, individuals can excel in their field, make significant contributions, and achieve long-term success.

Various Avenues for Gaining Expertise

There are several avenues for gaining expertise in a specialty area as a nurse. Here are some common avenues to consider:

- Continuing education programs: Many professional organizations and educational institutions offer continuing education programs specifically designed for nurses in various specialty areas. These programs provide in-depth knowledge and skills development through workshops, seminars, conferences, and online courses. They often cover the latest advancements, evidence-based practices, and emerging trends in the specialty.
- Specialty certification: Pursuing specialty certification is an excellent way to gain expertise and demonstrate proficiency in a specific area of nursing. Specialty certification programs are offered by professional organizations and require nurses to meet specific eligibility criteria and pass an examination. Certification not only enhances knowledge and skills but also validates expertise and can lead to career advancement opportunities.
- Mentorship and preceptorship: Seeking mentorship or working with a preceptor who is experienced in the specialty area can provide valuable guidance and support. Mentors and preceptors can share their expertise, provide insights into the specialty, and offer advice on professional development. They can help new nurses navigate the challenges of the specialty and accelerate their learning process.
- Clinical experience and practice: Gaining hands-on clinical experience in the specialty area is crucial for developing expertise. Seek opportunities to work in units or departments that specialize in the area of interest. Actively participate in patient care, observe experienced nurses, and engage in reflective practice to enhance knowledge and skills. The more exposure and practice you have in the specialty, the more expertise you will gain.
- Research- and evidence-based practice: Engaging in research- and evidence-based practice activities can deepen your understanding of the specialty area. Stay updated with the latest research studies, guidelines, and best practices relevant to the specialty. Participate in research projects, quality improvement initiatives, or journal clubs to contribute to the advancement of knowledge in the field and gain expertise through evidence-based practice.
- Professional networking: Building a professional network within the specialty area can provide opportunities for learning and collaboration. Attend specialty-specific conferences, seminars, and workshops to connect with experts and peers in the field. Join professional organizations or specialty-specific nursing associations to access resources, educational opportunities, and networking events.
- Self-study and independent learning: Take initiative in self-study and independent learning to gain expertise in the specialty area. Utilize textbooks, journals, online resources, and reputable websites to expand your knowledge. Engage in self-directed learning by setting learning goals, seeking out relevant literature, and reflecting on your practice. Online forums and discussion boards can also be valuable platforms for learning from others in the specialty.
- Clinical practice guidelines and protocols: Familiarize yourself with clinical practice guidelines and protocols specific to the specialty area. These guidelines provide evidence-based recommendations for the management of various

conditions or procedures. Adhering to these guidelines ensures that your practice aligns with the latest evidence and best practices in the specialty.

Gaining expertise in a specialty area is a continuous process. It requires dedication, ongoing learning, and practical experience. By actively pursuing these avenues for gaining expertise, you can enhance your knowledge, skills, and confidence in the specialty area and become a valuable asset to your healthcare team.

The Significance of Staying up to Date with the Latest Advancements and Evidence-Based Practices in the Specialty Area

Staying up to date with the latest advancements and evidence-based practices in a specialty area is of utmost significance for several reasons:

- Improved patient outcomes: Keeping abreast of the latest advancements and evidence-based practices ensures that healthcare professionals are providing the most effective and efficient care to their patients. By staying up to date, nurses can implement the latest techniques, treatments, and interventions that have been proven to enhance patient outcomes. This leads to improved quality of care, better patient satisfaction, and potentially better patient outcomes.
- Enhanced safety: Advancements in technology, procedures, and protocols often aim to improve patient safety. By staying current with the latest developments, nurses can implement safety measures and best practices that reduce the risk of errors, complications, and adverse events. This helps create a safer healthcare environment for patients and healthcare providers alike.
- Professional growth and development: Staying up to date with the latest advancements and evidence-based practices demonstrates a commitment to professional growth and development. It allows nurses to expand their knowledge and skills, making them more valuable assets to their healthcare team. Continuous learning and staying current with the latest research and practices can also open up opportunities for career advancement and specialization within the specialty area.
- Adherence to standards and guidelines: Many specialty areas have specific standards and guidelines that healthcare professionals are expected to follow. Staying up to date with the latest advancements ensures that nurses are aware of and adhere to these standards. This helps maintain consistency and quality of care within the specialty area and ensures that patients receive care that meets the highest standards.
- Collaboration and communication: Staying current with the latest advancements and evidence-based practices facilitates effective collaboration and communication within the healthcare team. When nurses are knowledgeable about the latest research and practices, they can contribute to discussions, share insights, and collaborate with other healthcare professionals to develop and implement the best care plans for their patients. This interdisciplinary collaboration leads to improved patient outcomes and a more cohesive healthcare team.
- Ethical responsibility: As healthcare professionals, nurses have an ethical responsibility to provide the best possible care to their patients. Staying up to date with the latest advancements and evidence-based practices is essential to fulfill this responsibility. It ensures that nurses are providing care that is based on the best

available evidence and aligns with ethical principles of beneficence and non-maleficence.

- Keeping pace with rapidly evolving healthcare landscape: The healthcare landscape is constantly evolving, with new research, technologies, and practices emerging regularly. Staying up to date allows nurses to keep pace with these changes and adapt their practice accordingly. It helps them remain relevant and competent in their specialty area and ensures that they are providing care that is in line with current best practices.

Staying up to date with the latest advancements and evidence-based practices in a specialty area is crucial for improving patient outcomes, enhancing safety, promoting professional growth, adhering to standards, facilitating collaboration, fulfilling ethical responsibilities, and keeping pace with the rapidly evolving healthcare landscape. By staying current, nurses can provide the highest quality of care and contribute to the advancement of their specialty area.

10.5   Professional Network and Establishing Relationships within the Specialty Area

Building a professional network within a specific specialty area is crucial for career growth and success. By connecting with like-minded professionals, one can gain access to valuable resources, opportunities, and support in their field. Establishing relationships with industry experts can provide mentorship, guidance, and insights that can help one navigate their career path more effectively. Networking also allows for collaboration, knowledge-sharing, and the exchange of innovative ideas that can elevate one's work and impact within their specialty area. Ultimately, investing time and effort into cultivating a strong professional network can open doors to new possibilities and enhance one's reputation in the industry.

Strategies for Building a Professional Network and Establishing Relationships within the Specialty Area

Building a professional network and establishing relationships within your specialty area are crucial for career growth and opportunities. Here are some strategies to help you:

- Attend institution and profession related events: Attend conferences, seminars, workshops, and networking events related to your specialty area. These events provide opportunities to meet professionals in your field, exchange ideas, and build connections.
- Join professional associations: Join industry-specific professional associations and organizations. These groups often host events, provide resources, and offer networking opportunities with professionals in your specialty area.
- Utilize social media: Use social media platforms like LinkedIn, Twitter, and Facebook to connect with professionals in your field. Join relevant groups and participate in discussions to establish your presence and build relationships.

- Volunteer or mentor: Offer your expertise by volunteering for industry-related projects or mentoring programs. This allows you to connect with professionals and demonstrate your skills and knowledge.
- Attend webinars and online events: Participate in webinars, online workshops, and virtual conferences related to your specialty area. These platforms provide opportunities to interact with professionals and expand your network.
- Seek informational interviews: Reach out to professionals in your specialty area and request informational interviews. These interviews allow you to learn from experienced individuals, gain insights, and build relationships.
- Collaborate on projects: Collaborate with professionals in your field on projects, research, or publications. This not only helps you establish relationships but also enhances your professional reputation.
- Stay active on professional forums: Engage in online forums and discussion boards related to your specialty area. Share your knowledge, ask questions, and connect with professionals who share similar interests.
- Attend workshops and training programs: Participate in workshops and training programs to enhance your skills and knowledge. These programs often attract professionals in your field, providing networking opportunities.
- Maintain relationships: Once you establish connections, maintain and nurture them. Stay in touch with your network through regular communication, sharing relevant information, and offering support when needed.

Building a professional network takes time and effort. Be genuine, show interest in others, and focus on building mutually beneficial relationships.

The Potential of Mentorship and Shadowing Opportunities to Gain Insights into the Unique Challenges and Best Practices of the Specialty Area

Mentorship and shadowing opportunities are invaluable tools for gaining insights into the unique challenges and best practices of a specialty area. By learning from seasoned professionals in the field, individuals can acquire firsthand knowledge and experience that may not be taught in a traditional classroom setting. Mentors can provide valuable guidance, advice, and support as mentees navigate their career path and strive to excel in their chosen specialty area. Shadowing allows individuals to observe professionals in action, witnessing firsthand the day-to-day tasks, responsibilities, and challenges they may face. By participating in mentorship and shadowing opportunities, individuals can gain a deeper understanding of their specialty area and develop the skills and knowledge needed to succeed in their chosen field.

The Importance of Adapting to the Culture and Dynamics of the Specialty Area

Adapting to the culture and dynamics of your specialty area is crucial for several reasons:

- Establishing credibility: Adapting to the culture and dynamics of your specialty area helps you establish credibility among your peers and colleagues. It shows that you understand and respect the norms and values of the field, which enhances your professional reputation.

- Building trust and relationships: Adapting to the culture and dynamics of your specialty area helps build trust and positive relationships with colleagues, clients, and stakeholders. When you align with the expectations and practices of the field, it becomes easier to collaborate, communicate effectively, and work together toward common goals.
- Effective communication: Each specialty area has its own jargon, terminology, and communication styles. Adapting to these specific communication practices allows you to effectively convey your ideas, understand others, and avoid misunderstandings. It facilitates clear and concise communication within your specialty area.
- Enhancing teamwork: Adapting to the culture and dynamics of your specialty area promotes effective teamwork. When team members share a common understanding of the field's expectations and norms, they can collaborate more seamlessly, leverage each other's strengths, and achieve better outcomes.
- Embracing innovation: Specialty areas often have unique challenges and opportunities. Adapting to the culture and dynamics of your specialty area allows you to understand these nuances and identify innovative solutions. By embracing the culture and dynamics, you can contribute to the advancement and growth of your field.
- Career advancement: Adapting to the culture and dynamics of your specialty area is essential for career advancement. It demonstrates your commitment to the field, your ability to adapt to new environments, and your willingness to learn and grow. Employers and industry leaders value professionals who can seamlessly integrate into the culture and dynamics of their specialty area.
- Professional development: Adapting to the culture and dynamics of your specialty area encourages continuous professional development. It motivates you to stay updated with the latest trends, technologies, and practices in your field. This ongoing learning and adaptation contribute to your professional growth and expertise.

Adapting to the culture and dynamics of your specialty area is vital for establishing credibility, building trust and relationships, facilitating effective communication and teamwork, embracing innovation, advancing your career, and fostering continuous professional development. By understanding and aligning with the culture and dynamics of your specialty area, you position yourself for success in your field.

Understanding the Expectations, Norms, and Values of the Specialty Area and Developing Effective Communication and Teamwork Skills within the Specialized Team

Understanding the expectations, norms, and values of your specialty area is essential for effective communication and teamwork within a specialized team. Here are some strategies to help you:

- Research and learn: Take the time to research and understand the specific expectations, norms, and values of your specialty area. This includes understanding the industry standards, best practices, and any unique aspects of your field.

- Seek guidance: Reach out to experienced professionals in your specialty area and seek their guidance. They can provide insights into the expectations and norms of the field and help you navigate any challenges.
- Observe and adapt: Pay attention to how professionals in your specialty area communicate and work together. Observe their behavior, communication styles, and problem-solving approaches. Adapt your own communication and teamwork skills to align with the norms of the field.
- Build relationships: Establish relationships with colleagues and team members within your specialty area. This allows you to learn from their experiences, gain insights into the expectations of the field, and develop effective communication and teamwork skills.
- Communicate clearly: Effective communication is crucial in any specialized team. Clearly convey your ideas, thoughts, and expectations to team members. Use appropriate terminology and be concise and specific in your communication.
- Active listening: Practice active listening skills to understand the perspectives and ideas of your team members. This helps build trust and fosters effective communication within the team.
- Collaborate and share knowledge: Foster a collaborative environment within your specialized team. Share your knowledge and expertise with others and be open to learning from your team members. This promotes effective teamwork and enhances the overall performance of the team.
- Respect differences: Recognize and respect the diverse perspectives and backgrounds of your team members. Embrace different ideas and approaches, as they can lead to innovative solutions and better outcomes.
- Seek feedback: Regularly seek feedback from your team members and supervisors. This helps you understand how your communication and teamwork skills are perceived and allows you to make improvements.
- Continuous learning: Stay updated with the latest developments and trends in your specialty area. Attend workshops, conferences, and training programs to enhance your skills and knowledge. This demonstrates your commitment to professional growth and contributes to effective communication and teamwork.

By understanding the expectations, norms, and values of your specialty area and developing effective communication and teamwork skills, new graduate nurses can contribute to the success of your specialized team and advance in your career.

10.6 Conclusion

In conclusion, this chapter highlights the importance of preparation, support, and ongoing education for new nurses entering specialty areas. It emphasizes the need for structured orientation programs, mentorship opportunities, and dedicated resources to help new graduates succeed in their chosen specialties. By providing a solid foundation and continuous support, healthcare organizations can ensure that new nurses feel confident, competent, and capable in their roles, ultimately leading to improved patient outcomes and job satisfaction. It is crucial for both new nurses and healthcare institutions to invest in a smooth transition process to specialty areas, as it sets the stage for long-term success and professional growth.

Review Questions
- Why is transitioning to a specialty area important in the healthcare profession?
- What are the key considerations new graduate nurses should consider when transitioning to a specialty area?
- Discuss the importance of self-assessment and reflection in identifying the right specialty area for an individual.
- What are the different avenues for gaining specialized knowledge and skills in a specific specialty area?
- How can new graduate nurses stay up to date with the latest advancements and evidence-based practices in their chosen specialty area?
- Explain the significance of building a professional network and establishing relationships within the specialty area.
- Discuss the benefits of joining professional organizations and attending conferences in the context of transitioning to a specialty area.
- How can mentorship and shadowing opportunities contribute to a successful transition to a specialty area?
- What challenges might new graduate nurses face when transitioning to a specialty area, and how can they be effectively managed?
- How can new graduate nurses adapt to the culture and dynamics of a specialty area?
- Discuss the importance of effective communication and teamwork skills in a specialized healthcare setting.
- How can new graduate nurses maintain a growth mindset and continue their professional development while transitioning to a specialty area?
- Provide examples of real-world experiences and lessons learned from new graduate nurses who have successfully transitioned to a specialty area.
- How does transitioning to a specialty area contribute to personal and professional growth in new graduate nurses?
- What are some strategies for new graduate nurses to thrive and excel in their chosen specialty area?

References

Giuffrida S, Silano V, Ramacciati N, Prandi C, Baldon A, Bianchi M (2023) Teaching strategies of clinical reasoning in advanced nursing clinical practice: a scoping review. Nurse Educ Pract 67:103548. https://doi.org/10.1016/j.nepr.2023.103548

Lee G, Roh YS (2023) Knowledge, barriers, and training needs of nurses working in delirium care. Nurs Crit Care 28(5):637–644. https://doi.org/10.1111/nicc.12724

Sustaining Clinical Competence

11

Contents

Test your learning and check your understanding of this book's contents: use the "Springer Nature Flashcards" app to access questions using ▶ https://sn.pub/pe441e. To use the app, please follow the instructions in Chap. 1.

11.1 What Is Sustaining Clinical Competence?

Sustaining clinical competence in nursing requires ongoing commitment to continued education, professional development, and practical experience. Sustaining clinical competence involves the ability to maintain the knowledge, skills, attitudes, and values required for the nurse the provide safe and effective patient care (Rahmah et al. 2022; Wu et al. 2018). New graduate nurses must stay current with the latest developments in healthcare practices, technology, and evidence-based research. This involves participating in workshops, seminars, and conferences to enhance their knowledge and skills (Hariyati et al. 2017). Additionally, nurses must continuously assess and reflect on their own performance, seeking feedback and opportunities for improvement. Consistent practice and exposure to diverse patient populations help nurses maintain their clinical skills and confidence in delivering high-quality care (Mlambo et al. 2021). Eventually, sustaining clinical competence in nursing is a lifelong journey of learning and growth that ensures nurses are able to provide safe and effective care to their patients.

Clinical Competence Is a Continuous Journey That Requires Ongoing Learning and Adaptation

It is important for new graduate nurses to remember that clinical competence is not a destination but a continuous journey that requires ongoing learning and adaptation. Therefore, they need to pay attention to the following key points in order to understand about the continuous nature of clinical competence:

- Evolving healthcare landscape: The healthcare field is constantly evolving with new research, technologies, and treatment modalities. New graduate nurses as members of the multidisciplinary team need to stay updated with the latest advancements and evidence-based practices to provide the best possible care. Ongoing learning ensures that professionals can adapt to changes in the healthcare landscape and incorporate new knowledge into their practice.
- Lifelong learning: Clinical competence requires a commitment to lifelong learning. New graduate nurses must actively seek out opportunities for professional development, such as attending conferences, workshops, and seminars, pursuing advanced degrees or certifications, and engaging in self-directed learning. By continuously expanding their knowledge and skills, professionals can adapt to emerging trends and advancements in their field.
- Evidence-based practice: Clinical competence is closely tied to evidence-based practice. As new research and evidence emerge, new graduate nurses need to update their knowledge and adjust their practice accordingly. Ongoing learning allows professionals to critically evaluate new evidence, integrate it into their decision-making process, and provide the most effective and up-to-date care to their patients.
- Continuous improvement: Clinical competence involves a commitment to continuous improvement. New graduate nurses should regularly reflect on their practice, identify areas for growth, and seek feedback from supervisors, mentors, colleagues, and patients. By actively seeking opportunities for improvement and making necessary adjustments, professionals can enhance their clinical competence over time.
- Adaptation to changing patient needs: Patient needs and expectations can change over time. New graduate nurses must be able to adapt their practice to meet these evolving needs. Ongoing learning helps professionals develop the skills and knowledge required to address new challenges, provide patient-centered care, and deliver positive outcomes.
- Interprofessional collaboration: Clinical competence extends beyond individual skills and knowledge. It also involves effective collaboration with other healthcare professionals. Ongoing learning provides opportunities for interprofessional education and collaboration, allowing new graduate nurses to develop a broader understanding of different roles and perspectives. This collaboration enhances

teamwork, communication, and coordination of care, ultimately improving patient outcomes.

- Professional growth and career advancement: Continuous learning and adaptation contribute to professional growth and career advancement. When new graduate nurses actively engage in ongoing education and development, they are more likely to be recognized for their expertise, take on leadership roles, and contribute to the advancement in their nursing career. Ongoing learning opens doors for new opportunities and allows them to stay competitive in their careers.

As clinical competence is a continuous journey that requires ongoing learning and adaptation, new graduate nurses must embrace lifelong learning, stay updated with the latest advancements, engage in evidence-based practice, continuously improve their skills, adapt to changing patient needs, collaborate with others, and pursue professional growth. By actively participating in this journey, new graduate can provide the highest quality of care and make a positive impact on patient outcomes.

11.2   The Importance of Sustaining Clinical Competence

It is crucial for new graduate nurses to maintain their clinical competence in order to provide safe, effective, and high-quality care to patients. As healthcare is constantly evolving with new technologies, treatment options, and protocols, it is imperative for nurses to stay up to date on the latest advancements and best practices in order to deliver evidence-based care. By continuously honing their clinical skills and staying current with new developments in the field, new graduate nurses can ensure that they are providing the best possible care to their patients and contributing to positive patient outcomes. Additionally, sustaining clinical competence can also help new nurses to build confidence in their abilities and fosters professional growth and development in their nursing careers.

The Critical Role of Clinical Competence in Providing Safe and Effective Patient Care

As it was previously discussed, clinical competence plays a critical role in providing safe and effective patient care. Therefore, sustaining clinical competence will be beneficial for these reasons:

- Patient safety: Clinical competence ensures that nursing practitioners have the necessary knowledge, skills, and abilities to deliver safe care to patients. Competent practitioners are able to accurately assess patients, make appropriate diagnoses, and develop effective treatment plans. By sustaining their clinical competence, new graduate nurses can maintain the understanding of the potential risks and complications associated with different interventions, and they can take necessary precautions to minimize harm.

- Quality of care: Clinical competence directly impacts the quality of care provided to patients. Competent practitioners are able to deliver evidence-based practices, follow established guidelines, and make informed decisions. Sustaining their clinical competence, new graduate nurses will ultimately have a strong foundation in clinical knowledge and can apply it effectively in their practice. This leads to improved outcomes, reduced errors, and enhanced patient satisfaction.
- Effective communication: Clinical competence includes effective communication skills, which are crucial for patient care. Competent practitioners can communicate clearly and empathetically with patients, their families, and other members of the multidisciplinary team. By sustaining their clinical competence, new graduate will be able to explain complex medical and nursing information in a way that patients can understand, actively listen to concerns, and address questions or doubts. Ultimately, effective communication promotes trust, collaboration, and patient engagement in their own care.
- Critical thinking and problem-solving: Clinical competence involves the ability to think critically and solve problems in complex clinical situations. Competent practitioners can analyze information, consider multiple perspectives, and make sound decisions. Sustaining their clinical competence, new graduate nurses can be able to identify potential risks, anticipate complications, and take appropriate actions to prevent or address them. This will ensure that patients receive timely and appropriate care, even in challenging circumstances.
- Continuity of care: Clinical competence contributes to the continuity of care for patients. Competent practitioners can effectively manage and coordinate care across different specialized areas within the multidisciplinary team members. By sustaining their clinical competence, new graduate nurses can accurately document patient information, share relevant data with other team members, and ensure that care plans are implemented consistently. This will promote seamless transitions and reduces the risk of errors or gaps in care.
- Professionalism and ethics: Clinical competence encompasses professionalism and ethical behavior. Competent practitioners adhere to ethical principles, maintain patient confidentiality, and respect cultural diversity. Sustaining their clinical competence, new graduate nurse will be able to demonstrate integrity, accountability, and a commitment to lifelong learning. Professionalism and ethical conduct build trust with patients and contribute to a positive healthcare environment.

Sustaining clinical competence is crucial for providing safe and effective patient care. It ensures patient safety, enhances the quality of care, promotes effective communication, fosters critical thinking and problem-solving, supports continuity of care, and upholds professionalism and ethics. New graduate nurses must continuously strive to develop and maintain their clinical competence to deliver the best possible care to their patients.

The Consequences of Not Sustaining Clinical Competence on New Graduate Nurses

The consequences of not sustaining clinical competence specifically for new graduate nurses can have significant impacts on their professional development as well as patient care. Here are some potential consequences:

- Increased risk to patient safety: New graduate nurses who do not sustain their clinical competence may be at a higher risk of making errors or providing suboptimal care. Inadequate knowledge, skills, or experience can lead to mistakes in medication administration, patient assessment, or treatment planning. This can compromise patient safety and result in adverse events or harm.
- Limited professional growth: Failing to sustain clinical competence can hinder the professional growth and development of new graduate nurses. Without ongoing learning and skill enhancement, they may struggle to keep up with advancements in healthcare practices and technologies. This can limit their career opportunities, specialization options, and potential for advancement within the nursing profession.
- Decreased confidence and job satisfaction: New graduate nurses who do not sustain their clinical competence may experience decreased confidence in their abilities. They may feel overwhelmed or uncertain in their practice, leading to decreased job satisfaction. This can impact their overall well-being and motivation to provide quality care.
- Difficulty transitioning to practice: New graduate nurses already face challenges in transitioning from the academic setting to the clinical practice environment. Not sustaining clinical competence can exacerbate these challenges. Inadequate competence can make it harder for new graduate nurses to adapt to the demands of their role, integrate into healthcare teams, and effectively manage patient care.
- Legal and ethical concerns: New graduate nurses have a professional and legal responsibility to provide safe and competent care to their patients. Failing to sustain clinical competence can raise legal and ethical concerns. If their lack of competence leads to patient harm or violates professional standards, they may face legal consequences or disciplinary actions.
- Impact on professional reputation: Inadequate clinical competence can impact the professional reputation of new graduate nurses. Colleagues, supervisors, and patients may perceive them as less competent or reliable. This can affect professional relationships, opportunities for mentorship, and future employment prospects.
- Missed learning opportunities: Not sustaining clinical competence can result in missed learning opportunities for new graduate nurses. Ongoing professional development allows nurses to stay updated with evidence-based practices, new research, and advancements in healthcare. Without actively engaging in learning, new graduate nurses may miss out on valuable knowledge and skills that can enhance their practice.

It is crucial for new graduate nurses to prioritize and actively engage in continuous learning and professional development. By seeking mentorship, participating in educational programs, and staying updated with best practices, new graduate nurses can enhance their clinical competence, provide safe and effective care, and thrive in their nursing careers.

11.3   The Key Components of Sustaining Clinical Competence for New Graduate Nurses

Sustaining clinical competence for new graduate nurses involves several key components that are essential for their growth and development in the healthcare setting. One of the main components is ongoing education and training, which helps new nurses stay updated on the latest healthcare practices and guidelines. Another crucial component is mentorship and support from experienced nurses, who can provide guidance, feedback, and encouragement. Reflective practice is also important for new graduate nurses to critically evaluate their performance and identify areas for improvement. Additionally, creating a supportive work environment that values learning and professional development is essential for sustaining clinical competence among new nurses. By focusing on these key components, healthcare organizations can help new graduate nurses thrive and continue to deliver high-quality care to their patients.

The Significance of Building a Solid Foundation Through Ongoing Education and Professional Development to Sustain Clinical Competence
Building a solid foundation through ongoing education and professional development is crucial for sustaining clinical competence in healthcare professionals. Here are some reasons why it is significant:

- Keeping up with advancements: The field of healthcare is constantly evolving with new research, technologies, and treatment modalities. Ongoing education and professional development allow healthcare professionals to stay updated with the latest advancements in their respective fields. This ensures that they are equipped with the knowledge and skills necessary to provide the most current and evidence-based care to their patients.
- Enhancing clinical skills: Ongoing education and professional development provide opportunities for healthcare professionals to enhance their clinical skills. Through workshops, conferences, and specialized training programs, professionals can learn new techniques, procedures, and best practices. This allows them to expand their repertoire of clinical skills and apply them effectively in their practice.
- Fostering critical thinking: Continuing education encourages healthcare professionals to engage in critical thinking and problem-solving. By exploring new concepts, research findings, and case studies, professionals can analyze complex clinical scenarios and develop innovative solutions. This fosters a mindset of

continuous learning and encourages professionals to think critically about their practice.

- Adapting to changing healthcare landscape: The healthcare landscape is constantly evolving, with changes in policies, regulations, and healthcare delivery models. Ongoing education and professional development help healthcare professionals adapt to these changes. By staying informed about healthcare reforms, quality improvement initiatives, and patient safety guidelines, professionals can adjust their practice to meet the evolving needs of the healthcare system.
- Expanding interprofessional collaboration: Ongoing education and professional development provide opportunities for healthcare professionals to collaborate with colleagues from different disciplines. Interprofessional education and collaborative practice enhance teamwork, communication, and coordination of care. By engaging in shared learning experiences, professionals can gain a broader perspective and develop a more holistic approach to patient care.
- Promoting personal and professional growth: Continuous education and professional development contribute to personal and professional growth. By seeking out new learning opportunities, professionals can challenge themselves, expand their knowledge base, and develop new areas of expertise. This not only enhances their clinical competence but also opens doors for career advancement and leadership roles.
- Meeting regulatory and certification requirements: Many healthcare professions have regulatory bodies or certification requirements that mandate ongoing education and professional development. By fulfilling these requirements, professionals ensure that they meet the standards set by their respective regulatory bodies. This helps maintain professional credibility and ensures compliance with professional standards of practice.

Building a solid foundation through ongoing education and professional development is essential for sustaining clinical competence. It allows healthcare professionals to keep up with advancements, enhance their clinical skills, foster critical thinking, adapt to changes in the healthcare landscape, expand interprofessional collaboration, promote personal and professional growth, and meet regulatory and certification requirements. By investing in continuous learning, professionals can provide the highest quality of care to their patients and contribute to the advancement of their respective fields.

Reflecting Experiences, Identifying Areas for Improvement, Seeking Feedback from Supervisors, Mentors, Colleagues, and Patients

New graduate nurses can use reflection, identification of areas for improvement, and seeking feedback from supervisors, mentors, colleagues, and patients as measures to sustain their clinical competence. Here's how they can incorporate these practices:

- Reflection: Reflection involves taking the time to think critically about one's experiences and actions. New graduate nurses can reflect on their clinical experiences by asking themselves questions such as the following: What went well during a particular patient interaction? What challenges did I face? What could I have done differently? Reflecting on experiences allows nurses to gain insights into their strengths and weaknesses, identify areas for improvement, and make adjustments in their practice.

- Identifying areas for improvement: Through reflection, new graduate nurses can identify specific areas where they feel they need to improve their clinical competence. This could include skills such as medication administration, wound care, or communication with patients and colleagues. By recognizing these areas, nurses can take proactive steps to seek out additional education, training, or mentorship to enhance their skills and knowledge in those specific areas.
- Seeking feedback from supervisors, mentors, colleagues, and patients: Feedback from others is invaluable in sustaining clinical competence. New graduate nurses can actively seek feedback from their supervisors, mentors, colleagues, and even patients. They can request regular performance evaluations, engage in open and honest conversations about their strengths and areas for improvement, and ask for specific feedback on their clinical practice. Feedback from others provides valuable insights, helps identify blind spots, and guides nurses in making necessary improvements.
- Engaging in peer learning and collaboration: New graduate nurses can benefit from engaging in peer learning and collaboration with their colleagues. This can involve participating in case discussions, sharing experiences, and seeking advice from more experienced nurses. Peer learning allows for the exchange of knowledge, insights, and best practices, which can contribute to the development of clinical competence.
- Utilizing mentors and preceptors: New graduate nurses can seek out mentors or preceptors who can provide guidance and support in their professional development. Mentors can offer advice, share their own experiences, and provide constructive feedback. Preceptors, who are experienced nurses assigned to guide new graduates during their transition to practice, can provide hands-on support, help navigate challenging situations, and offer guidance on clinical competence development.
- Embracing continuous learning: Sustaining clinical competence requires a commitment to lifelong learning. New graduate nurses can engage in ongoing education; attend conferences, workshops, and seminars; and stay updated with the latest research and evidence-based practices. They can also join professional organizations and take advantage of the resources and educational opportunities they offer.
- Actively seeking opportunities for growth: New graduate nurses can actively seek out opportunities to expand their clinical competence. This can include volunteering for challenging assignments, participating in quality improvement projects, or pursuing additional certifications or advanced training in specific areas of interest. Actively seeking growth opportunities demonstrates a commitment to professional development and helps sustain clinical competence.

New graduate nurses can sustain their clinical competence by incorporating reflection; identifying areas for improvement; seeking feedback from supervisors, mentors, colleagues, and patients; engaging in peer learning and collaboration; utilizing mentors and preceptors; embracing continuous learning; and actively seeking opportunities for growth. By actively engaging in these practices, new graduate nurses can continuously enhance their clinical competence and provide high-quality care to their patients.

11.4   Frameworks for Self-Assessment Assist New Graduate Nurses to Sustain Their Clinical Competence

Frameworks for self-assessment play a crucial role in assisting new graduate nurses to sustain their clinical competence. These frameworks provide a structured approach for nurses to reflect on their practice, identify areas for improvement, and set goals for professional development. By regularly evaluating their own performance, new graduate nurses can pinpoint any gaps in their knowledge or skills and take proactive steps to address them. This continuous cycle of self-assessment helps nurses to stay current with best practices, build confidence in their abilities, and ultimately enhance the quality of patient care. Additionally, frameworks for self-assessment foster a culture of lifelong learning, promoting ongoing growth and development in the nursing profession. Overall, these tools are invaluable for new graduate nurses as they navigate the complexities of the healthcare environment and strive to excel in their roles.

The Importance of Performance Evaluations and Self-Reflection Exercises in Gauging Clinical Competence and Identifying Arears for Growth
Performance evaluations and self-reflection exercises play a crucial role in gauging clinical competence and identifying areas for growth in healthcare professionals. Here are some reasons why they are important:

- Assessing clinical competence: Performance evaluations provide an objective assessment of a healthcare professional's clinical skills, knowledge, and abilities. They help determine if the individual is meeting the required standards of practice and delivering quality patient care. Evaluations can include observations of clinical interactions, review of medical records, and feedback from colleagues and patients.
- Identifying strengths and weaknesses: Performance evaluations help identify the strengths and weaknesses of healthcare professionals. By assessing their performance, supervisors can identify areas where the individual excels and areas that need improvement. This information can be used to create targeted development plans and training opportunities to enhance clinical competence.
- Promoting continuous learning: Self-reflection exercises encourage healthcare professionals to critically analyze their own performance and identify areas for improvement. By reflecting on their clinical practice, professionals can identify

gaps in knowledge, skills, or attitudes and take steps to address them. This promotes a culture of continuous learning and professional growth.

- Enhancing patient safety: Performance evaluations and self-reflection exercises contribute to enhancing patient safety. By identifying areas for improvement, healthcare professionals can address any deficiencies in their clinical practice, reducing the risk of errors and adverse events. Regular evaluations also ensure that healthcare professionals stay up to date with the latest evidence-based practices and guidelines.
- Supporting career development: Performance evaluations provide valuable feedback that can support career development. By identifying areas for growth, healthcare professionals can set goals and work toward advancing their clinical competence. Evaluations can also help identify potential leadership or specialized roles that align with the individual's strengths and interests.
- Fostering accountability: Performance evaluations promote accountability among healthcare professionals. By regularly assessing their performance, professionals are held accountable for their clinical practice and are motivated to maintain high standards of care. Evaluations also provide a platform for open and honest communication between supervisors and healthcare professionals, fostering a culture of transparency and accountability.

Performance evaluations and self-reflection exercises are essential in gauging clinical competence and identifying areas for growth in healthcare professionals. They support continuous learning, enhance patient safety, and contribute to career development. By providing feedback and promoting accountability, these practices help ensure the delivery of high-quality patient care.

When Is It Expected for New Graduate Nurses to Sustain Their Clinical Competence?

New graduate nurses are expected to sustain their clinical competence throughout their entire nursing career. However, there is a particular emphasis on maintaining competence in the early years of practice. It is crucial for new graduate nurses to continuously engage in ongoing education and training, seek mentorship from experienced professionals, and actively reflect on their practice to ensure they are providing safe and high-quality care to their patients. Many healthcare facilities also provide additional support and resources for new graduate nurses to help them transition into their roles successfully and keep up with the latest evidence-based practices. Ultimately, sustaining clinical competence is a lifelong commitment for all nurses that is essential for providing excellent patient care.

Who Is Responsible for New Graduate Nurses in Sustaining Their Clinical Competence?

New graduate nurses have a responsibility to take ownership of their own learning and development in order to sustain their clinical competence. However, it is also important for healthcare institutions, preceptors, and experienced colleagues to support and mentor new nurses as they transition into their roles. Preceptors play a crucial role in guiding new nurses, providing feedback, and offering opportunities for hands-on learning. In addition, ongoing education and training programs within healthcare organizations can help new nurses stay current with best practices and emerging technologies. Ultimately, sustaining clinical competence is a collaborative effort between the new graduate nurse and the various individuals and institutions that support their professional growth.

How Can New Graduate Nurses Sustain Their Clinical Competence?
New graduate nurses can sustain their clinical competence by actively participating in continuing education and professional development opportunities. This can include attending seminars, workshops, and conferences to stay updated on the latest advancements in healthcare and nursing practice. Seeking out mentorship from experienced nurses can also be beneficial in gaining practical skills and knowledge. Additionally, new graduate nurses should actively seek feedback from their supervisors and colleagues to identify areas for improvement and work on enhancing their clinical skills. Engaging in reflective practice and self-assessment can also help new nurses identify their strengths and weaknesses, allowing them to focus on areas that need improvement. By taking these proactive measures, new graduate nurses can continue to grow and develop their clinical competence throughout their nursing career.

The Role of Preceptorship and Mentorship Programs in Sustaining Clinical Competence of New Graduate Nurses
Preceptorship and mentorship programs play a crucial role in sustaining the clinical competence of new graduate nurses. These programs provide invaluable support, guidance, and hands-on experience to help bridge the gap between classroom knowledge and real-world clinical practice. Preceptors and mentors are experienced nurses who serve as role models, offering feedback, advice, and encouragement to help new nurses develop their skills, confidence, and critical thinking abilities. Through personalized one-on-one interactions, new graduate nurses can learn essential clinical skills, enhance their communication and teamwork abilities, and navigate the complexities of patient care effectively. By engaging in preceptorship and mentorship programs, new nurses can accelerate their professional growth, improve their clinical performance, and ultimately deliver safe, high-quality care to their patients.

The Benefits of Seeking Out Mentorship and Guidance from Experienced Nurses to Enhance Their Clinical Skills and Knowledge
Seeking out mentorship and guidance from experienced nurses can provide numerous benefits for new graduate nurses in enhancing their clinical skills and knowledge. Here are some of the benefits:

- Practical application of knowledge: Experienced nurses can help new graduate nurses bridge the gap between theoretical knowledge gained in nursing school and its practical application in the clinical setting. They can provide guidance on how to apply evidence-based practices, navigate complex patient care situations, and make sound clinical judgments.

- Skill development: Mentors can assist new graduate nurses in developing and refining their clinical skills. They can provide hands-on training, demonstrate procedures, and offer constructive feedback to help new graduates improve their technical abilities. This can enhance their confidence and competence in performing various nursing tasks.
- Clinical decision-making: Experienced nurses can share their expertise in clinical decision-making with new graduate nurses. They can help them develop critical thinking skills, prioritize patient care needs, and make informed decisions in complex situations. This guidance can improve the new graduates' ability to provide safe and effective care.
- Professional role modeling: Mentors serve as role models for new graduate nurses, demonstrating professionalism, ethical behavior, and effective communication skills. By observing experienced nurses in action, new graduates can learn how to interact with patients, collaborate with healthcare teams, and navigate challenging situations with professionalism and integrity.
- Emotional support and encouragement: Transitioning from student to professional nurse can be challenging and overwhelming. Mentors can provide emotional support and encouragement to new graduate nurses, helping them navigate the emotional aspects of patient care, cope with stress, and build resilience. This support can contribute to improved job satisfaction and overall well-being.
- Networking and professional connections: Mentors can introduce new graduate nurses to professional networks and connections within the healthcare industry. They can facilitate opportunities for new graduates to engage with other healthcare professionals, attend conferences, and participate in professional organizations. This networking can open doors for career advancement and future opportunities.
- Continued learning and growth: Mentors can inspire and motivate new graduate nurses to pursue lifelong learning and professional development. They can recommend relevant educational resources, encourage participation in continuing education programs, and guide new graduates in setting goals for their ongoing learning. This fosters a culture of continuous improvement and ensures that new graduates stay updated with current practices.

Seeking mentorship and guidance from experienced nurses can provide invaluable support and guidance to new graduate nurses as they navigate the transition into professional practice. It enhances their clinical skills, knowledge, confidence, and overall professional growth, ultimately leading to improved patient care outcomes.

11.5 Conclusion

Sustaining clinical competence is of utmost importance for new graduate nurses as they transition from the academic setting to the clinical practice environment. This chapter has highlighted the consequences of not sustaining clinical competence and the benefits of seeking out mentorship and guidance from experienced nurses. Not sustaining clinical competence can have significant consequences for new graduate nurses, including increased risk to patient safety, limited professional growth, decreased confidence and job satisfaction, and legal and ethical concerns. It can also hinder their ability to effectively transition to practice and impact their professional reputation. On the other hand, seeking mentorship and guidance from experienced nurses offers numerous benefits. It allows new graduate nurses to bridge the gap between theory and practice, develop and refine their clinical skills, enhance their clinical decision-making abilities, and learn from professional role models. Mentors also provide emotional support, encourage ongoing learning and growth, and facilitate networking and professional connections. By actively engaging in mentorship and seeking guidance from experienced nurses, new graduate nurses can enhance their clinical competence, provide safe and effective care, and thrive in their nursing careers. It is crucial for new graduate nurses to recognize the value of continuous learning, professional development, and the guidance of experienced mentors in order to excel in their clinical practice and deliver high-quality patient care.

Review Questions
- What are the key factors that contribute to sustaining clinical competence for new graduate nurses?
- How can new graduate nurses continue to develop and enhance their clinical skills and knowledge?
- What are some strategies for maintaining clinical competence in a rapidly changing healthcare environment?
- How can new graduate nurses effectively manage their time and prioritize tasks to ensure clinical competence?
- What role does ongoing education and professional development play in sustaining clinical competence for new graduate nurses?
- How can new graduate nurses seek and utilize feedback from colleagues and mentors to improve their clinical competence?
- What are some challenges that new graduate nurses may face in sustaining clinical competence, and how can they overcome these challenges?
- How can new graduate nurses effectively collaborate with interdisciplinary healthcare teams to enhance their clinical competence?
- What are the ethical considerations that new graduate nurses should be aware of in order to maintain clinical competence?
- How can new graduate nurses ensure they are providing safe and quality care while sustaining their clinical competence?

References

Hariyati RTS, Igarashi K, Fujinami Y, Susilaningsih FS, Prayenti F (2017) Correlation between career ladder, continuing professional development and nurse satisfaction: a case study in Indonesia. Int J Caring Sci 10(3):1490–1497. https://www.proquest.com/scholarly-journals/correlation-between-career-ladder-continuing/docview/1988003496/se-2

Mlambo M, Silén C, McGrath C (2021) Lifelong learning and nurses' continuing professional development, a metasynthesis of the literature. BMC Nurs 20:1–13. https://doi.org/10.1186/s12912-021-00579-2

Rahmah NM, Hariyati RTS, Sahar J (2022) Nurses' efforts to maintain competence: a qualitative study. J Public Health Res 11(2):jphr-2021. https://doi.org/10.4081/jphr.2021.2736

Wu XV, Chan YS, Tan KHS, Wang W (2018) A systematic review of online learning programs for nurse preceptors. Nurse Educ Today 60:11–22. https://doi.org/10.1016/j.nedt.2017.09.010

Part IV

Technology Integration

In this section, we explore the integration of technology in healthcare, specifically focusing on electronic health records (EHRs) and telehealth with remote monitoring. Technology has revolutionized the way healthcare is delivered, providing new opportunities to enhance patient care, improve efficiency, and increase access to healthcare services. The section highlights the importance of electronic health records (EHRs) in modern healthcare systems (Chap. 12). It discusses how EHRs have replaced traditional paper-based records, enabling healthcare providers to store, manage, and access patient information electronically. By utilizing EHRs, healthcare professionals can streamline workflows, improve accuracy, and enhance communication and collaboration among the healthcare team. It explores how advancements in technology have made it possible to deliver healthcare services remotely (Chap. 13), bridging the gap between patients and healthcare providers, which will be beneficial to enhancing clinical competence of new graduate nurses as members of the multidisciplinary team.

Electronic Health Records

12

Contents

> Test your learning and check your understanding of this book's contents: use the "Springer Nature Flashcards" app to access questions using ▶ https://sn.pub/pe441e. To use the app, please follow the instructions in Chap. 1.

12.1 An Overview of Electronic Health Records (EHRs)

Electronic health records (EHRs) are digital versions of a patient's paper chart that contain their medical history, diagnoses, medications, treatment plans, immunization dates, allergies, radiology images, and laboratory test results (Callahan et al. 2020; Tsai et al. 2020). EHRs provide a comprehensive overview of a patient's health information that can be accessed by healthcare providers at any point of care (Kruse et al. 2018; Fennelly et al. 2020). They are designed to improve the quality, safety, and efficiency of healthcare delivery by streamlining communication between providers and facilitating the sharing of patient information across different healthcare settings. EHRs also offer opportunities for patients to actively participate in their own healthcare by accessing their records online, scheduling appointments, and communicating with their providers (Birinci 2023; Zanaboni et al. 2020). Despite the many benefits of EHRs, there are challenges associated

© The Author(s), under exclusive license to Springer Nature Switzerland AG 2024   243
K. Matlhaba, *Enhancing Clinical Competence of Graduate Nurses*,
https://doi.org/10.1007/978-3-031-81407-5_12

with privacy and security concerns, interoperability issues, and the time and resources needed for implementation and training.

Benefits of EHRs in Improving Patient Care

EHRs are designed to improve patient care by providing healthcare professionals with easy access to comprehensive and up-to-date patient information. Here is an overview of EHRs and their benefits in improving patient care:

- EHRs consolidate all patient information into a single electronic record, making it easily accessible to healthcare providers. This allows for a more comprehensive view of the patient's medical history, enabling better informed decision-making and coordinated care. .
- EHRs facilitate seamless communication and collaboration among healthcare providers. Different healthcare professionals involved in a patient's care can access and update the EHR, ensuring that everyone has the most current information. This leads to better coordination and continuity of care.
- EHRs help improve patient safety by reducing errors and adverse events. With EHRs, healthcare providers can easily access information about a patient's allergies, medications, and previous treatments, reducing the risk of medication errors and adverse drug interactions. EHRs also provide decision support tools, such as alerts and reminders, to help healthcare providers make safer and more effective treatment decisions.
- EHRs automate various administrative tasks, such as appointment scheduling, billing, and documentation, leading to streamlined workflow and increased efficiency. Healthcare providers can spend less time on paperwork and more time on direct patient care. .
- EHRs enable the collection and analysis of large amounts of patient data, which can be used for population health management and research purposes. By analyzing aggregated data from EHRs, healthcare organizations can identify trends, patterns, and risk factors, leading to improved public health strategies and better patient outcomes.
- EHRs can empower patients to actively participate in their own healthcare. Patients can access their EHRs online, review their medical information, and communicate with their healthcare providers. This promotes patient engagement, shared decision-making, and better adherence to treatment plans.
- EHRs facilitate seamless information exchange between different healthcare settings, such as hospitals, clinics, and pharmacies. This ensures continuity of care and improves care coordination, especially during transitions of care, such as hospital discharge or referral to a specialist.
- EHRs promote accuracy in patient care. By using electronic documentation, new graduate nurses can avoid errors caused by illegible handwriting or miscommunication.
- EHRs also facilitate efficiency in patient care by providing quick and easy access to patient information, reducing the time spent searching for paper charts or deciphering handwritten notes.

- Enhance the ability to access comprehensive patient information in real time. With just a few clicks, nurses can view a patient's medical history, lab results, medications, and treatment plans, allowing for quicker decision-making and improved patient outcomes.
- EHRs promote continuity of care by allowing multiple healthcare providers to access and update the same patient record. This ensures that all members of the healthcare team are on the same page regarding the patient's condition and treatment plan.
- EHRs has the ability to generate alerts and reminders for important tasks, such as medication administration, vital sign monitoring, and follow-up appointments. This helps new graduate nurses stay organized and on top of their tasks, preventing potential errors and improving patient safety.
- EHRs help to reduce errors and improve coordination of care among healthcare providers.

EHRs have the potential to significantly improve patient care by providing healthcare professionals with timely and accurate information, promoting collaboration and communication, enhancing patient safety, and enabling data-driven decision-making.

The Importance of EHRs in Promoting Accuracy, Efficiency, and Continuity of Care

Electronic health records (EHRs) play a crucial role in promoting accuracy, efficiency, and continuity of care in healthcare. Here is the key importance of EHRs in these areas:

- Accuracy: EHRs improve the accuracy of patient information by eliminating the need for paper-based records, which are prone to errors, illegibility, and loss. With EHRs, healthcare providers can easily access and update patient information, reducing the risk of errors in diagnosis, treatment, and medication management.
- Efficiency: EHRs streamline healthcare processes and improve efficiency in several ways. They eliminate the need for manual paperwork, reducing administrative tasks and allowing healthcare providers to focus more on patient care. EHRs also enable quick and easy access to patient information, including medical history, test results, and treatment plans, which saves time and improves decision-making.
- Continuity of care: EHRs facilitate seamless communication and information sharing among healthcare providers, ensuring continuity of care. With EHRs, different healthcare professionals involved in a patient's care can access and update the same set of records, leading to better coordination and collaboration. This promotes continuity of care, especially during transitions between different healthcare settings or providers.
- Decision support: EHRs often include decision support tools, such as clinical guidelines, alerts, and reminders, which assist healthcare providers in making

informed decisions. These tools can help identify potential drug interactions, allergies, or other critical information, improving patient safety and reducing medical errors.

- Data analysis and research: EHRs provide a wealth of data that can be analyzed to identify trends, patterns, and outcomes. This data can be used for research purposes, quality improvement initiatives, and population health management. EHRs enable healthcare organizations to generate insights and make evidence-based decisions to improve patient outcomes and healthcare delivery.

EHRs play a vital role in promoting accuracy, efficiency, and continuity of care in healthcare. They enhance patient safety, streamline processes, improve communication, and provide valuable data for analysis and research.

The Potential Challenges and Concerns Associated with the Implementation of EHRs

While electronic health records (EHRs) offer numerous benefits, their implementation also comes with potential challenges and concerns. Here are some of the key challenges associated with EHR implementation:

- Implementing EHR systems can be expensive, requiring significant investments in software, hardware, training, and ongoing maintenance. Small healthcare practices or organizations with limited resources may find it challenging to afford the upfront costs and ongoing expenses.
- EHR systems can encounter technical issues, such as system downtime, slow response times, or compatibility problems with existing systems. These technical challenges can disrupt workflow, affect productivity, and lead to frustration among healthcare providers.
- EHRs store sensitive patient information, making data security and privacy a significant concern. There is a risk of unauthorized access, data breaches, or cyberattacks, which can compromise patient confidentiality and trust. Healthcare organizations must implement robust security measures and adhere to strict privacy regulations to mitigate these risks.
- Transitioning from paper-based records to EHRs requires healthcare providers and staff to adapt to new workflows and technologies. Resistance to change, lack of computer literacy, and inadequate training can hinder user adoption and lead to inefficiencies in utilizing EHR systems effectively.
- EHR systems from different vendors may have interoperability challenges, making it difficult to exchange patient information seamlessly between different healthcare organizations or systems. Lack of standardized data formats and protocols can hinder data sharing and care coordination, impacting the continuity of care.
- Implementing EHRs can initially disrupt workflow and productivity as healthcare providers and staff adjust to new processes and documentation requirements. It may take time to optimize workflows and integrate EHRs seamlessly into existing clinical practices.

- EHR implementation requires compliance with various legal and regulatory requirements, such as data protection laws, health information exchange regulations, and documentation standards. Ensuring compliance can be complex and time-consuming for healthcare organizations. .

Addressing these challenges requires careful planning, adequate resources, and effective change management strategies. It is essential to involve stakeholders, provide comprehensive training, prioritize data security, and address workflow concerns to maximize the benefits of EHR implementation while minimizing potential challenges.

Strategies to Overcome Challenges and Concerns Associated with Their Implementation of EHRs in Healthcare
To overcome challenges and concerns associated with the implementation of electronic health records (EHRs) in healthcare, organizations can adopt the following strategies:

- Comprehensive planning and preparation: Thorough planning is crucial before implementing EHRs. This includes conducting a needs assessment, defining goals and objectives, and developing a detailed implementation plan. Engage key stakeholders, including healthcare providers, IT staff, and administrators, to ensure their input and buy-in throughout the process.
- Adequate resources and support: Allocate sufficient resources, both financial and human, to support the EHR implementation. This includes budgeting for hardware, software, training, and ongoing maintenance. Provide dedicated IT support and training staff to assist healthcare providers and staff during the transition and address any technical issues or user concerns.
- User training and education: Comprehensive training programs should be provided to healthcare providers and staff to ensure they are proficient in using the EHR system. Training should cover system navigation, data entry, documentation workflows, and privacy/security protocols. Offer ongoing training opportunities to keep users updated with system updates and enhancements. .
- Change management and communication: Implementing EHRs involves significant change for healthcare providers and staff. Employ effective change management strategies, including clear communication, to address concerns, manage expectations, and foster a positive attitude toward the new system. Involve key stakeholders in decision-making and keep them informed throughout the implementation process.
- Workflow analysis and optimization: Conduct a thorough analysis of existing workflows and identify areas where EHR implementation can streamline processes and improve efficiency. Redesign workflows to align with the capabilities of the EHR system, ensuring that it supports the needs of healthcare providers and enhances patient care. Involve end users in workflow design to ensure their input and acceptance.
- Interoperability and data exchange: Prioritize interoperability by selecting EHR systems that adhere to industry standards and promote seamless data exchange.

Collaborate with other healthcare organizations and vendors to establish data sharing agreements and protocols. Participate in health information exchange initiatives to facilitate the exchange of patient information across different systems.

- Data security and privacy measures: Implement robust security measures to protect patient data and ensure compliance with privacy regulations. This includes encryption, access controls, regular system audits, and staff training on data security best practices. Conduct risk assessments and develop incident response plans to address potential security breaches. .

- Continuous evaluation and improvement: Regularly evaluate the effectiveness of the EHR system and address any identified issues or areas for improvement. Seek feedback from healthcare providers and staff to identify user satisfaction, usability concerns, and opportunities for system enhancements. Stay updated with industry trends and advancements to leverage new features and functionalities.

By implementing these strategies, healthcare organizations can overcome challenges and concerns associated with EHR implementation, leading to successful adoption and utilization of EHRs in improving patient care and outcomes.

12.2   The Role and Benefits of EHRs in Enhancing the Clinical Competence of New Graduate Nurses

- EHRs are digital versions of a patient's paper chart that contain all of their medical history, diagnoses, medications, treatment plans, immunization dates, allergies, radiology images, and laboratory test results.
- With EHRs, healthcare providers have access to all of this information at their fingertips, enabling them to make more informed decisions about patient care.
- EHRs can serve as valuable educational tools for new graduate nurses. By using EHRs, nurses can familiarize themselves with documenting patient information accurately, managing medications safely, and accessing critical data in a timely manner. These skills are essential for providing high-quality patient care and are crucial for the development of clinical competence.
- By utilizing EHRs, new graduate nurses can also improve their efficiency and effectiveness in providing patient care. They can develop essential skills in data entry, organization, and retrieval, which will ultimately enhance their ability to deliver safe and effective care to their patients.
- EHRs can also help new graduate nurses make informed decisions, enhance their critical thinking skills, and deliver evidence-based care.
- Through EHRs, new graduate nurses can efficiently input and retrieve patient data, track medication administration, and review vital signs and lab results. This hands-on experience not only enhances their understanding of healthcare documentation and medication management but also helps them develop essential skills for providing high-quality patient care.

- By utilizing EHRs as educational tools, new graduate nurses can become more proficient in utilizing technology to improve patient outcomes and streamline healthcare processes.

Challenges That May Arise with Utilization of EHRs in Nursing Practice
The utilization of EHRs in nursing practice can bring about several challenges. Here are some of the key challenges that may arise:

- Technical competence: Nurses need to develop technical competence to effectively navigate and utilize EHR systems. Some nurses may have limited computer literacy or experience with technology, which can hinder their ability to efficiently use EHRs. Adequate training and support are essential to ensure nurses can effectively utilize EHRs in their practice.
- Workflow disruptions: Implementing EHRs can disrupt nursing workflows initially as nurses adapt to new documentation processes and electronic charting. It may take time for nurses to become proficient in using EHRs, which can temporarily impact productivity and patient care. Organizations should provide adequate training and support to minimize workflow disruptions.
- Time constraints: Nurses often face time constraints in their practice, and the introduction of EHRs can add additional documentation and data entry tasks. Nurses may feel overwhelmed by the increased time required for EHR documentation, which can potentially impact the time available for direct patient care. Streamlining documentation processes and providing efficient EHR interfaces can help address this challenge.
- Interoperability issues: Interoperability challenges can arise when EHR systems from different vendors do not seamlessly exchange information. Nurses may face difficulties in accessing complete patient records or sharing information with other healthcare providers. Lack of interoperability can hinder care coordination and continuity. Standardization and interoperability efforts are necessary to address this challenge.
- Data entry and accuracy: Accurate and timely data entry is crucial for EHRs to be effective. Nurses may face challenges in entering data accurately and efficiently, especially during busy clinical settings. Incomplete or incorrect data entry can impact patient care and compromise the integrity of the EHR system. Adequate training, user-friendly interfaces, and clinical decision support tools can help address this challenge.
- Privacy and security concerns: Nurses must adhere to strict privacy and security protocols when accessing and documenting patient information in EHRs. Maintaining patient confidentiality and preventing unauthorized access or breaches are essential. Nurses need to be knowledgeable about privacy regulations and follow best practices to ensure data security.
- Transition from paper-based to electronic documentation: Some nurses may have been accustomed to paper-based documentation systems, and the transition to EHRs can be challenging. Adjusting to electronic documentation methods,

including templates, drop-down menus, and structured data entry, may require a learning curve for nurses. Ongoing training and support can facilitate a smooth transition.

Addressing these challenges requires a collaborative effort between nurses, healthcare organizations, and EHR vendors. Adequate training, user-friendly interfaces, streamlined workflows, and ongoing support are crucial to ensure successful utilization of EHRs in nursing practice. .

Strategies for New Graduate Nurses to Optimize Their Use of EHRs to Improve Their Clinical Competence

EHRs have revolutionized the way healthcare professionals manage patient care. For new graduate nurses, the use of EHRs can significantly enhance their clinical competence and improve patient outcomes. By effectively utilizing EHRs, new graduate nurses can streamline their workflow, access comprehensive patient information, and enhance communication with other members of the healthcare team.

- Training and orientation in the EHR system: This training should cover the basics of navigating the EHR system, documenting patient information accurately, and utilizing the various features and functions of the EHR software. By familiarizing themselves with the EHR system, new graduate nurses can effectively integrate it into their daily practice and improve their efficiency in managing patient care.
- Utilize available support and resources: New graduate nurses should take advantage of any resources or support available to them, such as EHR user guides, online tutorials, or continuing education courses. By continuously learning and practicing with the EHR system, new graduate nurses can gradually build their confidence and proficiency in using this technology.
- Prioritize patient safety when using EHRs: This includes being diligent in documenting accurate and up-to-date information, double-checking entries for errors, and following proper protocols for documenting and accessing patient information. By maintaining a high level of accuracy and attention to detail in their use of EHRs, new graduate nurses can ensure that they are providing safe and effective care to their patients.
- Collaboration and teamwork: New graduate nurses should collaborate with more experienced members of the healthcare team to learn best practices for using EHRs. By seeking guidance and mentorship from experienced nurses, new graduate nurses can gain valuable insights and tips for maximizing the benefits of EHRs in their clinical practice. This collaborative approach can also help new graduate nurses build their confidence and competence in using EHRs to improve patient care.

EHRs are powerful tools that can enhance the clinical competence of new graduate nurses. By undergoing training, prioritizing patient safety, and seeking guidance from experienced colleagues, new graduate nurses can optimize their use of EHRs and improve their efficiency and effectiveness in managing patient care. Embracing the use of EHRs is essential for new graduate nurses to stay current in their practice and deliver high-quality care to their patients.

12.3 Conclusion

In conclusion, electronic health records play a crucial role in enhancing the clinical competence of new graduate nurses. By effectively utilizing EHRs, nurses can streamline their workflow, improve patient care, and, ultimately, achieve better outcomes. With the right training, support, and perseverance, new graduate nurses can successfully navigate the challenges of EHRs and excel in their nursing practice.

Review Questions
- How do electronic health records (EHRs) contribute to the enhancement of clinical competence among new graduate nurses?
- What are the potential benefits and challenges associated with the implementation of EHRs in healthcare settings?
- How can EHR systems serve as educational tools for new graduate nurses, and what specific skills can they develop through their use?
- In what ways do EHRs facilitate evidence-based practice for new graduate nurses, and how can they access the latest research and clinical decision support tools?
- How does interoperability and data exchange in EHR systems promote collaboration and interdisciplinary care among healthcare providers, and how does this enhance the clinical competence of new graduate nurses? .
- What are the potential future developments and advancements in EHR technology, and how can new graduate nurses adapt and leverage these advancements to continuously enhance their clinical skills?
- How can the integration of telehealth, remote monitoring, and artificial intelligence in EHR systems impact the clinical competence of new graduate nurses?
- What are the ethical considerations and privacy concerns related to the use of EHRs, and how can new graduate nurses navigate these issues while ensuring patient confidentiality?
- How can new graduate nurses effectively utilize EHR systems to improve efficiency, accuracy, and continuity of care?
- What are some best practices and strategies for new graduate nurses to maximize the benefits of EHRs in enhancing their clinical competence and providing high-quality patient care?

References

Birinci Ş (2023) A digital opportunity for patients to manage their health: Turkey national personal health record system (The e-Nabız). Balkan Med J 40(3):215. https://doi.org/10.4274/balkan-medj.galenos.2023.2023-2-77

Callahan A, Shah NH, Chen JH (2020) Research and reporting considerations for observational studies using electronic health record data. Ann Intern Med 172(11_Supplement):S79–S84. https://doi.org/10.7326/M19-0873

Fennelly O, Cunningham C, Grogan L, Cronin H, O'Shea C, Roche M, Lawlor F, O'Hare N (2020) Successfully implementing a national electronic health record: a rapid umbrella review. Int J Med Inform 144:104281. https://doi.org/10.1016/j.ijmedinf.2020.104281

Kruse CS, Stein A, Thomas H, Kaur H (2018) The use of electronic health records to support population health: a systematic review of the literature. J Med Syst 42(11):214. https://doi.org/10.1007/s10916-018-1075-6

Tsai CH, Eghdam A, Davoody N, Wright G, Flowerday S, Koch S (2020) Effects of electronic health record implementation and barriers to adoption and use: a scoping review and qualitative analysis of the content. Life 10(12):327. https://doi.org/10.3390/life10120327

Zanaboni P, Kummervold PE, Sørensen T, Johansen MA (2020) Patient use and experience with online access to electronic health records in Norway: results from an online survey. J Med Internet Res 22(2):e16144. https://doi.org/10.2196/16144

Telehealth and Remote Monitoring

13

Contents

13.1 Definition of Telehealth and Remote Monitoring

Telehealth refers to the use of digital communication technologies to provide healthcare services remotely (Maleka and Matli 2024), and it provides and facilitates healthcare services such as provider and patient education, medical care, health-related information services, and self-care (Rajkumar et al. 2023). This can include video consultations, online appointments, and remote monitoring of patient vital signs. Remote monitoring, on the other hand, involves the collection and transmission of patient health data from a distance, allowing healthcare providers to track and monitor a patient's condition without the need for in-person visits. Both telehealth and remote monitoring play a crucial role in improving access to healthcare, especially for patients in rural or underserved areas. These technologies also allow for early detection of health issues, better management of chronic conditions, and increased convenience for both patients and healthcare providers. Overall, telehealth and remote monitoring are valuable tools in advancing the delivery of healthcare services in the modern world.

How Can Telehealth and Remote Monitoring Bridge the Gap Between Patients and Healthcare Providers?

Telehealth and remote monitoring can bridge the gap between patients and healthcare providers in several ways:

- Increased access to care: Telehealth allows patients to access healthcare services remotely, eliminating geographical barriers and reducing the need for in-person visits. Patients in rural or underserved areas can connect with healthcare providers without the need for long-distance travel. This increased access to care ensures that patients can receive timely interventions, follow-up appointments, and ongoing support, regardless of their location.
- Convenience and flexibility: Telehealth provides convenience and flexibility for both patients and healthcare providers. Patients can schedule virtual appointments at a time that suits them, reducing the need to take time off work or arrange transportation. Healthcare providers can also offer extended hours or after-hours consultations, accommodating patients' schedules. This flexibility improves patient satisfaction and engagement in their healthcare.
- Timely interventions and monitoring: Remote monitoring enables healthcare providers to continuously monitor patients' health conditions from a distance. Patients can use wearable devices, sensors, or mobile apps to collect and transmit their vital signs, symptoms, or other health data to healthcare providers. This real-time data allows healthcare providers to detect early signs of deterioration, intervene promptly, and adjust treatment plans as needed. Timely interventions can prevent complications, reduce hospitalizations, and improve patient outcomes.
- Chronic disease management: Telehealth and remote monitoring are particularly beneficial for managing chronic diseases. Patients with conditions like diabetes, hypertension, or heart disease can use remote monitoring devices to track their vital signs, medication adherence, or lifestyle factors. Healthcare providers can remotely review this data, provide feedback, and make necessary adjustments to treatment plans. This proactive approach to chronic disease management improves patient outcomes, reduces hospitalizations, and enhances patients' quality of life.
- Patient education and self-management: Telehealth platforms can be used to provide patient education materials, resources, and interactive tools. Patients can access information about their conditions, medications, or lifestyle modifications, empowering them to actively participate in their own care. Telehealth also enables healthcare providers to conduct virtual education sessions or counseling, supporting patients in self-management and promoting healthier behaviors.
- Continuity of care: Telehealth and remote monitoring facilitate seamless continuity of care. Patients can have virtual follow-up appointments with their healthcare providers, ensuring ongoing monitoring, medication adjustments, or treatment plan modifications. This reduces the risk of gaps in care and improves care coordination between different healthcare settings.

- Cost savings: Telehealth can lead to cost savings for both patients and healthcare systems. Patients can save on transportation costs, parking fees, and time away from work. Healthcare systems can reduce the burden of unnecessary emergency room visits or hospitalizations by providing remote consultations and monitoring. Telehealth can also help prevent disease progression or complications, leading to long-term cost savings.

By leveraging telehealth and remote monitoring technologies, patients and healthcare providers can overcome barriers of distance, time, and resources. These tools enhance access to care, enable timely interventions, support chronic disease management, promote patient education and self-management, ensure continuity of care, and contribute to cost savings. Ultimately, telehealth and remote monitoring bridge the gap between patients and healthcare providers, improving healthcare outcomes and patient experiences.

The Role of Remote Monitoring in Healthcare
Remote monitoring plays a significant role in healthcare by enabling healthcare providers to monitor patients' health status and vital signs remotely, outside of traditional healthcare settings. Here are some key roles of remote monitoring in healthcare:

- Continuous monitoring: Remote monitoring allows healthcare providers to continuously monitor patients' health conditions, even when they are not physically present in a healthcare facility. This is particularly beneficial for patients with chronic conditions or those who require close monitoring, as it provides real-time data on their vital signs, symptoms, and overall health status.
- Early detection and intervention: Remote monitoring helps in the early detection of changes or abnormalities in patients' health conditions. By continuously monitoring vital signs and other relevant data, healthcare providers can identify potential issues or deterioration in a patient's health and intervene promptly. This can help prevent complications, reduce hospitalizations, and improve patient outcomes.
- Chronic disease management: Remote monitoring is particularly valuable for managing chronic diseases such as diabetes, hypertension, and heart disease. It allows healthcare providers to remotely monitor patients' blood glucose levels, blood pressure, heart rate, and other relevant parameters. This enables timely adjustments to treatment plans, medication management, and lifestyle interventions, leading to better disease control and improved quality of life for patients.
- Postoperative care: Remote monitoring can enhance postoperative care by allowing healthcare providers to monitor patients' recovery progress remotely. Vital signs, wound healing, medication adherence, and other relevant parameters can be monitored, reducing the need for frequent in-person visits and enabling early detection of complications or issues that may arise after surgery.
- Aging in place: Remote monitoring enables older adults to age in place and receive healthcare services in the comfort of their own homes. By monitoring

vital signs, mobility, falls, and other relevant data, healthcare providers can ensure the well-being of older adults and provide timely interventions when needed. This promotes independence, reduces hospitalizations, and improves the overall quality of life for older adults.
- Telehealth and virtual care: Remote monitoring is an essential component of telehealth and virtual care. It allows healthcare providers to remotely assess and monitor patients' health conditions during virtual consultations. By integrating remote monitoring devices with telehealth platforms, healthcare providers can gather real-time data and make informed decisions about patient care without the need for in-person visits.

Overall, remote monitoring plays a crucial role in healthcare by enabling continuous monitoring, early detection of health issues, chronic disease management, postoperative care, aging in place, and supporting telehealth and virtual care. It enhances patient care, improves outcomes, and increases access to healthcare services, particularly for individuals with chronic conditions or limited mobility.

Remote Monitoring and Improvement of Patient Care Outcomes
Remote monitoring has the potential to significantly improve patient care outcomes in the following ways:

- Early detection of health issues: Remote monitoring allows healthcare providers to continuously monitor patients' vital signs, symptoms, and other relevant health data. This enables early detection of changes or abnormalities in a patient's health condition. By identifying potential issues at an early stage, healthcare providers can intervene promptly, preventing complications and improving patient outcomes.
- Timely intervention and treatment adjustments: With remote monitoring, healthcare providers can receive real-time data on patients' health status. This enables them to make timely interventions and adjustments to treatment plans. For example, if a patient's blood glucose levels are consistently high, healthcare providers can adjust their medication or recommend lifestyle changes to better manage their diabetes. Timely interventions can prevent exacerbations, reduce hospitalizations, and improve overall health outcomes.
- Improved chronic disease management: Remote monitoring is particularly beneficial for managing chronic diseases such as diabetes, hypertension, and heart disease. By remotely monitoring patients' vital signs, medication adherence, and other relevant parameters, healthcare providers can closely monitor disease control and make necessary adjustments to treatment plans. This leads to better disease management, reduced complications, and improved quality of life for patients with chronic conditions.
- Enhanced patient engagement and self-management: Remote monitoring empowers patients to actively participate in their own care. By providing patients with access to their own health data, such as blood pressure readings or glucose levels, they can become more engaged in managing their health. This can lead to

improved self-management, better adherence to treatment plans, and ultimately, improved patient outcomes.

- Reduced hospitalizations and emergency room visits: Remote monitoring can help reduce the need for hospitalizations and emergency room visits. By continuously monitoring patients' health conditions, healthcare providers can detect early signs of deterioration and intervene before the situation becomes critical. This proactive approach can prevent complications, reduce the need for hospital-based care, and improve patient outcomes.
- Improved access to care: Remote monitoring enables patients to receive care from the comfort of their own homes, eliminating the need for frequent in-person visits. This is particularly beneficial for individuals with limited mobility, those living in remote areas, or those with transportation challenges. Improved access to care ensures that patients receive timely interventions and follow-up, leading to better care outcomes.

Remote monitoring improves patient care outcomes by enabling early detection of health issues, facilitating timely interventions and treatment adjustments, enhancing chronic disease management, promoting patient engagement and self-management, reducing hospitalizations and emergency room visits, and improving access to care. It enhances the quality of care, improves patient outcomes, and contributes to a more patient-centered healthcare approach.

13.2   The Benefits of Incorporating Telehealth and Remote Monitoring into Nursing Practice

Incorporating telehealth and remote monitoring into nursing practice offers numerous benefits for both healthcare providers and patients. Here are some of the key benefits:

- Telehealth and remote monitoring technologies break down geographical barriers and increase access to healthcare services. Patients in remote or underserved areas can receive care from healthcare providers without the need for travel. This is particularly beneficial for patients with limited mobility or transportation challenges or those living in rural areas.
- Telehealth allows patients to receive care from the comfort of their own homes, eliminating the need for travel and reducing waiting times. It offers flexibility in scheduling appointments, making it easier for patients to access healthcare services at their convenience. This is especially beneficial for individuals with busy schedules or those who require frequent monitoring.
- Telehealth and remote monitoring technologies enable patients to actively participate in their own healthcare. Patients can access their health data, monitor their vital signs, and receive educational resources remotely. This promotes patient engagement and self-management and empowers individuals to take control of their health.

- Telehealth and remote monitoring facilitate seamless communication and collaboration between healthcare providers, ensuring continuity of care. Providers can easily share patient information, consult with specialists, and coordinate care plans. This leads to improved care coordination, reduced medical errors, and better patient outcomes.
- Remote monitoring technologies allow healthcare providers to continuously monitor patients' vital signs, symptoms, and health data. This enables early detection of changes or deterioration in a patient's condition, allowing for timely intervention and prevention of complications. Remote monitoring is particularly valuable for patients with chronic conditions or those requiring postoperative care.
- Incorporating telehealth and remote monitoring can lead to cost savings for both patients and healthcare systems. Patients can save on transportation costs, time off work, and childcare expenses associated with in-person visits. Healthcare systems can reduce hospital readmissions, emergency department visits, and unnecessary healthcare utilization through proactive remote monitoring and timely interventions.
- Telehealth and remote monitoring technologies streamline healthcare processes and improve efficiency. Providers can manage a larger patient population, reduce wait times, and optimize resource allocation. This allows healthcare organizations to deliver care more efficiently and effectively.
- Telehealth and remote monitoring provide opportunities for healthcare providers to engage in professional development and collaboration. Providers can participate in virtual conferences, access online educational resources, and consult with colleagues from different locations. This fosters knowledge sharing, enhances clinical skills, and promotes interdisciplinary collaboration.

Incorporating telehealth and remote monitoring into nursing practice offers numerous benefits, including increased access to healthcare, convenience for patients, improved patient engagement, enhanced continuity of care, early detection of health changes, cost savings, improved healthcare efficiency, and opportunities for professional development and collaboration. These technologies have the potential to transform healthcare delivery and improve patient outcomes.

Telehealth Platforms and Facilitation of Virtual Consultations

Telehealth platforms can facilitate virtual consultations that enable nurses to assess and provide care to patients remotely in the following ways:

- Symptom assessment: Nurses can use telehealth platforms to conduct symptom assessments with patients. They can ask targeted questions about the patient's symptoms, medical history, and current condition. Based on the patient's responses, nurses can make preliminary assessments, provide initial recommendations, and determine the urgency of further care or interventions.
- Vital sign monitoring: Some telehealth platforms integrate with remote monitoring devices that allow patients to measure and transmit their vital signs from

home. Nurses can remotely access this data during virtual consultations, enabling them to monitor the patient's health status. By reviewing vital signs such as blood pressure, heart rate, or oxygen saturation, nurses can make informed decisions about the patient's care and provide appropriate guidance.

- Medication management: Telehealth platforms can support medication management by allowing nurses to review the patient's medication list, dosage instructions, and adherence. Nurses can discuss medication-related concerns, provide education on medication use, and address any questions or side effects the patient may be experiencing. They can also use the platform to send electronic prescriptions or coordinate medication refills.
- Wound assessment: Telehealth platforms can facilitate wound assessments by allowing patients to capture and share images or videos of their wounds. Nurses can remotely review these images during virtual consultations, assess the wound's healing progress, and provide recommendations for wound care. They can also guide patients on proper wound dressing techniques and monitor for any signs of infection or complications.
- Patient education: Telehealth platforms provide a means for nurses to deliver patient education remotely. Nurses can share educational materials, videos, or interactive tools through the platform, ensuring that patients receive the necessary information to manage their condition or follow self-care instructions. They can also address any questions or concerns the patient may have, promoting patient understanding and engagement.
- Care coordination: Telehealth platforms enable nurses to collaborate and coordinate care with other healthcare providers involved in the patient's treatment. Nurses can use the platform to communicate with physicians, pharmacists, or other members of the healthcare team, sharing information, discussing treatment plans, and seeking input or advice. This ensures that the patient receives comprehensive and coordinated care, even in a remote setting.

By leveraging telehealth platforms, nurses can conduct virtual consultations that allow for comprehensive assessments, care provision, and patient education. These platforms enable visual assessments, symptom evaluations, vital sign monitoring, medication management, wound assessments, patient education, and care coordination. Virtual consultations through telehealth platforms provide a valuable means for nurses to remotely assess and provide care to patients, ensuring continuity of care and promoting patient well-being.

13.3   The Benefits of Telehealth and Remote Monitoring in Enhancing the Clinical Competence of New Graduate Nurses

The role of telehealth and remote monitoring in enhancing the clinical competence of new graduate nurses is a topic of increasing importance in the healthcare industry. With the rapid advancement of technology, telehealth has become a valuable tool in providing remote patient care and monitoring, allowing for more efficient and effective healthcare delivery.

- Telehealth platforms enable new graduate nurses to bridge the gap between patients and healthcare providers by facilitating virtual consultations and assessments. This enables nurses to provide care to patients in remote locations, beyond the confines of traditional healthcare settings. By utilizing telehealth technologies, new graduate nurses can develop essential skills in tele triage, patient assessment, and remote care management, ultimately enhancing their clinical competence in delivering patient-centered care.
- In addition to telehealth, remote monitoring plays a crucial role in healthcare by allowing healthcare providers to monitor patients' vital signs and health status in real time. This enables new graduate nurses to track and manage patients' health conditions more effectively, leading to improved patient outcomes and reduced healthcare costs.
- Patient education and self-management are also key components of telehealth and remote monitoring. New graduate nurses can use these technologies to educate patients on self-care practices, medication management, and lifestyle modifications, empowering patients to take an active role in their own healthcare. By promoting patient engagement and self-management, new graduate nurses can enhance their clinical competence in patient education and support, ultimately improving overall patient outcomes.
- Telehealth platforms have revolutionized the way healthcare is delivered, particularly for nurses who can now access and provide care to patients remotely through virtual consultations. These platforms have provided nurses with the tools and technology necessary to connect with patients from a distance, offering convenient and efficient care without the need for an in-person visit.
- Nurses can conduct assessments, provide medical advice, and even prescribe medications through telehealth platforms, improving access to care for patients who may have difficulty traveling to a healthcare facility. With the increasing popularity and functionality of telehealth platforms, nurses are able to expand their reach and impact by providing quality care to patients wherever they may be.
- Telehealth and remote monitoring can empower new graduate nurses to provide high-quality care and improve patient outcomes by giving them access to real-time data and resources that can enhance their decision-making skills. Through telehealth platforms, nurses can consult with healthcare professionals and specialists, receive training and support, and access patient information quickly and efficiently.
- Remote monitoring technologies allow nurses to track patient vital signs, medication adherence, and symptom progression from a distance, enabling them to intervene early and prevent potential complications. By utilizing these tools, new graduate nurses can deliver proactive, personalized care that is based on evidence and best practices, ultimately leading to better patient outcomes and increased satisfaction.

The integration of telehealth and remote monitoring into nursing practice is a crucial step toward advancing the clinical competence of new graduate nurses and improving healthcare delivery for patients. By embracing these technologies and leveraging their benefits, new graduate nurses can enhance their skills, improve patient outcomes, and provide more personalized and effective care to their patients.

Tele Triage, Patient Assessment, and Remote Care Management
Tele triage, patient assessment, and remote care management are essential components of healthcare delivery that involve the use of technology and remote communication to assess and manage patients' health conditions. Here's a brief explanation of each:

- Tele triage: Tele triage refers to the process of assessing and determining the urgency of a patient's healthcare needs remotely (Haimi and Wheeler 2024), typically through telephone or video consultations. Trained healthcare professionals, such as nurses or physicians, use standardized protocols and guidelines to gather information about the patient's symptoms, medical history, and current condition. Based on this information, they make decisions regarding the appropriate level of care needed, whether it's self-care advice, referral to a healthcare facility, or emergency intervention.
- Patient assessment: Patient assessment involves gathering comprehensive information about a patient's health status, including their medical history, current symptoms, vital signs, and other relevant data. Traditionally, patient assessments are conducted in-person by healthcare professionals. However, with the advancement of telehealth technologies, patient assessments can now be performed remotely through video consultations or remote monitoring devices. Healthcare professionals use their clinical expertise to interpret the collected data and make informed decisions about diagnosis, treatment plans, and ongoing care.
- Remote care management: Remote care management involves providing ongoing care and support to patients remotely, outside of traditional healthcare settings. It encompasses various aspects of healthcare, including monitoring patients' health conditions, managing chronic diseases, providing education and counseling, and coordinating care. Remote care management utilizes telehealth technologies, remote monitoring devices, and communication platforms to remotely assess patients' health, provide interventions, and ensure continuity of care. It aims to improve patient outcomes, enhance patient engagement, and reduce the need for in-person visits.

These three components, tele triage, patient assessment, and remote care management, are interconnected and rely on technology to enable healthcare professionals to remotely assess, manage, and support patients' health needs. They are particularly valuable in situations where in-person visits are not feasible or necessary, such as during emergencies, for patients with chronic conditions, or in remote areas with limited access to healthcare facilities. By leveraging telehealth technologies, healthcare providers can deliver timely and effective care, improve patient outcomes, and enhance the overall healthcare experience for patients.

How Can New Graduate Nurses Develop Skills in Tele Triage, Patient Assessment, and Remote Care Management, Which Will Ultimately Be Enhancing Their Clinical Competence in Delivering Patient-Centered Care?

New graduate nurses can develop their skills in tele triage, patient assessment, and remote care management through the following:

- Education and training: New graduate nurses can start by seeking out education and training programs that focus on telehealth, tele triage, and remote care management. These programs can provide them with the necessary knowledge and skills to effectively assess and manage patients remotely.
- Continuing education: It is important for new graduate nurses to stay updated with the latest advancements in telehealth and remote care. They can attend conferences, workshops, and webinars related to telehealth and remote care management to enhance their knowledge and skills.
- Mentorship and preceptorship: New graduate nurses can seek mentorship or preceptorship opportunities with experienced nurses who have expertise in telehealth and remote care. Learning from experienced practitioners can provide valuable insights and guidance in developing these skills.
- Practice and experience: New graduate nurses can actively seek opportunities to practice tele triage, patient assessment, and remote care management. This can be done through clinical rotations, volunteering in telehealth programs, or seeking employment in healthcare organizations that offer telehealth services.
- Utilize technology: Familiarizing themselves with the technology used in telehealth and remote care is crucial. New graduate nurses should learn how to effectively use telehealth platforms, remote monitoring devices, and other digital tools to provide patient-centered care.
- Collaborate with interdisciplinary teams: Telehealth and remote care often involve collaboration with other healthcare professionals. New graduate nurses should actively engage with interdisciplinary teams to learn from their expertise and develop effective communication and collaboration skills.
- Reflect and seek feedback: Reflecting on their tele triage, patient assessment, and remote care management experiences is important for continuous improvement. New graduate nurses should seek feedback from patients, colleagues, and supervisors to identify areas for growth and further development.

By following these steps, new graduate nurses can develop their skills in tele triage, patient assessment, and remote care management, ultimately enhancing their clinical competence in delivering patient-centered care.

Strategies to Effectively Utilize Telehealth and Remote Monitoring to Enhance Their Competence and Deliver Optimal Patient Care

- New graduate nurses can utilize telehealth and remote monitoring effectively by first familiarizing themselves with the technology and tools available.
- They should attend training sessions and seek guidance from experienced colleagues to learn how to navigate the platforms and systems effectively. It is important for them to communicate clearly with patients during virtual consultations and make use of visual aids if necessary.
- Regularly reviewing patient data and reports from remote monitoring devices will enable them to track progress and make informed decisions about patient care.
- Collaborating with other healthcare team members and specialists through telehealth platforms will also enhance their competence and enable them to deliver optimal patient care.

By staying organized and proactive in using telehealth and remote monitoring, new graduate nurses can improve their skills and provide effective care to their patients.

The Importance of Patient Education and Self-Management in Telehealth and Remote Monitoring

In the world of telehealth and remote monitoring, patient education and self-management are imperative for ensuring the success of these technologies. Patients must be educated on how to properly use the tools provided to them and understand the importance of monitoring their own health. By being actively involved in their own care, patients can better manage their conditions and make informed decisions regarding their health. Through education and self-management, patients can take control of their health and improve their overall well-being. Additionally, by understanding how to effectively use telehealth and remote monitoring tools, patients can communicate more effectively with their healthcare providers, leading to better outcomes and more personalized care. Ultimately, patient education and self-management are crucial components in maximizing the benefits of telehealth and remote monitoring.

Utilization of Telehealth and Remote Monitoring for Patient Education

New graduate nurses can utilize telehealth technologies to educate patients on self-care, medication management, and lifestyle modifications in the following ways:

- Virtual education sessions: New graduate nurses can conduct virtual education sessions with patients using telehealth platforms. They can use video conferencing to provide one-on-one or group education sessions, discussing topics such as medication management, self-care techniques, and lifestyle modifications. These sessions can include interactive presentations, demonstrations, and question and answer sessions to engage patients and ensure understanding.

- Telehealth apps and portals: New graduate nurses can recommend and guide patients to use telehealth apps and portals that provide educational resources and tools. These platforms may offer information on medication management, self-care practices, and lifestyle modifications. Nurses can help patients navigate these apps, access relevant educational materials, and track their progress in self-care activities.
- Remote monitoring devices: New graduate nurses can educate patients on the use of remote monitoring devices for self-care and medication management. They can explain how to properly use devices such as blood pressure monitors, glucose meters, or wearable fitness trackers. Nurses can guide patients on how to interpret the data collected by these devices and make informed decisions about their health and medication adherence.
- Multimedia resources: New graduate nurses can create or curate multimedia resources, such as videos, infographics, or interactive modules, to educate patients on self-care, medication management, and lifestyle modifications. These resources can be shared with patients through telehealth platforms, email, or patient portals. Nurses can also use these resources during virtual education sessions to enhance patient understanding and engagement.
- Telephonic support: New graduate nurses can provide telephonic support to patients, answering their questions, clarifying doubts, and reinforcing education on self-care, medication management, and lifestyle modifications. They can schedule regular check-in calls with patients to assess their progress, address concerns, and provide ongoing guidance. Telephonic support ensures that patients have access to a nurse's expertise and support even when in-person visits are not possible.
- Collaborative care planning: New graduate nurses can collaborate with patients and other healthcare team members through telehealth platforms to develop personalized care plans. They can involve patients in goal setting, discuss medication management strategies, and explore lifestyle modifications that align with the patient's preferences and capabilities. Collaborative care planning ensures that patients are actively involved in their care and have a clear understanding of their self-care responsibilities.
- Follow-up virtual visits: New graduate nurses can conduct follow-up virtual visits with patients to assess their progress, address any challenges, and reinforce education on self-care, medication management, and lifestyle modifications. These visits provide an opportunity to review the patient's adherence to the care plan, make necessary adjustments, and provide ongoing support and guidance.

By utilizing telehealth technologies, new graduate nurses can overcome barriers of distance and time and effectively educate patients on self-care, medication management, and lifestyle modifications. These technologies enable personalized education, remote monitoring, ongoing support, and collaborative care planning, empowering patients to take an active role in their health and well-being.

13.4 Conclusion

Telehealth and remote monitoring offer new graduate nurses opportunities to expand their clinical skills and knowledge beyond traditional in-person care settings. These technologies enable nurses to provide care and monitor patients remotely, bridging geographical barriers and increasing access to healthcare services. The integration of telehealth and remote monitoring technologies in the clinical practice of new graduate nurses offers numerous benefits in enhancing their clinical competence. By embracing these technologies, new graduate nurses can expand their clinical experience, improve communication and collaboration, engage in continuous learning, and adapt to future healthcare trends. It is essential for new graduate nurses to embrace and leverage these technologies to provide high-quality, patient-centered care in the digital age.

Review Questions
- How does telehealth contribute to the enhancement of clinical competence among new graduate nurses?
- What are the potential benefits and challenges associated with the implementation of telehealth and remote monitoring in healthcare settings?
- How can telehealth platforms facilitate virtual consultations and enable new graduate nurses to assess and provide care to patients remotely?
- In what ways does remote monitoring empower new graduate nurses to make informed decisions and provide proactive care to patients?
- How can new graduate nurses utilize telehealth and remote monitoring technologies to educate patients on self-care, medication management, and lifestyle modifications?
- What are the potential ethical and privacy considerations related to the use of telehealth and remote monitoring, and how can new graduate nurses navigate these issues effectively?
- How can new graduate nurses develop skills in tele triage, patient assessment, and remote care management with telehealth platforms?
- What are some best practices and strategies for new graduate nurses to ensure the secure and ethical use of telehealth and remote monitoring technologies?
- How can remote monitoring technologies, such as wearable devices and sensors, provide real-time data to new graduate nurses for trend analysis and early detection of potential health issues?
- What are the prospects and advancements in telehealth and remote monitoring, and how can new graduate nurses stay informed and adaptable to these emerging trends?

References

Haimi M, Wheeler SQ (2024) Safety in teletriage by nurses and physicians in the United States and Israel: narrative review and qualitative study. JMIR Hum Factors 11(1):e50676. https://doi.org/10.2196/50676

Maleka NH, Matli W (2024) A review of telehealth during the COVID-19 emergency situation in the public health sector: challenges and opportunities. J Sci Technol Policy Manag 15(4):707–724. https://doi.org/10.1108/JSTPM-08-2021-0126

Rajkumar E, Gopi A, Joshi A, Thomas AE, Arunima NM, Ramya GS, Kulkarni P, Rahul P, George AJ, Romate J, Abraham J (2023) Applications, benefits and challenges of telehealth in India during COVID-19 pandemic and beyond: a systematic review. BMC Health Serv Res 23(1):7. https://doi.org/10.1186/s12913-022-08970-8

Part V

Practical Applications/Activities

In this section, there is a selection of interactive and engaging activities to enhance new graduate nurses' learning experience. One of the activities you will find here is online flash card learning. Flash cards are a proven method for improving memory retention and recall (Chap. 14). These flash cards provide a convenient way for new graduate nurses to review and reinforce key concepts, definitions, and facts. Additionally, this section offers case studies to further enhance new graduate nurses' practical knowledge and critical thinking skills (Chap. 15). Case studies provide real-world scenarios that allow them to apply theoretical concepts to practical situations. By analyzing and solving these cases, they will develop a deeper understanding of how concepts and theories are applied in various industries and contexts. Both the flash card learning activities and case studies are designed to be interactive and self-paced, allowing new graduate nurses to learn at their own convenience. These activities provide a hands-on approach to learning, enabling them to actively engage with the material and deepen the new graduate nurses' understanding.

Online Flashcards Learning Activities

14

Contents

Test your learning and check your understanding of this book's contents: use the "Springer Nature Flashcards" app to access questions using ▶ https://sn.pub/pe441e. To use the app, please follow the instructions in Chap. 1.

Online Flashcards Learning Activities
Flashcards below are developed based on the identified learning needs for new graduate nurses as reported by Matlhaba and Nkoane (2022).
Flashcards for Ethical Considerations and Professional Conduct in Nursing
Front of flashcard: Question—What are some examples of ethical considerations and professional conduct in nursing?
Back of flashcard: Answers

1. Definition: Ethical considerations and professional conduct in nursing refer to the principles, values, and behaviors that guide nurses in providing safe, compassionate, and ethical care to patients while upholding professional standards (Ilkafah et al. 2021).
2. Patient autonomy: Nurses should respect and promote the autonomy of patients, allowing them to make informed decisions about their care and treatment. This includes obtaining informed consent, respecting confidentiality, and involving patients in their care planning.

© The Author(s), under exclusive license to Springer Nature Switzerland AG 2024 269
K. Matlhaba, *Enhancing Clinical Competence of Graduate Nurses*,
https://doi.org/10.1007/978-3-031-81407-5_14

3. Beneficence: Nurses have a duty to act in the best interest of their patients, promoting their Well-being and providing care that maximizes benefits and minimizes harm. This involves using evidence-based practice, advocating for patients, and ensuring their safety.

4. Non-maleficence: Nurses have a responsibility to do no harm to their patients. This includes avoiding actions or omissions that may cause harm, ensuring patient safety, and reporting any errors or adverse events promptly.

5. Confidentiality: Nurses must maintain patient confidentiality and privacy. This includes protecting patient information, only sharing information on a need-to-know basis, and following legal and ethical guidelines for the storage and transmission of patient data.

6. Professional boundaries: Nurses should establish and maintain professional boundaries with patients, ensuring that relationships remain therapeutic and focused on the patient's Well-being. This includes avoiding dual relationships and refraining from personal or inappropriate involvement with patients.

7. Integrity: Nurses should demonstrate honesty, integrity, and accountability in their professional practice. This includes being truthful in all interactions, taking responsibility for their actions, and adhering to professional standards and ethical codes.

8. Cultural sensitivity: Nurses should respect and value the cultural beliefs, values, and practices of their patients. This includes being aware of cultural differences, avoiding stereotypes, and providing culturally competent care that is sensitive to the patient's cultural background.

9. Collaboration and interprofessionalism: Nurses should collaborate effectively with other healthcare professionals, respecting their expertise and contributions. This includes effective communication, teamwork, and a commitment to interprofessional collaboration for the benefit of the patient.

10. Professional development: Nurses should engage in continuous professional development to enhance their knowledge, skills, and ethical decision-making abilities. This includes staying updated on current evidence-based practices, participating in educational opportunities, and seeking mentorship and guidance.

Note: These flashcards provide key points on ethical considerations and professional conduct in nursing. Use them as a study tool to reinforce understanding and promote awareness of the importance of ethical practice and professional conduct in nursing.

Flashcards for Management and Leadership Skills

Front of flashcard: Question—What are some key management and leadership skills required in nursing?

Back of flashcard: Answers

1. Definition: Management and leadership skills refer to the ability to effectively coordinate and organize resources, guide, and motivate a team, and make decisions to achieve optimal patient outcomes and organizational goals (Patel et al. 2024).
2. Communication: Effective communication is essential for nurse managers and leaders. It involves active listening, clear and concise verbal and written communication, and the ability to convey information and expectations to the healthcare team.
3. Decision-making: Nurse managers and leaders must possess strong decision-making skills. This includes the ability to analyze information, consider various options, weigh risks and benefits, and make timely and informed decisions for the benefit of patients and the organization.
4. Problem-solving: Nurse managers and leaders should be skilled in problem-solving. This involves identifying issues, gathering relevant information, generating creative solutions, and implementing and evaluating the effectiveness of interventions.
5. Team building: Nurse managers and leaders play a crucial role in building and fostering effective healthcare teams. This includes promoting collaboration, establishing clear roles and responsibilities, and creating a positive and supportive work environment.
6. Conflict resolution: Conflict is inevitable in healthcare settings, and nurse managers and leaders should be skilled in resolving conflicts. This involves active listening, facilitating open communication, and finding mutually beneficial solutions to promote a harmonious work environment.
7. Time management: Nurse managers and leaders must have strong time management skills to effectively prioritize tasks, delegate responsibilities, and ensure efficient use of resources. This helps maintain productivity and meet deadlines.
8. Emotional intelligence: Emotional intelligence is important for nurse managers and leaders to understand and manage their own emotions and effectively navigate interpersonal relationships. It involves empathy, self-awareness, and the ability to motivate and inspire others.
9. Change management: Nurse managers and leaders should be adept at managing change in healthcare settings. This includes anticipating and planning for change, effectively communicating changes to the team, and supporting staff through the transition process.
10. Continuous learning: Nurse managers and leaders should have a commitment to continuous learning and professional development. This involves staying updated on best practices, seeking opportunities for growth, and promoting a culture of lifelong learning within the team.

Note: These flashcards provide key points on management and leadership skills for nurses. Use them as a study tool to reinforce understanding and promote awareness of the important skills needed for effective management and leadership in nursing practice.

Flashcards for Assessment and Observation Skills in Nursing

Front of flashcard: Question—What are some important assessment and observation skills that are essential for nursing practice?

Back of flashcard: Answers

1. Definition: Assessment and observation skills in nursing refer to the systematic, continuous collection and interpretation of data about a patient's health status, using various techniques and tools, to identify actual or potential health problems (Toney-Butler and Unison-Pace 2018).
2. Purpose: The purpose of assessment and observation skills is to gather comprehensive and accurate information about a patient's physical, psychological, social, and cultural aspects to make informed clinical decisions and provide appropriate care.
3. Types of assessment: There are different types of assessments in nursing, including comprehensive assessments, focused assessments, ongoing assessments, and emergency assessments. Each type serves a specific purpose and is conducted at different times during the patient's care.
4. Physical assessment: Physical assessment involves the systematic examination of a patient's body systems, including inspection, palpation, percussion, and auscultation. It helps identify abnormalities, changes in health status, and potential risks.
5. Vital signs: Vital signs, such as temperature, pulse, blood pressure, and respiratory rate, are essential indicators of a patient's physiological status. Accurate measurement and interpretation of vital signs are crucial for monitoring and detecting changes in health.
6. Subjective and objective data: Assessment involves gathering both subjective data (information provided by the patient) and objective data (observable and measurable data). Both types of data are important for a comprehensive understanding of the patient's health status.
7. Documentation: Accurate and timely documentation of assessment findings is essential for effective communication among healthcare providers and continuity of care. It should include detailed and objective descriptions of the patient's condition, observations, and any abnormalities.
8. Communication and collaboration: Assessment and observation skills require effective communication and collaboration with patients, their families, and the healthcare team. Clear and open communication helps gather accurate information and ensures a holistic approach to care.
9. Critical thinking: Assessment and observation skills require critical thinking to analyze and interpret data, identify patterns, and make clinical

judgments. Critical thinking helps nurses prioritize care, anticipate potential problems, and initiate appropriate interventions.

10. Ongoing assessment: Assessment is an ongoing process that continues throughout a patient's care. Regular reassessment and observation are necessary to monitor changes in health status, evaluate the effectiveness of interventions, and modify the care plan as needed.

Note: These flashcards provide key points on assessment and observation skills in nursing. Use them as a study tool to reinforce understanding and promote awareness of the importance of accurate and comprehensive assessment in nursing practice.

Flashcard for Documentation and Recordkeeping in Nursing

Front of flashcard: Question—What are the aspects of documentation and recordkeeping, and is it important in nursing practice?

Back of flashcard: Answers

1. Definition: Documentation and recordkeeping in nursing refers to the systematic and accurate recording of patient clinical information, assessments, interventions, and outcomes; and it is used as a legal communication among nurses and other healthcare professionals for continued management of patients (Mutshatshi et al. 2018; Tasew et al. 2019).

2. Purpose: The purpose of documentation and recordkeeping is to provide a legal and professional record of the care provided, facilitate communication among healthcare providers, ensure continuity of care, and support quality improvement and research.

3. Legal and ethical considerations: Documentation must adhere to legal and ethical standards, including privacy and confidentiality regulations. It should be objective, accurate, and timely and reflect the nursing process and interventions provided.

4. Types of documentation: Common types of documentation in nursing include admission assessments, progress notes, nursing care plans, medication administration records, incident reports, and discharge summaries.

5. Content of documentation: Documentation should include relevant patient information, such as demographic data, medical history, allergies, vital signs, assessments, interventions, patient responses, and any changes in condition. It should be concise, clear, and organized.

6. Timeliness: Documentation should be completed in a timely manner, following the facility's policies and procedures. It is important to document interventions and assessments as soon as possible after they occur to ensure accuracy and prevent omission.

7. Communication and collaboration: Documentation serves as a means of communication and collaboration among healthcare providers. It allows

for the sharing of information, coordination of care, and continuity of treatment across different shifts and disciplines.

8. Accuracy and completeness: Documentation should be accurate, complete, and objective. It should reflect the patient's condition, interventions provided, and outcomes observed. Avoid using vague or subjective language and ensure all entries are signed and dated.

9. Documentation tools and technology: Nursing documentation can be done using paper-based systems or electronic health records (EHRs). Familiarity with documentation tools and technology is essential for efficient and effective recordkeeping.

10. Auditing and quality improvement: Documentation is subject to audits and quality improvement initiatives to ensure compliance with standards of care, identify areas for improvement, and promote patient safety and positive outcomes.

Note: These flashcards provide key points on documentation and recordkeeping in nursing. Use them as a study tool to reinforce understanding and promote awareness of the importance of accurate and comprehensive documentation in nursing practice.

Flashcards for Cultural Sensitivity When Rendering Patients Care

Front of flashcard: Question—Why is cultural sensitivity important when providing care to patients?

Back of flashcard: Answers

1. Definition: Cultural sensitivity refers to the awareness, understanding, and respect for the cultural beliefs, values, practices, and needs of patients from diverse backgrounds (Young and Guo 2016).

2. Importance: Cultural sensitivity is crucial in-patient care as it promotes effective communication, builds trust, and ensures the provision of culturally competent and patient-centered care.

3. Communication: Cultural sensitivity involves using appropriate language, tone, and nonverbal cues when communicating with patients from different cultures. It also includes being aware of cultural differences in communication styles and adapting accordingly.

4. Respect for diversity: Cultural sensitivity requires recognizing and respecting the diversity of patients' cultural backgrounds, including their beliefs, traditions, and customs. It involves avoiding stereotypes and biases and treating each patient as an individual.

5. Awareness of health beliefs: Healthcare providers should be aware of and respect patients' cultural health beliefs and practices. This includes understanding their views on illness, treatment, and healing and incorporating these beliefs into the care plan when appropriate.

6. Dietary and religious considerations: Cultural sensitivity involves being aware of dietary restrictions and religious practices that may affect a patient's care. Healthcare providers should accommodate these needs and work collaboratively with patients to find suitable solutions.

7. Body language and touch: Cultural sensitivity includes being mindful of cultural norms regarding personal space, touch, and body language. Healthcare providers should adapt their approach to respect patients' comfort levels and cultural preferences.

8. Collaboration and shared decision-making: Cultural sensitivity involves engaging patients and their families in shared decision-making and care planning. It recognizes the importance of involving patients in their own care and respecting their autonomy.

9. Continuous learning: Cultural sensitivity requires healthcare providers to engage in ongoing education and self-reflection to enhance their cultural competence. This includes seeking opportunities to learn about different cultures, traditions, and healthcare practices.

10. Addressing health disparities: Cultural sensitivity aims to address health disparities by recognizing and addressing the social, economic, and cultural factors that contribute to inequities in healthcare access and outcomes.

Note: These flashcards provide key points on cultural sensitivity in patient care. Use them as a study tool to reinforce understanding and promote awareness of the importance of cultural sensitivity in healthcare practice.

Flashcard for Evidence-Based Practice and Research in Nursing

Front of flashcard: Question—What is the significance of evidence-based practice and research in nursing?

Back of flashcard: Answers

1. Definition: Evidence-based practice (EBP) and research in nursing involve the integration of the best available evidence, clinical expertise, and patient preferences to guide nursing practice and improve patient outcomes (Mackey and Bassendowski 2017).

2. Importance of EBP and research: EBP and research help ensure that nursing care is based on the most current and reliable evidence. They promote the delivery of safe, effective, and high-quality care, improve patient outcomes, and contribute to the advancement of nursing knowledge.

3. Steps of EBP: EBP involves a systematic process that includes five steps: (1) formulating a clinical question, (2) searching for the best available evidence, (3) critically appraising the evidence, (4) applying the evidence to practice, and (5) evaluating the outcomes.

4. Types of research: Nursing research can be categorized into quantitative, qualitative, and mixed methods research. Each type of research provides unique insights and contributes to the evidence base for nursing practice.
5. Research process: The research process typically involves identifying a research question or problem, conducting a literature review, designing a study, collecting and analyzing data, interpreting the findings, and disseminating the results.
6. Sources of evidence: Nurses can access evidence from various sources, including research studies, systematic reviews, clinical practice guidelines, and expert opinions. It is important to critically evaluate the quality and relevance of the evidence.
7. Research ethics: Nursing research must adhere to ethical principles, such as respect for autonomy, beneficence, non-maleficence, and justice. Researchers must obtain informed consent, protect participant confidentiality, and ensure the ethical conduct of their studies.
8. Research utilization: Research utilization involves the application of research findings to inform and improve nursing practice. It involves translating research into practice guidelines, protocols, and interventions that can be implemented in healthcare settings.
9. Evidence-based practice guidelines: Evidence-based practice guidelines are recommendations based on the best available evidence. They provide nurses with standardized approaches to care and help guide clinical decision-making.
10. Continuous learning: EBP and research require nurses to engage in continuous learning and professional development. This includes staying updated on current research, attending conferences, participating in journal clubs, and seeking opportunities for further education.

Note: These flashcards provide key points on evidence-based practice and research in nursing. Use them as a study tool to reinforce understanding and promote awareness of the importance of integrating evidence, clinical expertise, and patient preferences, as well as conducting and utilizing research in nursing practice.

Suggestions for Further Reading

1. Zung I, Imundo MN, Pan SC (2022) How do college students use digital flashcards during self-regulated learning? Memory 30(8):923–941. https://doi.org/10.1080/09658211.2022.2058553

2. Kristanto B, Glomjai T, Putri D (2024) Enhancing nursing students' long-term retention and engagement in medical terminology through mnemonic-enhanced multimedia mobile learning. J Adv Health Inform Res 2(1):12–23. https://doi.org/10.59247/jahir.v2i1.178

3. Lu M, Farhat JH, Beck Dallaghan GL (2021) Enhanced learning and retention of medical knowledge using the mobile flash card application Anki. Med Sci Educ 31(6):1975–1981. https://doi.org/10.1007/s40670-021-01386-9

4. Chandrasoma J, Chu LF (2016) Teaching the twenty-first century learner: innovative strategies and practical implementation. Int Anesthesiol Clin 54(3):35–53. https://journals.lww.com/anesthesiaclinics/toc/2016/05430

5. Tan AJ, Davies JL, Nicolson RI, Karaminis T (2023) A technology-enhanced learning intervention for statistics in higher education using bite-sized video-based learning and precision teaching. Res Pract Technol Enhanced Learn https://doi.org/10.58459/rptel.2023.18001

6. Wanda D, Fowler C, Wilson V (2016) Using flash cards to engage Indonesian nursing students in reflection on their practice. Nurse Educ Today 38:132–137. https://doi.org/10.1016/j.nedt.2015.11.029

Note: These suggestions for further reading provide a starting point for exploring the use of online flashcards in nursing education to enhance clinical competence.

14.1 Conclusion

In conclusion, incorporating online flashcards learning activities into the training of new graduate nurses has proven to be a valuable tool in enhancing their clinical competence. By utilizing this interactive and engaging method of studying, nurses are able to reinforce their knowledge and skills in a more efficient and effective manner. This chapter has demonstrated the numerous benefits of using online flashcards, including improved retention of information, increased critical thinking abilities, and enhanced problem-solving skills. As new graduate nurses continue to face the challenges of a dynamic healthcare environment, the integration of online flashcards learning activities will undoubtedly play a crucial role in their ongoing professional development and success in providing high-quality patient care.

References

Ilkafah I, Mei Tyas AP, Haryanto J (2021) Factors related to implementation of nursing care ethical principles in Indonesia. J Public Health Res 10(2):jphr-2021. https://doi.org/10.4081/jphr.2021.2211

Mackey A, Bassendowski S (2017) The history of evidence-based practice in nursing education and practice. J Prof Nurs 33(1):51–55. https://doi.org/10.1016/j.profnurs.2016.05.009

Matlhaba KL, Nkoane NL (2022) Understanding the learning needs to enhance clinical competence of new professional nurses in public hospitals of South Africa: a qualitative study. Belitung Nurs J 8(5):414. https://doi.org/10.33546/bnj.2180

Mutshatshi TE, Mothiba TM, Mamogobo PM, Mbombi MO (2018) Record-keeping: challenges experienced by nurses in selected public hospitals. Curationis 41(1):1–6. https://hdl.handle.net/10520/EJC-105228f905

Patel NA, Nayak SN, Bariya BR, Patel MN (2024) Analysis of leadership and team management skills of middle-level healthcare managers of Valsad district, Gujarat. J Fam Med Prim Care 13(2):498–504

Tasew H, Mariye T, Teklay G (2019) Nursing documentation practice and associated factors among nurses in public hospitals, Tigray, Ethiopia. BMC Res Notes 12:1–6. https://doi.org/10.1186/s13104-019-4661-x

Toney-Butler TJ, Unison-Pace WJ (2018) Nursing, admission assessment and examination. StatPearls, pp 1–12. https://doi.org/10.4103/jfmpc.jfmpc_2434_22

Young S, Guo KL (2016) Cultural diversity training: the necessity of cultural competence for health care providers and in nursing practice. Health Care Manager 35(2):94–102. https://doi.org/10.1097/hcm.0000000000000294

Online Case Studies

15

Contents

> Test your learning and check your understanding of this book's contents: use the "Springer Nature Flashcards" app to access questions using ▶ https://sn.pub/pe441e. To use the app, please follow the instructions in Chap. 1.

A case study refers to an intensive study about a person, group of people, or units, which is aimed to generalize over several units (Gustafsson 2017; Heale and Twycross 2018; Goodrick 2020). Online case studies are detailed analysis of real-world situations or scenarios which are presented in an online platform.

> **Online Case Studies**
>
> **Case Study 1: Ethical Considerations and Professional Conduct**
>
> *Scenario*: B*alancing patient autonomy and beneficence*
>
> *You are a new graduate nurse working in a busy medical-surgical unit. Your patient, Mr. Brown, aged 45 years, has been admitted with end-stage renal disease on dialysis and needs a kidney transplant. He has been on the transplant waiting list for several years and has recently received news that a potential donor match has been found. However, Mr. Brown is hesitant and*

expresses concerns about the risks and potential complications of the transplant surgery.

Your task is to navigate the ethical considerations and provide patient-centered care while upholding professional conduct.

Learning Objectives

1. Understand the ethical principles of patient autonomy and beneficence.
2. Recognize the importance of respecting patient autonomy and involving patients in their care decisions.
3. Demonstrate effective communication skills to address patient concerns, and provide information about the risks and benefits of transplant surgery.
4. Apply ethical decision-making frameworks to balance patient autonomy and beneficence in complex clinical situations.

Case Study Details

- Mr. Brown expresses concerns about the risks and potential complications of the kidney transplant surgery. He is unsure whether he should proceed with the transplant or continue with hemodialysis.
- The healthcare team believes that a kidney transplant would significantly improve Mr. Brown's quality of life and increase his chances of long-term survival.
- The transplant surgeon emphasizes the benefits of the transplant and the success rates of similar procedures.
- Mr. Brown's family members have mixed opinions about the transplant, with some supporting his decision and others urging him to proceed with the surgery.
- The hospital ethics committee is consulted to provide guidance on the ethical considerations involved in this case.

Discussion Points

- Balancing autonomy and beneficence: Discuss the ethical principles of patient autonomy and beneficence and how they apply to this case. Explore the potential conflicts between respecting Mr. Brown's autonomy and promoting his overall Well-being.
- Informed consent: Discuss the importance of informed consent in this situation. How can you ensure that Mr. Brown has all the necessary information to make an informed decision about the transplant surgery?
- Communication and shared decision-making: Explore strategies for effective communication with Mr. Brown and his family members. How can you address their concerns, provide accurate information, and involve them in the decision-making process?

- Ethical decision-making frameworks: Apply ethical decision-making frameworks, such as the four principles approach or the ethical decision-making model, to analyze the case and determine the most ethically justifiable course of action.
- Collaboration and interprofessionalism: Discuss the importance of collaboration with the healthcare team including nurses and nephrologists, the transplant surgeon, social worker, and ethics committee, to ensure a comprehensive and ethical approach to patient care.

Note: This online case study is designed to enhance the clinical competence of new graduate nurses in ethical considerations and professional conduct. It provides a realistic scenario and learning objectives to help nurses navigate complex ethical situations and make informed decisions while upholding professional standards. The case study can be accessed online, allowing nurses to engage in interactive learning and self-assessment.

Case Study 2: Management and Leadership Skills for New Graduate Nurses

Scenario: Effective Communication and team collaboration

You are a new graduate nurse working on a busy medical-surgical unit. Your team consists of registered nurses, enrolled/staff nurses, nursing assistants, and other healthcare professionals. One day, you encounter a challenging situation where a patient had cardiac arrest and needed resuscitation. Your task is to demonstrate effective management and leadership skills to ensure efficient communication and team collaboration.

Learning Objectives

1. Understand the importance of effective communication and team collaboration in healthcare settings.
2. Demonstrate leadership skills, such as clear and assertive communication, delegation, and conflict resolution.
3. Apply critical thinking and decision-making skills to prioritize patient care and allocate resources effectively.
4. Foster a positive and collaborative work environment that promotes teamwork and enhances patient outcomes.

Case Study Details

- The patient's condition deteriorates rapidly, requiring immediate intervention and coordination among the healthcare team.
- The team consists of nurses, nursing assistants, respiratory therapists, and a physician.
- The workload is high, and there is a need to delegate tasks effectively while ensuring patient safety and quality care.

- Communication barriers, such as language differences or conflicting schedules, may arise within the team.

Discussion Points

- Effective communication: Discuss the importance of effective communication in healthcare settings. How can you ensure clear and assertive communication among team members during a critical situation?
- Leadership skills: Explore leadership skills, such as delegation, decision-making, and conflict resolution, that are essential for effective management. How can you delegate tasks while considering the skills and capabilities of team members?
- Critical thinking and prioritization: Apply critical thinking skills to prioritize patient care and allocate resources effectively. How can you make informed decisions in a time-sensitive situation?
- Team collaboration: Discuss strategies to foster a positive and collaborative work environment. How can you promote teamwork, respect, and open communication among team members?
- Reflection and continuous improvement: Reflect on the case study and identify areas for improvement in your management and leadership skills. How can you enhance your skills to become a more effective leader in the future?

Case Study 3: Assessment and Observation Skills in Nursing
Scenario: *Recognizing and responding to deteriorating patient condition*
You are a new graduate nurse working on a medical-surgical unit. Your patient, Mrs. Brown, has been admitted with pneumonia. Throughout your shift, you notice subtle changes in her condition, including increased respiratory rate, decreased oxygen saturation, and restlessness. Your task is to demonstrate effective assessment and observation skills to recognize these changes and respond appropriately.
Learning Objectives

1. Understand the importance of thorough assessment and observation skills in nursing practice.
2. Demonstrate proficiency in conducting a comprehensive physical assessment, including vital signs, respiratory assessment, and neurological assessment.
3. Recognize early signs of patient deterioration and respond promptly to prevent further complications.
4. Communicate effectively with the healthcare team and collaborate in the patient's care.

Case Study Details

- Mrs. Brown is admitted with pneumonia and is receiving antibiotic therapy.
- Throughout your shift, you notice increased respiratory rate, decreased oxygen saturation, and restlessness in Mrs. Brown.
- You perform a thorough assessment, including vital signs, respiratory assessment, and neurological assessment.
- You communicate your findings to the healthcare team and collaborate in the development of a care plan.

Discussion Points

- Assessment and observation skills: Discuss the importance of thorough assessment and observation skills in nursing practice. How can you ensure a comprehensive assessment of the patient's condition?
- Vital signs assessment: Explore the significance of vital signs in monitoring patient status. How can you accurately measure and interpret vital signs to identify changes in the patient's condition?
- Respiratory assessment: Discuss the components of a respiratory assessment and the importance of monitoring respiratory status in patients with pneumonia. How can you recognize early signs of respiratory distress?
- Neurological assessment: Explore the components of a neurological assessment and their relevance in assessing patient deterioration. How can you identify changes in the patient's level of consciousness or neurological function?
- Prompt response and collaboration: Discuss the importance of prompt response to changes in the patient's condition. How can you effectively communicate your findings to the healthcare team and collaborate in the patient's care?

Case Study 4: Documentation and Recordkeeping in Nursing

Scenario: *Ensuring accurate and comprehensive documentation*

You are a new graduate nurse working in a busy surgical unit. You have just completed a complex dressing change for a postoperative patient, Mr. Davids. Your task is to demonstrate effective documentation and recordkeeping skills to ensure accurate and comprehensive documentation of the procedure and the patient's condition.

Learning Objectives

1. Understand the importance of accurate and comprehensive documentation in nursing practice.
2. Demonstrate proficiency in documenting nursing assessments, interventions, and patient responses.

3. Apply critical thinking skills to prioritize and organize information for documentation.
4. Adhere to legal and ethical standards in documentation and recordkeeping.

Case Study Details

- Mr. Davids has undergone a surgical procedure, and he requires a complex dressing change.
- You perform the dressing change, ensuring proper technique and infection control measures.
- You document the procedure, including the assessment findings, the dressing change process, and the patient's response to the intervention.
- You adhere to legal and ethical standards in documentation, ensuring confidentiality and accuracy.

Discussion Points

- Importance of documentation: Discuss the importance of accurate and comprehensive documentation in nursing practice. How does documentation contribute to patient safety, continuity of care, and legal protection?
- Documentation standards: Explore the documentation standards and guidelines in your healthcare setting. How can you ensure that your documentation meets these standards?
- Critical thinking and prioritization: Apply critical thinking skills to prioritize and organize information for documentation. How can you determine the most relevant and important details to include in the documentation?
- Legal and ethical considerations: Discuss the legal and ethical standards in documentation and recordkeeping. How can you ensure confidentiality, accuracy, and accountability in your documentation?
- Documentation challenges: Identify common challenges in documentation and recordkeeping. How can you overcome these challenges and ensure accurate and timely documentation?

Case Study 5: Cultural Sensitivity in Patient Care
Scenario: Providing culturally sensitive care to a diverse patient population
You are a new graduate nurse working in a hospital that serves a diverse patient population. One day, you are assigned to care for a patient, Mrs. Zulu, who is from a different cultural background than your own. Your task is to demonstrate cultural sensitivity and provide patient-centered care that respects Mrs. Zulu's cultural beliefs, values, and preferences.
Learning Objectives

1. Understand the importance of cultural sensitivity in nursing practice.

2. Demonstrate proficiency in assessing and addressing cultural factors that may influence patient care.
3. Apply cultural competence skills to provide patient-centered care that respects cultural beliefs, values, and preferences.
4. Communicate effectively with patients from diverse cultural backgrounds and collaborate in their care.

Case Study Details

- Mrs. Zulu is from a different cultural background and has specific cultural beliefs and practices.
- You assess Mrs. Zulu's cultural background, beliefs, and preferences through effective communication and active listening.
- You incorporate Mrs. Zulu's cultural beliefs and preferences into her care plan, ensuring that it aligns with her cultural values.
- You collaborate with the healthcare team to provide culturally sensitive care and address any cultural barriers that may arise.

Discussion Points

- Cultural sensitivity in nursing: Discuss the importance of cultural sensitivity in nursing practice. How does cultural sensitivity contribute to patient-centered care, trust, and improved patient outcomes?
- Cultural assessment: Explore the components of a cultural assessment and the importance of assessing cultural factors that may influence patient care. How can you effectively assess a patient's cultural background, beliefs, and preferences?
- Cultural competence skills: Discuss the skills and knowledge required for cultural competence in nursing practice. How can you apply these skills to provide patient-centered care that respects cultural beliefs, values, and preferences?
- Communication and collaboration: Explore strategies for effective communication with patients from diverse cultural backgrounds. How can you overcome language barriers, use interpreters effectively, and promote open dialog with patients?
- Addressing cultural barriers: Discuss common cultural barriers that may arise in patient care. How can you address these barriers and ensure that patients receive culturally sensitive care?

Case Study 6: Evidence-Based Practice and Research in Nursing
Scenario: *Implementing evidence-based practice in wound care*
You are a new graduate nurse working in a wound care clinic. Your task is to enhance your clinical competence in evidence-based practice and research

by implementing the latest evidence-based guidelines in the care of patients with chronic wounds.

Learning Objectives

1. Understand the importance of evidence-based practice and research in nursing.
2. Demonstrate proficiency in searching for and critically appraising relevant research articles.
3. Apply evidence-based guidelines and interventions in the care of patients with chronic wounds.
4. Collaborate with the healthcare team to implement evidence-based practice and evaluate patient outcomes.

Case Study Details

- You are assigned to care for a patient with a chronic wound that has not been healing effectively.
- You conduct a literature search to identify relevant research articles and evidence-based guidelines on wound care.
- You critically appraise the selected articles to determine their validity and applicability to the patient's condition.
- Based on the evidence, you develop a care plan that incorporates evidence-based interventions and guidelines for wound care.
- You collaborate with the healthcare team to implement the care plan and evaluate the patient's response to evidence-based interventions.

Discussion Points

- Importance of evidence-based practice: Discuss the importance of evidence-based practice and research in nursing. How does evidence-based practice contribute to improved patient outcomes, quality of care, and professional growth?
- Searching for research articles: Explore strategies for conducting a literature search to identify relevant research articles. How can you use databases and search terms effectively to find the most current and reliable evidence?
- Critical appraisal of research articles: Discuss the process of critically appraising research articles. How can you evaluate the validity, reliability, and applicability of research findings to clinical practice?
- Implementing evidence-based practice: Explore strategies for implementing evidence-based practice in nursing care. How can you integrate evidence-based guidelines and interventions into your care plan?

- Collaboration and evaluation: Discuss the importance of collaboration with the healthcare team in implementing evidence-based practice. How can you evaluate patient outcomes and continuously improve your practice based on the evidence?

Suggestions for Further Reading

1. Bowman K (2017) Use of online unfolding case studies to foster critical thinking. J Nurs Educ 56(11):701–702. https://doi.org/10.3928/01484834-20171020-13
2. Craig SL, McInroy LB, Bogo M, Thompson M (2017) Enhancing competence in health social work education through simulation-based learning: strategies from a case study of a family session. J Soc Work Educ 53(sup1):S47–S58. https://doi.org/10.1080/10437797.2017.1288597
3. Fung JTC, Zhang W, Yeung MN, Pang MTH, Lam VSF, Chan BKY, Wong JYH (2021) Evaluation of students' perceived clinical competence and learning needs following an online virtual simulation education programme with debriefing during the COVID-19 pandemic. Nurs Open 8(6):3045–3054. https://doi.org/10.1002/nop2.1017
4. Kennedy S (2017) Designing and teaching online courses in nursing. Springer Publishing Company
5. Seshan V, Matua GA, Raghavan D, Arulappan J, Al Hashmi I, Roach EJ, Prince EJ (2021) Case study analysis as an effective teaching strategy: perceptions of undergraduate nursing students from a middle eastern country. SAGE Open Nurs 7:23779608211059265. https://doi.org/10.1177/23779608211059265
6. Nicoll P, MacRury S, Van Woerden HC, Smyth K (2018) Evaluation of technology-enhanced learning programs for health care professionals: systematic review. J Med Internet Res 20(4):e9085. https://doi.org/10.2196/jmir.9085

Note: These suggestions for further reading provide a starting point for exploring the use of online case studies in nursing education to enhance clinical competence.

15.1   Conclusion

In conclusion, online case studies have proven to be a valuable tool for enhancing the clinical competence of new graduate nurses. By simulating real-life patient scenarios and providing opportunities for critical thinking and decision-making, online case studies help bridge the gap between theory and practice. They allow new nurses to apply their knowledge in a safe and controlled environment, helping them build confidence and skills that are essential for providing high-quality patient care. As technology continues to advance, incorporating online case studies into nursing education will be crucial in preparing new graduate nurses for the challenges they will face in the clinical setting. It is evident that online case studies offer a convenient and effective way to support the ongoing development of nursing professionals.

References

Goodrick D (2020) Comparative case studies, vol 9. SAGE Publications, Thousand Oaks
Gustafsson J (2017) Single case studies vs. multiple case studies: a comparative study
Heale R, Twycross A (2018) What is a case study? Evid Based Nurs 21(1):7–8. https://doi.
    org/10.1136/eb-2017-102845

Conclusion

This book "Enhancing Clinical Competence of New Graduate Nurses" serves as a comprehensive guide and valuable resource for new graduate nurses embarking on their professional journey. Throughout the chapters, various essential skills and strategies that contribute to the development and enhancement of clinical competence were explored. From the foundation of clinical knowledge and skills to the cultivation of effective communication and interpersonal skills, this book has provided new graduate nurses with the necessary tools to excel in their practice. Then emphasis on the importance of patient-centered care, critical thinking, and problem-solving abilities in navigating complex situations and delivering safe and quality care. The book has also highlighted the significance of ongoing education, professional development, and self-reflection in sustaining clinical competence. By encouraging new graduate nurses to seek feedback, engage in interdisciplinary collaboration, and embrace a lifelong learning mindset, we have aimed to empower them to continuously grow and adapt in the ever-evolving healthcare landscape. Furthermore, ethical considerations have been woven throughout the book, reminding new graduate nurses of the importance of upholding ethical principles, advocating for patients, and maintaining professionalism in their practice. As new graduate nurses embark on their careers, they will face challenges, uncertainties, and opportunities for growth. This book aims to provide them with a solid foundation and a roadmap to success. By embracing the knowledge, skills, and strategies presented within these pages, new graduate nurses can enhance their clinical competence, provide exceptional patient care, and make a positive impact in the lives of those they serve. It is hopeful that this book serves as a valuable tool, guiding new graduate nurses through their early years of practice and beyond. May it inspire them to continuously strive for excellence, embrace lifelong learning, and become confident, competent, and compassionate healthcare professionals. It is important to note that the journey to clinical competence is ongoing, therefore, with dedication, perseverance, and a commitment to continuous improvement, new graduate nurses can truly make a difference in the lives of their patients and the healthcare community as a whole.

© The Editor(s) (if applicable) and The Author(s), under exclusive license to Springer Nature Switzerland AG 2024
K. Matlhaba, *Enhancing Clinical Competence of Graduate Nurses*,
https://doi.org/10.1007/978-3-031-81407-5

Glossary

Academic vs. workplace Contrasting environments of learning in a classroom (academic) and applying skills in a real-world setting (workplace).

Achievable Goals that are realistic and within one's reach.

Active listening A communication skill that involves fully engaging with the speaker, showing empathy, and seeking to understand their perspective through attentive listening and feedback.

Accuracy The quality of being correct and precise in collecting and documenting patient information.

Adaptation Adjusting to new challenges and experiences in the clinical setting to sustain and improve clinical competence.

Advanced education Further education and training beyond basic nursing qualifications to acquire specialized knowledge and skills.

Advocating Speaking out on behalf of others to promote awareness, understanding, and explaining change or amendments in practices that may impact their health and well-being.

Analytical approach A method of breaking down complex situations into smaller parts in order to understand and address them effectively.

Assertiveness The ability to express one's thoughts, feelings, and needs confidently and respectfully, while also being receptive to others' perspectives and input.

Bedside reporting A communication practice where nurses provide shift handoff information at the patient's bedside, involving the patient and family in the care planning and decision-making process.

Clinical competence The combination of knowledge, skills, attitudes, and behaviors that enable healthcare professionals to deliver high-quality care.

Clinical decision-making The process of selecting the best course of action among multiple options in patient care.

Clinical judgment The process of making decisions based on clinical knowledge and experience, taking into account the patient's condition and available evidence.

K. Matlhaba, *Enhancing Clinical Competence of Graduate Nurses*, https://doi.org/10.1007/978-3-031-81407-5

Clinical practice The application of theoretical knowledge and skills in real-world healthcare settings.

Clinical reasoning The cognitive process used by healthcare professionals to make decisions about patient care based on critical thinking and evidence.

Collaboration Working together with interdisciplinary team members to coordinate care and seek input from experts in complex cases.

Collaborative problem-solving Working together with others to identify, analyze, and solve problems through shared expertise, perspectives, and skills, promoting teamwork, communication, and critical thinking skills.

Communication The process of exchanging information, thoughts, and feelings between individuals or groups through verbal, non-verbal, or written means.

Communication competence The ability to effectively convey and receive messages demonstrates empathy and active listening skills and adapts communication style to meet the needs of diverse individuals in healthcare environments.

Competencies Specific abilities and knowledge required to perform tasks effectively in a clinical setting.

Conflict resolution The process of addressing and resolving disagreements or misunderstandings among team members through open communication, negotiation, and problem-solving techniques.

Continuity of care The seamless and coordinated delivery of healthcare services to ensure the best possible outcomes for patients.

Continuous growth The ongoing process of learning, developing skills, and improving clinical practice to provide optimal patient care.

Continuous learning The ongoing process of acquiring knowledge and skills to improve cultural competence and provide better care to diverse patient populations.

Critical thinking The ability to think clearly and rationally, analyze and evaluate information, and make sound decisions in clinical practice.

Cultural assessment The process of gathering information about an individual's cultural background, beliefs, and practices to provide more culturally sensitive care.

Cultural barriers Obstacles or challenges that may impede a nurse's ability to become culturally competent, such as language barriers or limited cultural awareness.

Cultural competence The ability to effectively interact with individuals from different cultures, while respecting and valuing their beliefs and practices.

Cultural diversity The existence of a variety of different cultures within a society or healthcare setting.

Cultural humility A mindset of recognizing and respecting the different cultural backgrounds and experiences of others, while being open to learning and growth.

Cultural immersion The process of fully immersing oneself in a different culture to gain a deeper understanding and appreciation for its customs, traditions, and values.

Cultural mentors Individuals who can provide guidance, support, and insights on cultural competence to help new graduate nurses navigate challenges and barriers.

Culturally appropriate care Healthcare that takes into consideration the cultural beliefs, traditions, values, and practices of patients in order to provide more effective and respectful care.

Data entry The act of inputting information into a computer system or database.

Decision-making process The steps involved in identifying and choosing a course of action to address a patient's needs and concerns.

Delegation Assigning tasks to appropriate team members to effectively manage complex situations and ensure timely interventions.

Educational tools Resources used for teaching and learning, such as EHR systems that help nurses develop clinical skills.

Efficiency in healthcare The ability to perform tasks in a timely and effective manner, minimizing waste of time and resources.

Effective communication The ability to convey information clearly and respectfully, while also actively listening and understanding others' perspectives.

Electronic health records Digital versions of patient charts that contain essential health information, such as medical history, medications, lab results, and treatment plans.

Emergency management The act of maintaining calmness, prioritizing tasks, and following established protocols in high-stress situations to ensure patient safety.

Empathy The ability to understand and share the feelings and experiences of another person, leading to a deeper connection and trust in therapeutic relationships.

Essential clinical skills Fundamental skills and competencies necessary for new graduate nurses to succeed in the clinical setting.

Evidence-based care Care that is based on scientific evidence and clinical expertise to improve patient outcomes.

Evidence-based practice The integration of best available evidence with clinical expertise and patient values to guide healthcare decisions.

Flashcard activities Learning exercises that involve creating or using flashcards to reinforce key concepts and information.

Goals Desired achievements or outcomes that one works toward.

Growth The process of continual development and improvement in one's personal and professional life.

Growth mindset An attitude of continuous learning, improvement, and resilience in the face of challenges and setbacks.

Healthcare disparities Differences in access to and quality of healthcare services, often based on factors such as race, ethnicity, income, and education level.

Healthcare providers Professionals who deliver healthcare services, including doctors, nurses, pharmacists, and other allied health professionals.

Health equity The concept of ensuring that all individuals have equal access to healthcare resources, regardless of their background, race, ethnicity, or socioeconomic status.

Implementation The process of putting a plan or system into effect.

Information retrieval The process of accessing stored information for reference or analysis.

Interdisciplinary teamwork   Collaboration among healthcare professionals from different disciplines to provide comprehensive and coordinated care for patients, involving effective communication, respect, and shared goals.

Interpersonal skills   The abilities and techniques used to effectively interact and communicate with others in a healthcare setting, including patients, families, and healthcare team members.

Introspection   A reflective process of looking inward to explore one's thoughts, emotions, and motivations.

Key concepts   Fundamental ideas or principles that are essential for understanding a topic.

Knowledge retention   The process of storing and recalling information over time.

Measurable   Goals that can be quantified or observed to track progress.

Mentor   An experienced and trusted advisor who provides guidance, support, and encouragement in a professional setting.

Mentorship   Guidance and support provided by experienced nurses or healthcare professionals to new graduate nurses in developing their clinical skills and knowledge.

Network   A group of professional contacts within the nursing field that can provide support, guidance, and opportunities for growth.

Networking   Building professional relationships and connections within the healthcare field.

Non-verbal communication/cues   Communication that occurs through gestures, facial expressions, body language, and tone of voice, often conveying more meaning than words alone.

Nursing education   Nursing education refers to the formal training and instruction provided to individuals seeking to become licensed nurses.

Nursing student   A student who is studying to become a nurse, acquiring knowledge and skills in a formal education setting.

Nursing practitioner   A qualified nurse who is actively practicing in the field, providing care to patients, and applying nursing knowledge in real-world situations.

Nursing skills   Essential abilities and knowledge that nurses must possess to provide effective care to patients and navigate the complexities of the healthcare system.

Ongoing growth and development   Continuous learning and adaptation to improve clinical skills and knowledge throughout a nurse's career.

Open-ended questions   Questions that require more than a yes or no answer and encourage patients to share their thoughts and perspectives.

Patient assessment   The evaluation of a patient's health status, including physical, emotional, and psychosocial factors, to guide the development of a care plan.

Patient care   The services provided to patients based on their individual needs and preferences to promote health, prevent illness, and treat medical conditions.

Patient-centered care   Providing care that is respectful of and responsive to individual patient preferences, needs, and values.

Patient-centered communication   A communication approach that focuses on the patient's needs, concerns, and preferences to promote patient satisfaction and optimal outcomes.

Patient engagement   The involvement of patients in their own care, including active participation in decision-making, treatment planning, and goal setting.

Patient outcomes   The results of healthcare interventions on patients' health and well-being.

Personal brand   The unique identity and reputation that a nurse develops through their work, skills, values, and interactions with others.

Practical application   The ability to apply theoretical knowledge and skills to real-world situations, demonstrating competency, problem-solving abilities, and critical thinking in clinical practice.

Practical learning activities   Interactive and hands-on exercises designed to enhance the clinical competence of new graduate nurses.

Problem-solving   The process of identifying, analyzing, and finding solutions to complex problems or challenges in a logical and systematic manner.

Problem-solving skills   The ability to identify, analyze, and solve complex problems in clinical practice.

Professional development   Continuing education and learning opportunities to build a solid foundation for clinical competence.

Professional identity   The unique identity and values that a nurse brings to their role, shaped by their experiences, skills, and personal beliefs.

Professional journey   The career progression and growth of an individual in the nursing field, marked by milestones such as transitioning from student to practitioner.

Quick recall   The ability to remember and retrieve information rapidly.

Real-world scenarios   Practical situations or problems that reflect the challenges and complexities of the professional environment, providing an opportunity for learners to apply their knowledge and skills in a realistic context.

Reflective practice   The process of analyzing and evaluating one's own actions and experiences to identify strengths and areas for improvement in clinical practice.

Reflective questioning   A technique used in active listening to clarify the speaker's thoughts and feelings, encourage further discussion, and deepen understanding.

Relevant   Goals that are meaningful and aligned with one's values and aspirations.

Remote patient monitoring   The practice of using technology to monitor patients' health remotely, allowing for early detection of health issues and improving patient outcomes.

Resilience   The ability to bounce back from difficult situations and maintain well-being while managing complex scenarios in healthcare settings.

Respects and values   Show regard and appreciation for the cultural backgrounds, beliefs, and practices of individuals, acknowledging their importance in shaping their health and well-being.

Self-assessment   Evaluating one's own performance and identifying areas for growth through tools like performance evaluations and self-reflection exercises.

Self-awareness   The ability to recognize and understand one's feelings, thoughts, and behaviors, leading to a greater sense of self.

Self-care   Practices and strategies that promote physical, mental, and emotional well-being and prevent burnout.

Self-reflection   The practice of examining one's thoughts, actions, and experiences to gain insight, self-awareness, and promote personal growth.

Shadowing   Observing and learning from experienced professionals in a specialty area to gain insights and knowledge.

Simulation exercises   Activities that simulate real-world clinical scenarios to help new graduate nurses practice and improve their clinical skills in a controlled environment.

Skill building   Developing and enhancing clinical skills through practice, education, and mentorship to excel in nursing practice.

SMART goals   Specific, measurable, achievable, relevant, time-bound goals that guide goal setting and achievement.

Specialty areas   Specific areas within the healthcare field that require specialized expertise and knowledge.

Specialized expertise   Knowledge and skills that are specific to a particular specialty area in healthcare.

Specific   Clearly defined and well-defined goals that are focused and measurable.

Stress management   Techniques and strategies to cope with and reduce stress in daily life.

Strengths   Positive attributes or qualities that contribute to one's effectiveness and success.

Support system   A network of people, including mentors, colleagues, and loved ones, who provide emotional and practical support in times of need.

Systematic approach   A methodical and structured way of assessing, analyzing, and prioritizing patient needs in rapidly changing environments.

Systemic barriers   Obstacles or challenges that are embedded within the healthcare system itself, which may prevent certain cultural groups from accessing quality care.

Technology advancements   Innovations in technology that improve healthcare delivery, such as telehealth platforms, remote monitoring devices, and health information systems.

Telehealth   The use of telecommunications technology to provide remote healthcare services, including virtual consultations and monitoring.

Tele triage   The process of assessing patient symptoms and determining the urgency of care needed, conducted remotely through telehealth platforms.

Theoretical knowledge   The foundational knowledge and concepts acquired through academic study, research, and professional development that inform clinical practice and decision-making.

Therapeutic relationships   Relationships that are built on trust, respect, empathy, and effective communication, enhancing patient outcomes and satisfaction in healthcare settings.

Time-bound   Goals that have a specific deadline or timeframe for completion.

Transition The process of moving from being a nursing student to becoming a nursing practitioner, involving a shift from theoretical learning to practical application.

Values Core beliefs and principles that guide one's behaviors and decisions.

Verbal communication Communication that involves the use of spoken or written words to convey information, emotions, and ideas.

Virtual learning environment An online platform or software that facilitates teaching and learning activities in a digital space, allowing for interaction, collaboration, and access to resources remotely.

Weaknesses Areas in which one may need improvement or development to reach their full potential.

Well-being The overall state of health, happiness, and satisfaction in one's life.

Work-life balance The balance between one's professional responsibilities and personal life, to ensure overall well-being and happiness.

Written communication Communication that is documented in writing, such as chart notes, reports, and emails, to ensure clarity, accuracy, and compliance with legal and ethical standards.

References

Ali JO, Ali AM, Ahmed LM, Yahya OA, Ali AH, Hasan HI (2024) The perfect nurse-patients' relationship and its impact on the care plan and patient's outcomes. J Biosci Appl Res 10(3):338–351. https://doi.org/10.21608/jbaar.2024.295122.1050

Atkins K, Lorelle S (2022) Cultural humility: lessons learned through a counseling cultural immersion. J Couns Prep Superv 15(1):9. https://research.library.kutztown.edu/jcps/vol15/iss1/9

Baciu A, Negussie Y, Geller A, Weinstein JN, National Academies of Sciences, Engineering, and Medicine (2017) The root causes of health inequity. In: Communities in action: pathways to health equity. National Academies Press (US). https://www.ncbi.nlm.nih.gov/books/NBK425845/

Backhouse A, Ogunlayi F (2020) Quality improvement into practice. BMJ 368. https://doi.org/10.1136/bmj.m865

Barrow JM, Sharma S (2024) Five rights of nursing delegation. In: StatPearls. StatPearls Publishing, Treasure Island, FL. https://www.ncbi.nlm.nih.gov/books/NBK519519/

Bella KMJ (2023) A STUDY ON BALANCING WORK AND PERSONAL LIFE. Int J Sci Res Modern Sci Technol 2(11):29–34. https://ijsrmst.com/index.php/ijsrmst/article/view/162

Bendriss R (2022) Multimodality in medical education: perspectives on medical shadowing from an experiential learning curriculum. Studies in technology enhanced. Learning 2(1). https://doi.org/10.21428/8c225f6e.304da1f8

Caprara L, Caprara C (2022) Effects of virtual learning environments: a scoping review of literature. Educ Inf Technol 27(3):3683–3722. https://doi.org/10.1007/s10639-021-10768-w

Falchenberg Å, Andersson U, Wireklint Sundström B, Bremer A, Andersson H (2021) Clinical practice guidelines for comprehensive patient assessment in emergency care: a quality evaluation study. Nordic J Nurs Res 41(4):207–215. https://doi.org/10.1177/20571585211006980

Farzandipour M, Nabovati E, Sharif R (2024) The effectiveness of tele-triage during the COVID-19 pandemic: a systematic review and narrative synthesis. J Telemed Telecare 30(9):1367–1375. https://doi.org/10.1177/1357633X221150278

Flaubert JL, Le Menestrel S, Williams DR, Wakefield MK, National Academies of Sciences, Engineering, and Medicine (2021) The role of nurses in improving health care access and quality. In: The future of nursing 2020–2030: charting a path to achieve health equity. National Academies Press (US). https://www.ncbi.nlm.nih.gov/books/NBK573910/

Foronda C (2020) A theory of cultural humility. J Transcult Nurs 31(1):7–12. https://doi.org/10.1177/1043659619875184

Hossain F, Kumasey AS, Rees CJ, Mamman A (2020) Public service ethics, values and spirituality in developing and transitional countries: challenges and opportunities. Public Adm Dev 40(3):147–155. https://doi.org/10.1002/pad.1890

Johansen ML, O'Brien JL (2016, January) Decision making in nursing practice: a concept analysis. Nurs Forum 51(1):40–48. https://doi.org/10.1111/nuf.12119

Koukourikos K, Tsaloglidou A, Kourkouta L, Papathanasiou IV, Iliadis C, Fratzana A, Panagiotou A (2021) Simulation in clinical nursing education. Acta Inform Med 29(1):15. https://doi.org/10.5455/aim.2021.29.15-20

Lee PA, Greenfield G, Pappas Y (2018) The impact of telehealth remote patient monitoring on glycemic control in type 2 diabetes: a systematic review and meta-analysis of systematic reviews of randomised controlled trials. BMC Health Serv Res 18:1–10. https://doi.org/10.1186/s12913-018-3274-8

Matlhaba KL, Khunou SH (2022) Transition of graduate nurses from student to practice during the COVID-19 pandemic: integrative review. Int J Afr Nurs Sci 17:100501. https://doi.org/10.1016/j.ijans.2022.100501

Nicholas S (2023) Defining goals. Cornerstone experience. https://fsw.pressbooks.pub/sls1515/chapter/defining-goals/. Accessed 7 Nov 2024

Philippa R, Ann H, Jacqueline M, Nicola A (2021) Professional identity in nursing: a mixed method research study. Nurse Educ Pract 52:103039. https://doi.org/10.1016/j.nepr.2021.103039

Posluns K, Gall TL (2020) Dear mental health practitioners, take care of yourselves: a literature review on self-care. Int J Adv Couns 42(1):1–20. https://doi.org/10.1007/s10447-019-09382-w

Ribeiro LFV, Silva JVJ (2021) Cultural diversity and implications in social environment. In: Reduced inequalities. Springer International Publishing, Cham, pp 1–12. https://doi.org/10.1007/978-3-319-71060-0_134-1

Ruggeri K, Garcia-Garzon E, Maguire Á, Matz S, Huppert FA (2020) Well-being is more than happiness and life satisfaction: a multidimensional analysis of 21 countries. Health Qual Life Outcomes 18:1–16. https://doi.org/10.1186/s12955-020-01423-y

South African Nursing Council, Nursing Act (Act no 33 of 2005) (2013) Regulation 786, regulations regarding the scope of practice of nurses and midwifes. (Government notice). 2013. Government Gazette, 38935 (2005), p 6. http://www.gov.za/sites/www.gov.za/files/36935_rg10037_gon786.pdf. Accessed 6 Nov 2024

Stewart V, McMillan SS, Hu J, Collins JC, El-Den S, O'Reilly CL, Wheeler AJ (2024) Are SMART goals fit-for-purpose? Goal planning with mental health service-users in Australian community pharmacies. Int J Qual Health Care 36(1):mzae009. https://doi.org/10.1093/intqhc/mzae009

Tennant K, Long A, Toney-Butler TJ (2017) Active listening. https://europepmc.org/article/nbk/nbk442015

Vahdat S, Hamzehgardeshi L, Hessam S, Hamzehgardeshi Z (2014) Patient involvement in health care decision making: a review. Iran Red Crescent Med J 16(1):e12454. https://doi.org/10.5812/ircmj.12454

Vermeir P, Vandijck D, Degroote S, Peleman R, Verhaeghe R, Mortier E, Hallaert G, Van Daele S, Buylaert W, Vogelaers D (2015) Communication in healthcare: a narrative review of the literature and practical recommendations. Int J Clin Pract 69(11):1257–1267. https://doi.org/10.1111/ijcp.12686

Weger H Jr, Castle GR, Emmett MC (2010) Active listening in peer interviews: the influence of message paraphrasing on perceptions of listening skill. The Intl Journal of Listening 24(1):34–49. https://doi.org/10.1080/10904010903466311

Williamson M, Harrison L (2010) Providing culturally appropriate care: a literature review. Int J Nurs Stud 47(6):761–769. https://doi.org/10.1016/j.ijnurstu.2009.12.012

World Health Organization (2006) Quality of care: a process for making strategic choices in health systems. World Health Organization. https://apps.who.int/iris/bitstream/handle/10665/43470/?sequence=1. Accessed 7 Nov 2024

Index

© The Editor(s) (if applicable) and The Author(s), under exclusive license to Springer Nature Switzerland AG 2024
K. Matlhaba, *Enhancing Clinical Competence of Graduate Nurses*,
https://doi.org/10.1007/978-3-031-81407-5